Updates on Hearing Loss and its Rehabilitation

Edited by Andrea Ciorba and Stavros Hatzopoulos

Published in London, United Kingdom

Updates on Hearing Loss and its Rehabilitation
http://dx.doi.org/10.5772/intechopen.110959
Edited by Andrea Ciorba and Stavros Hatzopoulos

Contributors
Alejandro Santiago Nazario, Soraya Abdul-Hadi, Antonio Riera March, Alenka Kravos, Charvi Malhotra, Peter Kullar, Guillermo Spitzmaul, Ezequiel Rías, Leonardo Dionisio, Manal Alkharji, Emma Broome, Clare Burgon, Eithne Heffernan, Tom Dening, Sian Calvert, Saima Rajasingam, Helen Henshaw, Karol Myszel, Piotr Henryk Skarżyński, Charlotte T. Jespersen, Qingwei Ruan, Jian Ruan, Xiuhua Hu, Aiguo Liu, Zhuowei Yu, Noriko Katsuya, Tomoko Sano, Tania Hanekom, Johan Hanekom, Werner Badenhorst, René Baron, Talita le Roux, André Uys

First published in London, United Kingdom, 2023 by IntechOpen
IntechOpen is the global imprint of INTECHOPEN LIMITED, registered in England and Wales, registration number: 11086078, 5 Princes Gate Court, London, SW7 2QJ, United Kingdom

British Library Cataloguing-in-Publication Data
A catalogue record for this book is available from the British Library

Additional hard and PDF copies can be obtained from orders@intechopen.com

Updates on Hearing Loss and its Rehabilitation
Edited by Andrea Ciorba and Stavros Hatzopoulos
p. cm.
Print ISBN 978-1-83769-778-6
Online ISBN 978-1-83769-777-9
eBook (PDF) ISBN 978-1-83769-779-3

Meet the editors

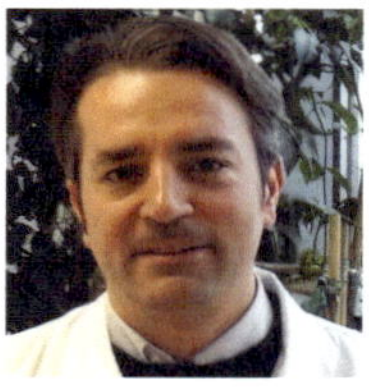

Prof. Andrea Ciorba, MD, has been a member of the Audiology and ENT Clinic, University of Ferrara, Italy, since 2004. He is the author of about 190 peer-reviewed papers and book chapters and a member of several journal editorial boards. His clinical field of interest is audiology and vestibology and he is involved in research activities in otoacoustic emissions and inner ear electrophysiology. Dr. Ciorba obtained an MD in 1999, a diploma in Otolaryngology and Head and Neck Surgery in 2003, and a Ph.D. in Audiology in 2008. He has been an Associate Professor of Audiology at the Audiology and ENT Clinic, University of Ferrara, since 2020.

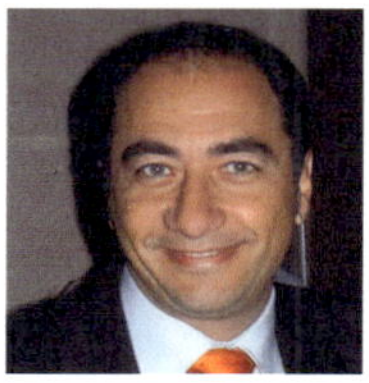

Dr. Stavros Hatzopoulos has been a faculty member of the Audiology and ENT Clinic, University of Ferrara, Italy, since 1994. His background is in biomedical engineering, audiological engineering, and hearing science. He obtained a BSc from the University of Southern California, an MSc from Texas A&M University, and a Ph.D. from Worcester Polytechnic Institute, Massachusetts, USA. He received his habilitation as an associate professor in 2014. He is the author of more than 225 book chapters, peer-reviewed papers, and congress presentations. He has participated in numerous European Concerted Action projects in otoacoustic emissions, genetics, and nanotechnologies. Dr. Hatzopoulos is the editor of the Otoacoustic Emissions Portal (www.otoemissions.org), the Audiology section editor for the *Journal of Hearing Science,* and the managing editor for *Hearing, Balance and Communication.*

Contents

Preface

This volume presents the latest information related to hearing loss, which is among the most prevalent chronic disabilities worldwide. Nowadays, adequate and prompt identification and rehabilitation of hearing impairment, whenever possible, is paramount because hearing loss can seriously interfere with psychosocial development, family dynamics, and social interactions. This book has been edited with a strong educational perspective and provides updates on hearing loss diagnosis and management. The book contains the valuable contributions of eleven authors, and its chapters are suitable for graduate students in audiology, otolaryngology, hearing science, and neurosciences. It is composed of two sections. Section 1 provides updates on hearing loss and its etiology, focusing on the problems associated with some specific types of hearing impairment. Section 2 discusses several rehabilitative techniques, providing some insights into precision medicine.

We would like to thank all the contributing authors for their excellent chapters. We also thank the staff at IntechOpen, especially Ms. Tea Jelaca for her continuous and generous assistance during the preparation of this volume.

Andrea Ciorba and Stavros Hatzopoulos
University of Ferrara,
Ferrara, Italy

Section 1

Hearing Loss and Its Etiology

Chapter 1

Congenital Hearing Loss – Overview, Diagnosis, and Management Strategies

Alejandro Santiago Nazario, Soraya Abdul-Hadi and Antonio Riera March

Abstract

Congenital hearing loss, i.e., hearing loss that presents during the perinatal period from the 20th week of gestation to the 28th day of birth, is a prevalent cause of physiological and social morbidity in pediatric patient development. Hearing loss may be hereditary or acquired, with the former including syndromic and nonsyndromic causes and the latter consisting of infections and ototoxic medication exposure. With the help of various diagnostic tools and universal newborn hearing screening programs, many of these patients may be identified early and intervened to improve long-term outcomes. Interventions may include amplification, otologic surgeries, cochlear implantation, and brainstem auditory implants.

Keywords: congenital hearing loss, non-syndromic hearing loss, syndromic hearing loss, neonatal hearing screening, hearing loss due to infections

1. Introduction

Hearing loss may result from disruption at any level of the auditory system. If the hearing loss results from abnormalities housed in the external ear (e.g., the auricle, the external acoustic canal) or the middle ear (e.g., the middle ear cavity, the ossicular chain, etc.), it is deemed a conductive hearing loss. On the other hand, if the abnormality is located in the inner ear (e.g., the cochlea, the spiral ganglion, or the distal afferent fibers of the cochlear nerve) or in proximal portions of the neural component of the auditory system (e.g., the cochlear nerve, higher-degree neurons in the brainstem projecting to cephalad parts of the auditory system), then it is called sensorineural hearing loss (SNHL). If both conductive and sensorineural components explain a patient's hearing loss, it is considered a mixed hearing loss. The severity of the loss is categorized by hearing thresholds recorded as decibels. In pediatric patients, mild hearing loss corresponds to 20–39 dB, moderate hearing loss from 4069 dB, severe hearing loss from 70 to 89 dB, and profound hearing loss from values equal to or higher than 90 dB. Congenital hearing loss, i.e., hearing loss that presents during the perinatal period from the 20th week of gestation to the 28th day of birth, is a prevalent cause of physiological and social morbidity in pediatric patient development. Early diagnosis and intervention are critical to optimize the patient's language and social development.

2. Epidemiology

Congenital hearing loss is considered the most common birth defect in the U.S., with estimates ranging from an average of 1.7 per 1000 infants [1]. However, not all infants are affected equally. Studies have shown that there are racial and ethnic disparities in the prevalence of congenital hearing loss, with higher rates disproportionately affecting minorities and infants from low-income neighborhoods compared to non-Hispanic white infants and those from more affluent communities [2].

3. Etiologies

Congenital hearing loss may be genetically inherited (50%) or acquired (50%) after exposure to infections or ototoxic medications. Hereditary hearing loss can be further divided into syndromic, i.e., as part of a condition involving a constellation of clinical symptoms affecting a patient, or non-syndromic, i.e., an isolated clinical finding in an otherwise healthy patient.

3.1 Inherited syndromic congenital hearing loss

3.1.1 Pendred syndrome

Pendred syndrome is one of the most common inherited syndromic forms of sensorineural hearing loss, accounting for 5–10% of cases of congenital hearing loss [3]. It results from mutations in the pendrin gene (SLC26A4/PDS) on chromosome 7q, which codes for a protein pump responsible for transporting chloride, iodine, and other anions in the cochlea and thyroid follicular cells [4]. Affected patients usually present during adolescence with bilateral, progressive, and profound SNHL with or without structural cochlear abnormalities (such as enlarged vestibular aqueduct and Mondini deformity) [5] and with diffuse thyroid goiter with or without hypothyroidism.

3.1.2 Waardenburg syndrome

The most common form of autosomal dominant syndromic congenital deafness is Waardenburg syndrome, accounting for 2–5% of congenital hearing loss cases [6]. Multiple genes have been described as responsible for the phenotype of this syndrome and involve the PAX3 gene (i.e., paired box 3 transcription factor) located on chromosome 2q37, MITF (microphthalmia-associated transcription factor), EDN3 (endothelin 3) and SOX10 (Sry bOX10 transcription factor).

The clinical features of Waardenburg syndrome include unilateral or bilateral SNHL, pigmentary changes in the skin, hair, or eyes, and craniofacial dysmorphic features [7]. The pigmentary changes may consist of the following:

- A white forelock (a patch of white hair on the scalp hair).

- Heterochromia irides (heterogenous coloration of the iris).
- Premature graying of hair.
- Vitiligo.

Additionally, the craniofacial dysmorphic features may include:

- Dystopia canthorum (abnormal position of the medial canthi of the eyes).
- A broad nasal root.
- Synophrys (unibrow).

There are four different variants of Waardenburg syndrome, as summarized in **Table 1**.

3.1.3 Usher syndrome

Another common syndrome causing inherited congenital sensorineural hearing loss is Usher syndrome. It is considered the most common cause of combined inherited vision and hearing loss, and up to 3–6% of cases of congenital hearing loss may be attributed to Usher syndrome [8, 9]. Mutations in several genes cause it; however, the most involved gene is MYO7A, which codes for a myosin protein in various tissues, most notably in the cochlea and retina [10]. Aside from SNHL, it is associated with retinitis pigmentosa (hereditary retinal dystrophy) and may be associated with or without vestibular system abnormalities. Retinitis pigmentosa initially manifested by nyctalopia (night blindness), progressing to peripheral vision impairment, and finally leading to blindness. Evaluation by an ophthalmologist is critical in the management of Usher syndrome.

There are four different types of Usher syndrome, as summarized in **Table 2**.

3.1.4 Branchio-oto-renal syndrome (Melnick-Fraser syndrome)

Branchio-oto-renal syndrome is an autosomal dominant inherited condition with complete penetrance and variable expressivity characterized by congenital hearing

Waardenburg syndrome types	Pattern of inheritance	Clinical features
Type I	Autosomal dominant	Sensorineural hearing loss, heterochromia irides, white forelock, patchy hypopigmentation, dystopia canthorum
Type II	Autosomal dominant	Type I, but without dystopia canthorum
Type III	Autosomal dominant	Type I with microcephaly, musculoskeletal abnormalities, intellectual disability
Type IV	Autosomal recessive	Type II with Hirschsprung disease

Table 1.
The four subtypes of Waardenburg syndrome.

Usher syndrome types	Pattern of inheritance	Clinical features
Type I	Autosomal dominant	Most severe phenotype, clinical presentation during childhood, sensorineural hearing loss, vestibulopathy, retinitis pigmentosa
Type II	Autosomal dominant	Most common subtype, clinical presentation during adolescence, no vestibulopathy, retinitis pigmentosa
Type III	Autosomal dominant	Similar clinical features as Type I Usher syndrome but with milder symptoms

Table 2.
The three major different subtypes of Usher syndrome.

loss (may be conductive, sensorineural, or mixed), external ear deformities, branchial cleft anomalies, and renal abnormalities [11, 12]. The genetic mutations involve the EYA1 gene, intimately involved with the embryonal development of the auditory system, branchial arches, and the genitourinary system.

3.1.5 Jervell and Lange-Nielsen syndrome

Jervell and Lange-Nielsen syndrome is a rare genetic disorder resulting from mutations in the KCNQ1 or KCNE1 genes affecting the β-subunit of connexin 26 located in the marginal cells of the stria vascularis and heart, leading to sensorineural hearing loss and long QT syndrome [13]. This syndrome accounts for less than 1% of cases of congenital hearing loss. Episodes of arrhythmias characterize this syndrome due to a defect in cardiac conduction that can even terminate with sudden death. The degree of hearing loss is variable; however, it is usually severe to profound.

3.1.6 Other syndromes

These are just a few examples of the syndromes that can cause congenital hearing loss. Other syndromes associated with hearing loss include Alport syndrome, Treacher-Collins syndrome, CHARGE syndrome, and Stickler syndrome, as detailed in **Table 3** [14, 15].

3.2 Inherited nonsyndromic congenital hearing loss

Non-syndromic hereditary hearing loss can result from a functional or structural abnormality. Loss of function commonly results from mutations in proteins involved in the processing of sound signals. These conditions are inherited in an autosomal recessive manner in 80% of cases, and the remaining 20% in an autosomal dominant manner. Mutations in GJB2, which encodes for connexin 26, a gap junction protein that facilitates communication between cells in the stria vascularis, cause 50% of all autosomal recessive cases, leading to severe-profound bilateral sensorineural hearing loss [16]. Mutations affecting otoferlin are another important cause of non-syndromic SNHL. This transmembrane protein plays a crucial role in inner hair cell glutamate exocytosis at the synapse with the cochlear nerve ends [17].

On the other hand, structural malformations lead to hearing loss by disrupting the pathway of soundwaves. These malformations can affect the external, middle, or inner ear and can occur in isolation or as part of a syndrome. Examples of structural

Clinical syndrome	Predominant pattern of inheritance	Clinical key points
Alport syndrome	X-linked pattern	Progressive, bilateral SNHL resulting from defective collagen type IV synthesis (present in the basement membranes of the inner ear and kidneys). Hearing loss occurs before the onset of kidney insufficiency. Renal disease results from progressive glomerulonephritis, mostly ending at end-stage renal disease.
Treacher-Collins syndrome (Mandibular Facial Dysostosis)	Autosomal dominant	Autosomal dominant craniofacial condition affecting the bones and tissues in the face leading to deformities of the ears, eyes, zygomatic bones, and chin, *i.e.*, structures derived from the first and second pharyngeal arches during embryologic development. Malformations of the ear may include microtia and aural meatal atresia leading to conductive hearing loss; however, bilateral SNHL may also be possible.
CHARGE syndrome	Sporadic (not inherited)	C (coloboma of the eye) H (heart disease) A (atresia of choanae) R (development and growth retardation) G (genitourinary abnormalities) E (ear abnormalities) The ear malformations may be associated with conductive or SNHL and are usually asymmetric.
Stickler syndrome	Autosomal dominant	Hearing loss, ocular abnormalities (*e.g.*, retinal detachment, cataracts, and myopia), bone and joint abnormalities (*e.g.*, arthritis and joint hypermotility), and Pierre Robin sequence. Hearing loss is usually progressive sensorineural but also can be conductive due to abnormalities in the middle ear. There are several types of Stickler syndrome (Type 1, type 2, and type 3) due to mutations in different genes.

Table 3.
Other syndromes associated with congenital hearing loss.

abnormalities leading to conductive hearing loss include: microtia, where the external ear is dysplastic or absent; stenosis or atresia of the external auditory canal; anomalies of the ossicular chain; and congenital cholesteatomas, which are benign tumors of keratinizing epithelium found in the middle ear cavity and can result in chronic inflammation. Sensorineural hearing loss can result from cochlear malformations such as enlarged vestibular aqueduct, cochlear hypoplasia, dysplasia, or aplasia. The most common cochlear anomaly is Mondini dysplasia, also known as type II dysplasia, where the cochlea has one and a half turns instead of the normal two and a half turns [18].

3.3 Acquired congenital hearing loss due to infections

Hearing loss can be caused by infections occurring before or after birth. Therefore, infections play a major causative role in acquired congenital hearing loss, particularly TORCH infections, which include Toxoplasmosis, Other (such as Syphilis, Varicella-Zoster virus, Hepatitis B virus), Rubella, Cytomegalovirus, and Herpes simplex virus. Although we will only mention a few examples, many other viruses are associated with congenital hearing loss, including Lymphocytic choriomeningitic virus, Measles, and Human immunodeficiency virus [19].

3.3.1 Cytomegalovirus infection

The most common cause of non-genetic congenital sensorineural hearing loss is congenital infection with cytomegalovirus (CMV), a member Herpesviridae family, which causes up to 40% of cases [19]. CMV infection in newborns is notorious for affecting the auditory system, as it is also the most common sequelae caused in this patient population. Contrary to other otologic viral pathogens (e.g., Rubella), maternal immunity does not confer immunity against vertical transmission to the fetus [20]. Thus, it may be transmitted through the placenta or by direct contact with infectious body fluids during labor or while breastfeeding. Hearing loss correlates with the degree of viral load and results from both, direct cytopathic effects of viral inclusions bodies and indirect effects induced by the host's inflammatory response to the virus in the inner ear and cochlear nerve [19].

Primary CMV infection during pregnancy poses a 40% risk of intrauterine transmission. Approximately 90% of infants are asymptomatic at birth, but approximately 15% will develop hearing loss eventually. Therefore, asymptomatic babies can develop hearing loss several years after birth, making the diagnosis of congenital CMV infection challenging. On the contrary, symptomatic babies at birth can have the following: microencephaly, low birth weight, premature birth, jaundice, development delay, hepatosplenomegaly, petechiae, chorioretinitis, thrombocytopenia, hyperbilirubinemia, anemia, and hearing loss. The diagnosis in newborns requires a high index of suspicion by the clinician and is made by detection of CMV DNA in the urine, saliva or blood during the first 3 weeks of life [21].

3.3.2 Toxoplasmosis infection

Toxoplasmosis is caused by an intracellular protozoan parasite, Toxoplasma gondii, that infects humans and animals. Toxoplasmosis is acquired by exposure to cat feces, meat, soil, and water contaminated with the parasite. Intrauterine transmission can result in congenital hearing loss due to damage caused by the inflammatory response in the cochlea and cochlear nerve. This response its mainly triggered by the tachyzoite form of the parasite during active infection [22]. The cystic form (dormant form) of the parasite is not associated with pathological findings. The risk of SNHL following congenital Toxoplasmosis infection has been reported to be 27%, with patients having a 5-fold increased risk of abnormal neonatal hearing screening results compared to non-infected patients [23].

The primary infection during pregnancy carries a 30–50% risk of intrauterine transmission. However, 85% of infants with congenital toxoplasmosis at birth are asymptomatic. The manifestations of congenital toxoplasmosis include micro/macrocephaly, hydrocephalus, cerebral calcification, chorioretinitis, hepatosplenomegaly, jaundice, anemia, thrombocytopenia, petechiae, and lymphadenopathy. The diagnosis will require a high index of clinical suspicion plus positive laboratory serologic findings. Although treatment is not standardized, it is recommended that children receive treatment with pyrimethamine and sulfadiazine [24].

3.3.3 Rubella infection

Rubella virus, a member of the Togaviridae family of viruses, is another pathogen responsible for causing sensorineural hearing loss. It occurs as part of the broader Congenital Rubella Syndrome, which involves cataract formation, cardiac anomalies, intellectual disability, a characteristic "blueberry muffin" rash, and SNHL. First, the primary infection of an unvaccinated mother occurs during pregnancy, with subsequent vertical transmission to the fetus through the placenta. Following viremia, the virus invades the inner ear and directly damages the stria vascularis and Organ of Corti in the cochlea leading to SNHL [19]. If the pregnant mother is infected during the first 11 weeks of pregnancy the chance of congenital rubella syndrome is approximately 90%. Fortunately, Congenital Rubella Syndrome has plummeted since widespread vaccination programs against the Rubella virus began [25]. The Centers for Disease Control and Prevention (CDC) in the United States suggests administering the rubella vaccine, as part of the combined measles, mumps, and rubella (MMR) vaccine, between 12 and 15 months, followed by a booster shot at 4 to 6 years old.

3.3.4 SARS-CoV-2 infection

Coronaviruses, a family of enveloped, single-stranded RNA viruses, have the ability to invade the cranial nervous system through both anterograde and retrograde transport from nerve endings [26]. The recent epidemic caused by SARS-CoV-2, which emerged in 2019, has been linked to hearing loss in certain adults [27]. However, the impact of intrauterine transmission of SARS-CoV-2 on the inner ear development in embryos is still unclear. Despite limited research in this area, several retrospective multicenter cohort studies have investigated whether exposure to COVID-19 in utero increases the risk of hearing loss in infants. To date, these studies suggest that intrauterine exposure to COVID-19 is not a risk factor to the development of hearing loss [27–29].

3.4 Acquired congenital hearing loss due to ototoxic medications

Another important cause of acquired congenital hearing loss is ototoxic medication exposure. For example, aminoglycosides (antibiotics commonly used to treat severe neonatal infections such as meningitis) are notorious for causing sensorineural hearing loss. Cochlear hair cells are terminally differentiated cells without the capability of regenerating following insults. Drugs may reach the inner ear through the blood-labyrinth barrier or topically through the middle ear and the round or oval windows. However, regardless of how they reach the inner ear, aminoglycosides tend to concentrate in the endolymph of the inner ear and cause direct cytotoxic damage through the chelation of iron, the increased signaling of NMDA receptors, and creation or reactive oxygen species, ultimately affecting the stria vascularis and outer hair cells [30]. As it more commonly affects the inner row and basilar turn of the cochlea first and later progresses towards the apex, ototoxicity caused by aminoglycosides manifests as high-frequency hearing loss. Other medications can also induce SNHL, such as systemic chemotherapy (*e.g.*, cisplatin), macrolides antibiotics, salicylates, and loop diuretics.

4. Screening and diagnostic approach

A child who is deaf or hard of hearing in infancy is at increased risk for delays in speech and language development, academic achievement, and social outcomes without early recognition [31]. Before the advent of universal neonatal screening programs, the average age of diagnosis of congenital hearing loss was two years old [32].

U.S. states and territories, as well as other international jurisdictions, have implemented Early Hearing, Detection, and Intervention (EHDI) programs to maximize the number of newborn patients screened for hearing loss [33]. The specific goals by age are summarized in the "1–3-6" guideline, i.e., screening all newborns within 1 month of age, evaluating and establishing a diagnosis in all newborns that failed the hearing screening tests within 3 months of age, and starting therapeutic hearing intervention within 6 months of age in those patients with confirmed hearing loss. These interventions have been correlated with improved language outcomes.

4.1 Neonatal hearing screening

The screening consists of two electrophysiological tests that must permit detecting hearing thresholds deficits of equal or more than 35 dB and that may be used in infants less than or equal to 3 months of age, e.g., Automated auditory brainstem responses (AABR) and Otoacoustic emissions (OAE) [34]. The most commonly used test for neonatal hearing screening is the AABR, which estimates the integrity of the entire auditory pathway by using a series of electrodes placed in the patient's skull to detect electrical signal changes recorded as a waveform in response to 35 dB click. In AABR, the generated waveform from the patient is compared to that of a standard control sample. Like the conventional auditory brainstem response (ABR) test, the generated waveform consists of a series of peaks corresponding to different events in the auditory pathway. However, the comparison in AABR is made in an all-or-none binary fashion, with a pass-fail type of result. Thus, even though the estimated accuracy for identifying patients with decreased hearing thresholds under 35 dB between an AABR and an Auditory Brainstem Response is 98% [35], further characterization of the hearing loss must be done after a neonate fails a test.

Otoacoustic emissions (OAE) is another commonly employed objective screening test, which registers changes in the tympanic membrane compliance in response to acoustic signals generated from the cochlea's outer hair cells. It is worth mentioning that the middle ear must be cleared of existing pathologies (e.g., middle ear effusion) to use OAE as an indicator for cochlear function. Both tests, AABR and OAE, are performed sequentially [34].

4.2 Evaluation of an infant after a failed hearing screening test

Providers must conduct a comprehensive audiological assessment for patients who do not pass the screening test, including otoscopic examination, audiometric tests, and Auditory Brainstem Responses.

The otoscopic evaluation may reveal important causes of hearing loss, including external ear canal stenosis or middle ear effusion. Concerning audiometric testing, providers must tailor these tests based on the patient's neurodevelopmental age. For instance, trained audiologists can conduct a Behavioral Audiological evaluation for patients younger than 6 months. During this examination, patients are placed in a sound-controlled room and are presented with various tone stimuli, such as speech and warbled tones, through an earphone. The audiologist records the patient's minimal response level (MRL), which may include behaviors like eye widening and head movements and traces the patient's response as a function of the frequency at which the stimuli were presented, which ranges from 500 Hz to 4000 Hz. However, due to the subjective nature of this evaluation and its inherent variability, other objective audiological assessments are more commonly utilized in this patient population, e.g., Auditory Brainstem Responses.

Visual Reinforcement Audiometry is another audiological evaluation used to screen for congenital hearing loss in children, although suitable for patients older than 6 months but younger than 30 months. This test involves placing the patient in a sound-controlled environment like a Behavioral Audiometric evaluation. However, operant conditioning is employed by associating different sound levels with a playing video or moving toy, creating a conditioned behavioral response (e.g., head movements).

Upon objective confirmation of hearing loss, patients require further investigations and ongoing monitoring [36]. It is imperative to conduct genetic testing to identify common genetic mutations associated with congenital hearing loss with an unknown etiology. Prompt screening for potential causative infections, such as cytomegalovirus, is also essential. Obtaining head and neck imaging studies, including Computerized Tomography (CT) and/or Magnetic Resonance Imaging (MRI), is highly recommended to assess the presence of structural ear abnormalities and other pertinent features (e.g., state of cochlear nerves to evaluate candidacy for cochlear implants, later detailed). Moreover, considering the increased likelihood of accompanying ophthalmological abnormalities, an ophthalmological evaluation is advised for individuals with congenital sensorineural hearing loss.

5. Management strategies

Management of congenital hearing loss is done by providing the best hearing amplification option personalized to the specific auditory necessity of a given patient. It is also primarily dictated by addressing what caused it in the first place. Early intervention with hearing amplification (ideally before 6 months of age) is critical for infants with congenital hearing loss for their language and communication development.

5.1 Nonsurgical management

5.1.1 Hearing amplification

Hearing aids are small electronic devices that amplify sound and deliver it to the ear, and in infants, they may be used as young as a few weeks old. They consist of a microphone, an amplifier, and a speaker. For infants with hearing loss, the behind-the-ear (BTE) hearing aid is preferred as it is cheaper (parents only need to change the ear mold as the external ear grows) and a safer (lower risk for swallowing) alternative to in-the-ear (ITE) hearing aids. Fitting should be done every 3 months during the first 2 years of use due to the relatively rapid remodeling that the external ear undergoes during development [37]. The clinician and the audiologist should be aware that infants (children younger than 2 years), children from mothers with no college education, and children with mild hearing loss have been known to report less compliance with hearing aid daily use. Thus, increased surveillance and intervention is required to avoid poor outcomes in these patients.

5.1.2 Assistive listening devices

Assistive-learning technologies (*e.g.*, personal amplifiers, FM systems) are devices consisting of a microphone and a speaker that aim to optimize the acoustic signal-to-noise ratio that patients experience during spoken language [38]. It may be particularly useful in specific situations like, for example, for children struggling in their academic performance due to poor comprehension. In these situations, the teacher would have a microphone and the student would possess the assisted listening device in the better hearing ear, in conjunction with his or her hearing aid.

5.1.3 Auditory-verbal therapy

Auditory-verbal therapy is a type of therapy that serves as adjuvant therapy to hearing aids, cochlear implants, or assistive listening devices to improve spoken language skills. It has been shown to increase receptive language skills and improve speech production in infants with hearing loss [39]. Therapies involve the patient and his or her family, which play a central role. A trained speech and language pathologist conducts the therapy, or other trained personnel (e.g., a teacher for the deaf, audiologist) excludes non-verbal means of communication (e.g., sign language) to achieve competency in spoken language.

5.2 Surgical management

5.2.1 Otologic surgeries

The appropriate management approach primarily of congenital conductive hearing loss revolves around addressing the underlying causes of the hearing loss [40]. For instance, in external auditory canal atresia without ossicular chain pathology, patients may benefit from remodeling the external canal shape through an atresiaplasty after they reach 6 years of age. For patients with microtia who have significant hearing loss and psychological distress from cosmetic deformity, surgical intervention can provide substantial benefit. Alloplastic implants, i.e., made from artificial materials, can be used as early as 3 years of age. If the option of using autologous rib harvest is being contemplated, it is generally preferred to wait until the patient's ear reaches full adult size, which typically occurs around the age of 6 years. If the tympanic membrane or ossicles house any abnormality that would deem them amenable for surgical correction (e.g., chronic suppurative otitis media, ossicular chain fixation), a tympanoplasty with or without ossicular chain reconstruction, for example, may be indicated to restore the function of the middle ear.

A common finding in neonates that fail newborn hearing screening is Otitis Media with Effusion. The Academy of Otolaryngology and Head and Neck Surgery recommends ensuring adequate follow-up for neonates failing the newborn hearing screening with Otitis Media with Effusion, as it does not necessarily rule out the possibility of another co-existing cause of hearing loss [41]. Usually, otitis media with effusion resolves by itself within three months. For those patients who do not resolve after such a period, tympanostomy with ventilation tube placement can be considered. Additionally, for patients with congenital aural atresia, other forms of congenital conductive hearing loss not amenable to the surgeries mentioned above, or sensorineural hearing loss not amenable to cochlear implants, a bone-anchored hearing aid (BAHA) provides an excellent alternative [42]. It involves an osseointegrated titanium implant inserted into the temporal bone and a percutaneous abutment for the bone-conduction hearing aid.

5.2.2 Cochlear implantation

Patients with profound bilateral sensorineural hearing loss and an intact cochlear nerve may be candidates for cochlear implantation [43]. In the United States, the Food and Drug Administration (FDA) has approved cochlear implants for patients as young as 9 months of age, with device-specific approval granted recently [44]. Lowering the minimum age for consideration is supported by evidence showing that early implantation enhances quality of life, improves language skills, and promotes auditory development. Bilateral cochlear implantation is advocated as it further improves language skills and sound localization. The anatomy and integrity of the vestibulocochlear nerve are confirmed through imaging, including Magnetic Resonance Imaging (MRI) and Computerized Tomography (CT) scans of the temporal bone. Prior to surgical consideration, patients should be up to date with their vaccinations.

5.2.3 Brainstem auditory implantation

In cases with profound sensorineural hearing loss in which the cochlear nerve is absent or damaged or in cases where cochlear implantation cannot be done, an auditory brainstem implant (ABI) can be considered [45]. The implant is placed along the lateral recess of the fourth ventricle, and its electrode directly stimulates the cochlear nucleus, effectively bypassing the vestibulocochlear nerve and more distal portions of the auditory apparatus. In the United States, ABIs are only approved for patients older than 12 years of age and suffer from Neurofibromatosis type 2, a rare condition caused by mutations in the Merlin protein gene located in chromosome 22 that results in multiple nerve tumors, including bilateral vestibular nerve schwannomas. However, in recent years other applications have been described, such as in post-meningitis bilateral total ossified cochlea, various inner ear malformations, and trauma.

6. Conclusions

Congenital hearing loss is a common factor contributing to both physical and social challenges in the development of pediatric patients. This type of hearing loss can be either inherited or acquired, with inherited causes encompassing syndromic and non-syndromic, while acquired causes include infections and exposure to ototoxic medications. Through the utilization of various diagnostic tools and the implementation of universal newborn hearing screening programs, many of these patients can be identified early on and receive appropriate interventions to enhance long-term outcomes.

Conflict of interest

The authors declare no conflict of interest.

Author details

Alejandro Santiago Nazario*, Soraya Abdul-Hadi and Antonio Riera March
Otolaryngology-Head and Neck Surgery, University of Puerto Rico, San Juan, Puerto Rico

*Address all correspondence to: alejandro.santiago4@upr.edu

References

[1] CDC. Summary of Diagnostics Among Infants Not Passing Hearing Screening [Internet]. Centers for Disease Control and Prevention. 2021. Available from: https://www.cdc.gov/ncbddd/hearingloss/2019-data/06-diagnostics.html [Accessed: May 14, 2023]

[2] Lantos PM, Maradiaga-Panayotti G, Barber X, Raynor E, Tucci D, Hoffman K, et al. Geographic and racial disparities in infant hearing loss. Otolaryngology–Head and Neck Surgery. 2018;**159**(6):1051-1057. Available from: https://www.ncbi.nlm.nih.gov/pmc/articles/PMC6456438

[3] Fraser GR. Association of congenital deafness with goitre (Pendred's syndrome): A study of 207 families. Annals of Human Genetics. 1964;**28**(13):201-250

[4] Dossena S, Nofziger C, Tamma G, Bernardinelli E, Vanoni S, Fall T, et al. Molecular and functional characterization of human pendrin and its allelic variants. Cellular Physiology and Biochemistry. 2011;**28**(3):451-466

[5] Phelps PD, Coffey R, Trembath RC, Luxon LM, Grossman AB, Britton KE, et al. Radiological malformations of the ear in pendred syndrome. Clinical Radiology. 1998;**53**(4):268-273

[6] Pingault V, Ente D, Dastot-Le Moal F, Goossens M, Marlin S, Bondurand N. Review and update of mutations causing Waardenburg syndrome. Human Mutation. 2010;**31**(4):391-406 Available from: https://pubmed.ncbi.nlm.nih.gov/20127975

[7] Read AP, Newton VE. Waardenburg syndrome. Journal of Medical Genetics. 1997;**34**(8):656-665 Available from: https://pubmed.ncbi.nlm.nih.gov/9279758/

[8] Bonnet C, El-Amraoui A. Usher syndrome (sensorineural deafness and retinitis pigmentosa). Current Opinion in Neurology. 2012;**25**(1):42-49

[9] Vernon M. Usher's syndrome—Deafness and progressive blindness. Journal of Chronic Diseases. 1969;**22**(3):133-151

[10] Jaijo T, Aller E, Beneyto M, Najera C, Graziano C, Turchetti D, et al. MYO7A mutation screening in Usher syndrome type I patients from diverse origins. Journal of Medical Genetics. 2007;**44**(3):e71. Available from: https://www.ncbi.nlm.nih.gov/pmc/articles/PMC2598023

[11] Lindau TA, Cardoso ACV, Rossi NF, Giacheti CM. Anatomical changes and audiological profile in branchio-oto-renal syndrome: A literature review. International Archives of Otorhinolaryngology. 2014;**18**(1):68-76. Available from: https://www.ncbi.nlm.nih.gov/pmc/articles/PMC4296951

[12] Fraser FC, Sproule JR, Halal F, Optiz JM. Frequency of the b=ranchio-oto-renal (BOR) syndrome in children with profound hearing loss. American Journal of Medical Genetics. 1980;**7**(3):341-349

[13] Matsuda S, Ohnuki Y, Okami M, Ochiai E, Yamada S, Takahashi K, et al. Jervell and Lange-Nielsen syndrome with novel KCNQ1 and additional gene mutations. Human Genome Variation. 2020;**7**(1):1-4

[14] Gettelfinger J, Dahl J. Syndromic hearing loss: A brief review of common

presentations and genetics. Journal of Pediatric Genetics. 2018;**07**(01):001-008

[15] Usman N, Sur M. Charge Syndrome. Treasure Island, FL: StatPearls Publishing; 2022. Available from: https://www.ncbi.nlm.nih.gov/books/NBK559199

[16] Snoeckx RL, Huygen PLM, Feldmann D, Marlin S, Denoyelle F, Waligora J, et al. GJB2 mutations and degree of hearing loss: A Multicenter study. The American Journal of Human Genetics. 2005;**77**(6):945-957 Available from: https://www.ncbi.nlm.nih.gov/pmc/articles/PMC1285178/

[17] Roux I, Safieddine S, Nouvian R, Grati M, Simmler MC, Bahloul A, et al. Otoferlin, defective in a human deafness form, is essential for exocytosis at the auditory ribbon synapse. Cell. 2006;**127**(2):277-289 Available from: https://www.sciencedirect.com/science/article/pii/S0092867406012189?via%3Dihub

[18] Feraco P, Piccinini S, Gagliardo C. Imaging of inner ear malformations: A primer for radiologists. La radiologia Medica. 2021;**126**(10):1282-1295

[19] Cohen BE, Durstenfeld A, Roehm PC. Viral causes of hearing loss: A review for hearing health professionals. Trends in Hearing. 2014;**18**:1-17

[20] Mussi-Pinhata MM, Yamamoto AY. Natural history of congenital cytomegalovirus infection in highly seropositive populations. The Journal of Infectious Diseases. 2020;**221**:S15-S22. Available from: https://www.ncbi.nlm.nih.gov/pmc/articles/PMC7057789/

[21] Akpan US, Pillarisetty LS. Congenital Cytomegalovirus Infection (Congenital CMV Infection). Treasure Island (FL): StatPearls Publishing; 2020. Available from: https://www.ncbi.nlm.nih.gov/books/NBK541003/

[22] Salviz M, Montoya JG, Nadol JB, Santos F. Otopathology in congenital toxoplasmosis. Otology & Neurotology. 2013;**34**(6):1165-1169

[23] Fontes AA, da Carvalho SA, de Andrade GM, Carellos EV, Romanelli RC, de Resende LM. Study of brainstem auditory evoked potentials in early diagnosis of congenital toxoplasmosis. Brazilian Journal of Otorhinolaryngology. 2019;**85**(4):447-455. Available from: https://pubmed.ncbi.nlm.nih.gov/29929810/

[24] CDC. Toxoplasmosis - resources for health professionals. www.cdc.gov. 2019. Available from: https://www.cdc.gov/parasites/toxoplasmosis/health_professionals/index.html

[25] Stanley FJ, Sim M, Wilson G, Worthington S. The decline in congenital rubella syndrome in Western Australia: An impact of the schoolgirl vaccination program? American Journal of Public Health. 1986;**76**(1):35-37

[26] Sharma A, Ahmad Farouk I, Lal SK. COVID-19: A review on the novel coronavirus disease evolution, transmission, detection, control and prevention. Viruses. 2021;**13**(2):202. Available from: https://pubmed.ncbi.nlm.nih.gov/33572857/

[27] Kirbac A et al. Is intrauterine exposure to COVID-19 infection a risk factor for infant hearing loss? American Journal of Otolaryngology. 2023;**44**(4):103859-103859. DOI: 10.1016/j.amjoto.2023.103859

[28] Goulioumis A et al. Hearing screening test in neonates born to COVID-19–positive mothers. European Journal

of Pediatrics. 2022;**182**(3):1077-1081. DOI: 10.1007/02 s00431-022-047 70-8

[29] Toker GT et al. Is gestational COVID-19 a risk factor for congenital hearing loss? Otology & Neurotology. 2023;**44**(2):115-120. DOI: 10.1097/mao.0000000000003761

[30] Fu X, Wan P, Li P, Wang J, Guo S, Zhang Y, et al. Mechanism and prevention of ototoxicity induced by aminoglycosides. Frontiers in Cellular Neuroscience. 2021;**15**:15

[31] Lieu JEC, Kenna M, Anne S, Davidson L. Hearing loss in children. Journal of the American Medical Association. 2020;**324**(21):2195

[32] Coplan J. Deafness: Ever heard of it? Delayed recognition of permanent hearing loss. Pediatrics. 1987;**79**(2):206-213

[33] Journal of Early Hearing Detection and Intervention. 2019;**4**(2):1-44. Available from: : https://digitalcommons.usu.edu/jehdi/vol4/iss2/1

[34] Gáborján A, Katona G, Szabó M, Muzsik B, Küstel M, Horváth M, et al. Universal newborn hearing screening with automated auditory brainstem response (AABR) in Hungary: 5-year experience in diagnostics and influence on the early intervention. European Archives of Oto-Rhino-Laryngology. 2022;**279**(12):5647-5654

[35] Straaten H. Automated auditory brainstem response in neonatal hearing screening. Acta Paediatrica. 2007;(88):76-79

[36] Korver AMH, Smith RJH, Van Camp G, Schleiss MR, Bitner-Glindzicz MAK, Lustig LR, et al. Congenital hearing loss. Nature Reviews Disease Primers [Internet]. 2017;**3**:16094. Available from: https://www.ncbi.nlm.nih.gov/pmc/articles/PMC5675031/

[37] Tharpe AM, Gustafson S. Management of children with mild, moderate, and moderately severe sensorineural hearing loss. Otolaryngologic Clinics of North America. 2015;**48**(6):983-994

[38] Walker EA, Spratford M, Moeller MP, Oleson J, Ou H, Roush P, et al. Predictors of hearing aid use time in children with mild-to-severe hearing loss. Language, Speech, and Hearing Services in Schools. 2013;**44**(1):73-88

[39] Brennan-Jones CG, White J, Rush RW, Law J. Auditory-verbal therapy for promoting spoken language development in children with permanent hearing impairments. Cochrane Database of Systematic Reviews. 2014;**2014**:4

[40] Zhang T, Bulstrode N, Chang KW, Cho YS, Frenzel H, Jiang D, et al. Functional ear reconstruction. The Journal of International Advanced Otology;**15**(2):204-208 Available from: https://www.ncbi.nlm.nih.gov/pmc/articles/PMC6750779

[41] Coggins R, Gagnon L, Hackell JM, et al. Clinical practice guideline. Otolaryngology–Head and Neck Surgery. 2016;**154**(2):201-214. Available from: https://journals.sagepub.com/doi/10.1177/0194599815624407

[42] Kiesewetter A, Ikari L, Brito R, Bento R. Bone-anchored hearing aid (BAHA): Indications, functional results, and comparison with reconstructive surgery of the ear. International Archives of Otorhinolaryngology. 2013;**16**(03):400-405

[43] Purcell PL, Deep NL, Waltzman SB, Roland JT, Cushing SL, Papsin BC, et al. Cochlear implantation in infants:

Why and how. Trends in Hearing. 2021;**25**:233121652110317

[44] Center for Devices and Radiological Health. Cochlear Implants. U.S. Food and Drug Administration; Silver Springs, MD 2019. Available from: https://www.fda.gov/medical-devices/implants-and-prosthetics/cochlear-implants

[45] Deep N, Choudhury B, Roland J. Auditory brainstem implantation: An overview. Journal of Neurological Surgery Part B: Skull Base. 2019;**80**(02):203-208

Chapter 2

Auditory Neuropathy

Alenka Kravos

Abstract

Some patients visit the doctor because of hearing problems in noise. The hearing examination, however, does not show any specifics. Only an extended and targeted investigation leads to the suspicion of auditory neuropathy, which means altered temporal coding of the acoustic signal and explains the problems. Additional investigations show pathology of the synapse between the inner auditory sense and the auditory nerve or the process of conduction along the nerve. The combination of otoacoustic emissions and the auditory brainstem evoked potentials investigations raises the suspicion of auditory neuropathy. Auditory neuropathy occurs in both children and adults. In children, the diagnostic procedure is quite difficult.

Keywords: auditory nerve, inner hearing cell, synapsis, auditory brainstem responses, otoacoustic emissions

1. Introduction

Auditory neuropathy (AN) is a hearing impairment which can be recognized by deteriorated speech perception, while pure-tone detection thresholds remain relatively preserved. Affected individuals usually performed abnormal or no auditory brainstem responses (ABR), but normal otoacoustic emissions (OAE). This numerous groups of disorders described as "auditory neuropathy" includes abnormal function of peripheral synaptic sound processing by inner hair cells (synaptopathy) and/or of the generation and spread of action potentials in the auditory nerve (neuropathy). Audiological attributes of AN suggest that it is most certainly caused by the disturbed function of inner hearing cells (IHC) and/or spiral ganglion neurons. Meanwhile, the function of outer hearing cells (OHC) remains normal. This leads to a divergence between the hearing level thresholds and speech audiogram [1].

In neonates, AN can be seen as congenital sensorineural hearing loss (SNHL) of various degrees, usually bilateral with absent or abnormal ABR and mostly preserved otoacoustic emissions (OAE) and/or cochlear microphonics (CM).

In older children, AN is considered as a state where speech understandability is worse than should be expected based on behavioral audiograms while speech comprehension/discernment is poor.

During later lifetime we can recognize AN in affected individuals as a dysfunction of hearing with moderately good results in hearing level measures and bad comprehension abilities especially in loud and/or noisy environments.

2. History

AN is a relatively new audiology disease because some worthwhile methods and electrophysiologic equipment had to be developed for the exact assessment of the auditory pathway. Research in this field started after ABR for assessment of the inner ear were invented. Researches started in 1974 by Hecox and Galambos [2].

The term AN was first used in audiology in the 1980s, following the observation of adult patients who had a feeling of deteriorated hearing level despite their measured hearing levels were within normal range. They had difficulty detecting the sounds, especially in a noisy environment [3]. The term "auditory neuropathy" was till then considered as a part of the clinical picture of hereditary sensorimotor neuropathy [4]. AN as an audiological dysfunction was an object of scientific investigation of Starr. He observed that some patients with hearing problems in noisy environment had normal OHC function but their transmission of sound was impaired [5]. He did some electrophysiologic research and found out that the main pathology was not represented at the level of sound detection, by its transduction through the auditory pathway.

Later AN was identified in the pediatric population a few years later on the basis of bad cochlear implantation results. That was after initiating neonatal hearing screening [6].

Infants and adults without central nervous system disease got the diagnosis confirmed by measuring OAE, ABR, and CM [6–8]. At that time, OAE began to be routinely used. Similar results have assessed the investigations were also carried out in children with delayed speech development.

Today ABR remains the gold standard for objective hearing assessment with a new function in diagnostic procedure in people with listening problems in noisy environments and children with delayed speech development. In modern audiological diagnostic procedure difunctional parts in auditory pathway, including internal hair cells, auditory nerve fibers, auditory neurons in the spiral ganglia, or a combination of these can be determined [9].

3. Spectrum disease

In the future, some authors propose to rename AN into auditory neuropathy spectrum disease (ANSD) regarding a wide range of possible etiologies. Most importantly, many specific etiologies are identified as causing AN [10, 11]. We do not agree with the nomenclature of spectrum disease regarding that the main pathologies come from synaptic dysfunction [12]. We suggest using the term postsynaptic and presynaptic AN regarding the site of the lesion.

4. Pathophysiology

Examination of temporal bones in subject's postmortem with diagnosed AN showed that the number, as well as appearance of inner and outer hair cells, remained normal. Auditory ganglion cells and nerve fibers, however, were both reduced in number and demyelinated [13]. Loss of auditory nerve fibers attenuated neural input while demyelination affected the synchrony of neural conduction. We suggest that the loss of auditory nerve fibers and altered neural transmission, due to the reduction of neural synchrony, contribute to the abnormalities of ABRs and hearing.

The conversion of mechanical energy into a molecular change by IHC is the catalyst that initiates an electrical signal which travels along the acoustic neuron. Mechanical energy is generated by the undulation of the tectorial membrane, which begins the process of binding calcium molecules to receptors. This causes the release of neurotransmitters in synapses [14]. The signal then travels further along the peripheral axon of the sensorineural ganglion (SNG) from the synapse towards the central nervous system (CNS) [15]. SNGs are bipolar neurons, frequency-tuned by IHC so that tonotopy is preserved even at higher levels during transmission to the CNS. The effectiveness of coding relies on fast and accurate signal generation in the auditory nerve [16]. The process is called transduction and an error at any stage of the transmission of the acoustic signal means AN.

5. Temporal processing

The auditory system can transmit and process temporal information. This is the so-called temporal processing of sound. Precise detection of the temporal features of sounds is basic for speech perception. This process takes a great metabolic demand because very short electrical phenomena are necessary to achieve the speed which is needed to conduct and transform all the information that is hidden in the incoming sound. Auditory nerve fibers are capable of processing phase-locked signal outcoming from the movement of IHC stereocilia. Two movements are possible, backward and forward. They open or close ionic canals for cation influx. That makes temporal fine structure processing possible. Studies of temporal processing abilities are done by measuring gap detection threshold by noise-burst stimuli. Gap detection is lowered in AN. Temporal processing takes a great metabolic consumption because very short electrical parameters are necessary to achieve rapid temporal processing. IHC and auditory neurons have such characteristics, they have high conductance in the resting state. Any structural deficit in this area enables this high conductance and leads to asynchrony. In AN temporal processing is disrupted mostly as a consequence of asynchronicity. That does not affect the sensation of tone. The temporal processing is important for speech comprehension, localization of sounds, and separating signals from ground noise [3]. The temporal envelope of a sound-how it changes over time is basic for speech perception. It is measured by noise-burst stimuli which represent a very sophisticated way of scientific research. It is measuring how sound changes in amplitude over time. Auditory evoked potentials measure the millisecond-by-millisecond activity of a population of neurons as a form of auditory perception. Time is a parameter to identify and dissolve auditory streams. Deficits in temporal processing were also detected in children with dyslexia and autism. It is also a part of age-related hearing deterioration.

Demielinisation is expressed to a greater extent than the loss of the number of axones [10, 17, 18]. This is the case of type I neuropathy [17], where a concomitant peripheral neuropathy exists which can be hereditary or inflammatory in origin [18]. Another option is type II where the hearing loss is isolated [19].

In AN temporal processing is the major defect and is the reason for the major events in AN. These are clear hearing in a noisy background, sound localization, and a good understanding of spoken language [20].

AN appears to consist of several varieties depending on the site of the lesion of temporal processing [1] presynaptic in inner hair cell ribbon synapses, [2] postsynaptic in auditory nerve dendrites, and [3] postsynaptic in auditory nerve axons.

6. Prevalence

The prevalence of ANSD in children diagnosed with severe to profound hearing loss is uncertain. It ranges from 1 to 14% of hearing-impaired persons, while the prevalence of auditory neuropathy in the non-risk population is unknown [21].

Among neonates from the intensive care unit, it is much higher and is assumed to be up to 30% of hearing-impaired neonates [22].

7. Etiologies

Because the auditory pathway is long and complexly constructed, there are potentially many possible sites for error in signal transmission and thus AN. Because AN is a transduction problem (temporal processing) the site of lesion must be somewhere post or presynaptic or in the nerve where transduction takes place. So there is a range of possible sites of pathology. Transduction in IHC means converting mechanical energy into a molecular signal for the entry of cations into IHC. After the invasion, the cell is depolarized, allowing calcium influx through calcium channels. The pairing of presynaptic ribbon synapse calcium channels between the IHC and the nerve releases glutamate into the synapse. Dysfunction at any level of transduction can disturb the coding of the acoustic signal.

Besides many possibilities of localization of pathological changes in anatomic structures and function in IHC, synapse, there are also many possible etiological factors. They can be divided according to the time of occurrence (prenatal, postnatal, later), the site of the defect according to the anatomy (presynaptic, postsynaptic, axonal), according to the origin of the nox (genetic or non-genetic). The distributions are mixed. 50–60% of children with AN will have significant birth histories. The remaining 40–50% of cases should be explained by a genetic disorder.

Birth histories are pre, peri, and postnatally.

Prenatally they are genetic, morphogenetic failures (cochlear malformations), fetal mumps infections, rubella and cytomegalovirus, and dysmaturity.

Perinatally they are hypoxia and mechanical ventilation.

Postnatally they are also genetic with a delayed onset of the clinical picture, prematurity, icterus, septicemia, ototoxic drugs and meningitis [23].

8. Genetic etiologies

Many gene defects (IHC, Synapses between IHC and auditory nerves) are responsible for the development of AN [24–26]. This diversity is also responsible for the diversity in the clinical presentations of AN and for variations in therapy success. Genetic analysis predisposes to predict c, as well as the variations in cochlear implantation (CI) success. By direct stimulation of the cochlear nerve, the CI enables the bypass of the defective synapse. However, if the defect is more centrally postsynaptic, CI supplementation may be less successful.

A. These may code some deficits in glutamate metabolism in synaptic vesicles, the influx of synaptic Ca, and can alter synaptic vesicle turnover.

1. OTOFERLIN (OF). OF can have a range of possible genetic mistakes because it is a very compleksly formed protein important in presynaptic membrane fusion. It is the most important mutation in synaptopathies [27]. Its role is in bindings ions in exocytosis of synaptic vesicles and fusion [28].

OF mutations are multiple and represent 3.5% of hearing impairments. Patients have normal OAE response, abnormal ABR, and normal balance. Clinical pictures in OF mutations with different clinical pictures and results of electrophysiological measurements.

OHC is normal, but IHC is dysfunctional regarding the malfunctioning ribbons in the synapse [29].

2. CACNA1D gene defines the structure of the Ca2+ channel important for the glutamate release in the synapse [30]. These channels are located in OHC, IHC, and cardiomyocytes and these gene defects present a syndrome called "sino-atrial node dysfunction and deafness" (SANDD syndrome) [31].

3. CABP2 gene is involved in Ca channel regulation for glutamate release. It can be a part of profound prelingual deafness and with Marfan phenotype expression [32].

4. SLC17A8 gene defines another vesicular glutamate transporter type 3 (VGluT3), which regulates glutamate uptake in synapses [33].

5. 12q22-q24 gene mutation defines congenital deafness at DFNA25 locus associated with mutations of SLC17A8 [34, 35]. Neonates have progressive SNHL located in high frequencies. CI demonstrates very good therapy decisions [36].

B. Postsynaptic genetic synaptopathy. Their clinical appearance can mimic neuropathies (dendritic), afferent nerve axons, or nerve demyelination problems. Transmission of nerve impulse is disrupted.

1. OPA1 mutations combine two options. As solitary nonsyndromic dominant optic atrophy (DOA) form [37] or the syndromic DOA form associated with hearing impairment due to the degeneration of the terminal nerve fiber [38].

Hearing loss is moderate to profound. DOA is in 60% as syndromic combining hearing loss, sensorimotor neuropathy, myopathy, and ataxia [39].

2. ROR1 gene defines the receptor tyrosine kinase-like orphan 1 located in plasma. It is important for neural growth. It is an important factor in lowered number of nerve fiber of the auditory nerve. It is XXX fan synaptopathy [40].

3. ATP1A3 gene defines the morphology of the transmembrane Na/K-ATPase pump. The patient has cerebellar ataxia, pes cavus, optic atrophy, areflexia, and SNHL, called CAPOS syndrome [41–43].

Overall in both synaptopathies, good CI outcomes were reported [43].

C. Neurone conduction neuropathies

AN easily occurs in the context of other peripheral nerve disorders, leading to various syndromic conditions.

1. Charcot–Marie-Tooth is the most common sensory-motor neurological disease, where it is a defect of myelination. Deafness is sensorineural with disproportionally worse speech understanding compared to the measured hearing threshold values. Histologically, the neuronal cell is normal, myelination is pathological. Assessment of hearing rehabilitation after CI gives as poor results [44, 45].

2. Spino-Cerebellar Ataxia (Friedreich's) Hereditary Motor and Sensory Neuropathy. Patients have ataxia with a range of progressive features including axonal degeneration of sensory nerves [46].

3. Synaptopathy and neuropathy Pejvakin, encoded by DFNB 59 gene in hair cells and neurons, acts as a sensor that activates autophagy in case of oxidative stress such as noise-induced damage [47].

Other etiologic factors besides genetics are multiple.

The most prevalent etiologic factor besides genetics is hyperbilirubinemia reported in 10–50% of cases in some studies [48]. Hyperbilirubinemia is the most common cause of AN, especially in its unbound form bilirubin (BR) is very neurotoxic. But fortunately, very high levels of BR can be neurotoxic. Anoxia, prematurity, and low birth weight can predispose to toxic effects of BR in even lower levels. AN can be also a transient one and the hearing level can become normal after the period of time (12–18 months), if BR are corrected to normal level and the child is not a carrier of gen for deafness [49].

Anoxia is the second most important factor in inducing AN. It affects IHC and OHC in different matters. Mild chronic hypoxia causes damage to the IHC, and acute anoxia affects them all. Prematurity is a typical state of mild chronic hypoxia, a well-known anamnestic data in evaluating children with AN [50].

Other etiologic factors may be morphologic developmental changes [51], toxic-metabolic disorders [52]; infections (e.g., meningitis), inflammation (e.g., siderosis), neoplasms (e.g., acoustic neuroma), genetic mutations affecting neural functions [13] and ribbon synapse function [12].

9. Hidden hearing loss (HHL)

It is a kind of hearing impairment by which the clinical picture of hearing dysfunction expresses only in challenging auditory conditions (noise, less or rapidly articulated speech). Audiograme and BERA are normal in a quiet environment. There is a defect in auditory fibers which have defects in responding to sounds of high-intensity sounds [53–55].

10. Clinical expression of AN

AN refers to a range of different audiological profiles. They are associated with specific changes in auditory perceptions depending on pathologic alteration of managing the spread of acoustic signals. These changes influence speech sensation, space localisation of sound, and perception of sounds in noise [56].

The typical clinical picture of the affected subjects presents speech discrimination difficulties, particularly in background noise, that is out of proportion compared to their pure-tone detection thresholds. AN is usually bilateral. The hearing levels in audiometric exam may very fluctuate as much as 40 dB. Fluctuations are more frequent in children than in adults and the improvement in AN or its disappearance is possible in children [57, 58].

Even in children, AN presents a whole spectrum of different clinical pictures. As the etiologies are very diverse, the clinical picture is also variable. In neonates it is a clinical picture of severe hearing loss. This form of AN neuropathy is mostly diagnosed before the first year of life, while the other milder clinical forms are identified only later, mostly after the first year of age. or later in the form of delayed speech development. In the period after the first year of age, AN manifests itself in the form of slowed speech development.

In those where the synapse is defective, the temporal processing of sound is impaired due to characteristic gaps in sound perception. Gaps are caused by impaired signal transduction and prevent the perception of sounds with multiple short stimuli and therefore require stronger sound intensities to detect changes in frequency. That's why background noise is extremely annoying for such people. Speech understanding is severely impaired in a noisy environment. Sound localization, which uses the interaural time difference for its functioning, is also impaired.

The clinical picture is slightly different for people with a normal synapse but disturbed conduction along the auditory nerve, as they do not have problems with time processing, but with longer latency times. Ambient noise does not bother them so much, but they have even more problems understanding speech, loud sounds bother them [59].

11. Comparison between SNHL and AN

Approximately 60% of patients with AN have severe or profound hearing loss. But the characteristics of hearing loss are different. Perception of pitch and temporal cues are very distinct [60]. Frequency resolution in AN is regarding the preserved outer hair cell quite good, but the temporal function is disrupted. In SNHL there is weak frequency resolution, temporal processing and listening in noise are normal.

12. Association with other diseases

AN can be associated with other syndromes or neurologic pathologies. We have already listed these neurological diseases, which are in the form of syndromes.

13. Transient AN

AN can be reversible. Some children with well-known AN have documented improvement in electrophysiologic findings over time. We can say that AN is unpredictable. So we recommend not to cure children too soon with cochlear implant, especially if they were from the group with low birth weight [61].

In case of high-risk infants (birth head trauma, ischemia, hyperbilirubinemia, metabolical diseases) ABR exams should be repeated and the time for observation should be prolonged because their ABR abnormalities can recover. Maturation of the nervous system is an ongoing process [62, 63].

14. Diagnostic procedure

Besides OAEs and ABRs, a basic audiological assessment may include stapedial reflex measurements, supraliminal psychoacoustic tests, electrocochleography (ECochG), and audiometry.

14.1 OAE

OAE are sounds produced by the movement of OHCs and their stereocilia. For the sound energy to be strong enough to be detected by the measuring probe in the ear canal, it must be amplified by external stimulation with additional sound. We do this in two ways: with transient stimulation (TOAE) and simultaneous stimulation with two different sounds (DPOAE). Kemp was the first who described the phenomena in 1978 [64]. He studied the sound coming out of OHC after transient stimulation or after two simultaneous tone stimuli [65]. Sound which was detected came from the moving OHC [66].

OHC contribute most of the potential measured in ABR before then I wave. This potential originates from mechanosensitive channels in the stereocilia of OHC cells, to a lesser extent they are also produced by IHC (OHC are more numerous). During movement, the basilar membrane opens and closes the transduction channels in the cilia of these cells. Polarization and depolarization are performed, which are generators of cochlear microphonics (CoM) [67]. These can be shown on an ABR examination using rarefaction and condensation methods. The summation of these two gives us the summation potential (SP) and the compound action potential (CAP). CAP represents wave I on ABR or it can be detected by electrocochleography (ECochG) [68].

In 20 to 80% of OAE, they may disappear. Cases have been described where an initially unsynchronized auditory pathway eventually becomes synchronized [63].

14.2 Electrocochleography (ECochG)

We can do this examination in two ways (extratympanic or transtympanic) to study cochlear microphonics (CoM), summating potential (SP), and cochlear action potential (CAP) [69, 70]. CoM and OAE are the results of the OHC function. SP serves for the assessment of IHC, especially for the study of ototoxine damage on IHC [71]. CoM can be prolonged in subjects with AN [72]. Amplitudes of CoM in AN are normal. CoM in persons with AN due to synaptopathy is not CAP, while CoM and SP are registered [72, 73]. In auditory synaptopathy, the CoM and the SP are preserved, while CAP is not detectable [12].

14.3 ABR investigation

It is an electrophysiologic diagnostic tool for objectively assessing the status of the auditory pathway from the cochlea to the central nervous system. We use it since the late 1960s as a diagnostic tool for adults and children. It was not meant to detect hearing levels, but to test the synchronicity of the auditory pathway. Before its invention patient with AN were hidden among those who were declared to be hard-of-hearing people with SNHL. The proportion of such patients among SNHL is approximately 10–15%, they were soonly named AN ones [74].

The most typical result of this investigation who confirmed AN diagnosis is an inversion of the ABR waveform in area I as a response to a change in a stimulus polarity (rarefaction and condensation cliks). Reversion of polarity is the only sign that helps us to separate AN from purely central processing disorders which have similar OAE and ABR results [75, 76].

Besides wave I which defines the state of IHC, 4 more waves are found during ABR measuring and each of it represents the transmission ability of the sound through a specific part of the auditory pathway.

If OHC is damaged, no atypical ABR patterns are found.

14.4 Audiometry

Audiometry does not show to what extent the auditory pathway is damaged, it is only an assessment of the functioning of the cochlea, better OHC. Audiometry can be in the range of normal to severe hearing loss. Speech audiometry is very poor. Stapedius reflex is pathological [4].

In adults with AN, hearing level threshold is usually pathologic in the low frequency range and quite normal in higher frequencies. It can be also perfectly normal, sometimes pathologic in entire curve or impaired only in high tones.

For children older than 4 years, the hearing threshold can be determined by audiometry, but up to the age of 4 children are not able to participate, so we use two methods. Both are based on observing the body's response to different intensities and pitches of sound [77].

The first is CBT (conditional behavioral threshold), and the second is VRA (visual reinforcement audiometry). We test children in an open field or through earphones with specific tonal stimulation in the range from 0.5 to 4 kHz.

In newborns, the level of hearing loss is 65% severe to very severe. The percentage is slightly higher because in this age period, we only manage to find more affected children, as neonatal screening is only performed based on OAE measurements immediately after birth, and ABR is performed routinely only in newborns from intensive care.

15. Therapy

The goal of the therapy in AN is to overcome synapse if synaptopathy is the reason for AN or to synchronize the sound transduction through the auditory nerve.

Conventional hearing aids (HA) amplify the signal but fail to overcome the neural dys-synchrony responsible for impaired speech comprehension. HA are recommended as the first step in rehabilitation process as the least harmful. HA have many disadvantages because they are not able to improve temporal processing. So infants need a precise behavioral observation for their fitting or switching to CI [78].

Some studies were done (Berlin) on the success of HA in AN and a good result was only in 3.5% of patients, 10.5% of them were only satisfied, 24.7% noticed only a bit of improvement, 61.1% had no benefit. CI was much more successful with 85% positive results [79].

CI can bypass the synapse and thus the auditory signal is directly transduced to the auditory nerve [23].

But in some cases of only moderate hearing loss or in nerve malformation AN or in syndromic AN, a HA can be a good solution in children. Later on, if their language development stagnates, CI may be suggested [23, 80–82].

In the rehabilitation process, the site of the lesion ver predisposes to a therapeutic outcome [83].

Despite technologically sophisticated HA or CI, patients with AN do not succeed in fully providing normal sensations of hearing sounds. Ever-new scientific research in the field of genetics has enabled us to very precisely determine the location of the error in the cell and thus the possibility of correcting this error with gene therapy which means a process of changing defective parts of DNK with new genes. It is a very promising procedure for the future. Specially for the field of neurodegeneration of auditory pathways [84].

16. Conclusion

AN is a modern disease, well known only in recent years. Presented in adults and children. The clinical picture in adults is much more benign than in children, by each can be very variable because of potentially many sites of origin, pre or postsynaptic or neurogenic. Multiple etiologic factors (genetic, infectious, environmental, toxic, metabolic) can induce AN in every part of life.

Rehabilitation is still a challenging area of investigation because there are still some deficiencies in rehabilitation in children with AN which have no proper level of hearing. That is why gene therapy promises a lot.

Author details

Alenka Kravos
University Clinical Centre Maribor, Slovenia

*Address all correspondence to: tomsunny54@gmail.com

References

[1] Ptok M. Otoakustische Emissionen, Hirnstammpotentiale, Tonschwellengehör und Sprachverständlichkeit bei auditorischer Neuropathie [otoacoustic emissions, auditory evoked potentials, pure tone thresholds, and speech intelligibility in cases of auditory neuropathy]. HNO. 2000;**48**(1):28-32

[2] Hecox K, Galambos R. Brain stem auditory evoked responses in human infants and adults. Archives of Otolaryngology. 1974;**99**(1):30-33

[3] Schulman, Galambos C, Galambos R. Brain stem evoked response audiometry in newborn hearing screening. Archives of Otolaryngology. 1979;**105**:86-90

[4] Starr A, Dong CJ, Michalewski HJ. Brain potentials before and during memory scanning. Electroencephalography and Clinical Neurophysiology. 1996;**99**:28-37

[5] Starr A, Picton TW, Sininger Y, Hood LJ, Berlin CI. Auditory neuropathy. Brain. 1996;**119**:741-753

[6] Bielecki I, Horbulewicz A, Wolan T. Prevalence and risk factors for auditory neuropathy spectrum disorder in a screened newborn population at risk for hearing loss. International Journal of Pediatric Otorhinolaryngology. 2012;**76.16**(1):75-79

[7] Gohari N, Farahani F. The proposed protocol for universal newborn hearing screening in Iran. Pajouhan Scientific Journal. 2013;**12**(1):61-63

[8] Sobhy OA, Asal S, Ragab F. Study of reversibility of auditory brainstem abnormalities in infants with high risk for hearing loss. Egyptian Journal of Ear, Nose, Throat and Allied Sciences. 2015;**16**(1):75-79

[9] Hood LJ. Auditory neuropathy/ Auditory Synaptopathy. Otolaryngologic Clinics of North America. 2021;**54**(6): 1093-1100

[10] Sininger Y, Starr A. Auditory neuropathy. A new perspective on hearing disorders. Singular. Thomson Learning. Audiological Medicine. 2001;**1**(2):151

[11] Santarelli R. Information from cochlear potentials and genetic mutations helps localize the lesion site in auditory neuropathy. Genome Medicine. 2010;**2**:1-10

[12] Moser T, Starr A. Auditory neuropathy—Neural and synaptic mechanisms. Nature Reviews. Neurology. 2016;**12**(3):135-149

[13] Starr A et al. Pathology and physiology of auditory neuropathy with a novel mutation in the MPZ gene (Tyr145→Ser). Brain. 2003;**126**(7):1604-1619

[14] Starr A, Sininger YS, Pratt H. The varieties of auditory neuropathy. Journal of Basic and Clinical Physiology and Pharmacology. 2000;**11**(3):215-230

[15] Zaaroor M, Starr A. Auditory brain-stem evoked potentials in the cat after kainic acid-induced neuronal loss. II. Cochlear nucleus. Electroencephalography and Clinical Neurophysiology. 1991;**80**(5):436-445

[16] Penido RC, Isaac ML. Prevalence of auditory neuropathy Spectrum disorder in an Auditory health care service.

Brazilian Journal of Otorhinolaryngology. 2013;**79**(4):429-433

[17] Kim KX, Rutherford MA. Maturation of nav and Kv Channel topographies in the Auditory nerve spike initiator before and after developmental onset of hearing function. The Journal of Neuroscience. 2016;**36**:2111-2118

[18] Nayagam BA, Muniak MA, Ryugo DK. The spiral ganglion: Connecting the peripheral and central Auditory systems. Hearing Research. 2011;**278**:2-20

[19] Fuchs PA. Time and intensity coding at the hair Cell's ribbon synapse. The Journal of Physiology. 2005;**566**:7-12

[20] Zeng GF, Oba S, Garde S, Sininger Y, Starr A. Temporal and speech processing deficits in auditory neuropathy. Neuroreport. 1999;**10**:3429-3435

[21] Kaga K, Nakamura M, Shinigami M, Tsuzuku T, Yamada K, Shindo M. Auditory nerve disease of both ears revealed by auditory brainstem response, electrocochleography, and otoacoustic emissions. Scandinavian Audiology. 1996;**25**:233-238

[22] Butinar D, Starr A, Zidar J, Koutsou P, Christodoulou K. Auditory nerve is affected in one of two different point mutations of the neurofilament light gene. Clinical Neurophysiology. 2008;**119**(2):367-375

[23] Ehrmann-Müller D, Cebulla M, Cancer K, Scheich M, Back D, Hagen R, et al. Evaluation and therapy outcome in children with Auditory neuropathy Spectrum disorder (ANSD). International Journal of Pediatric Otorhinolaryngology. 2019;**127**:109618

[24] Jung S, Maritzen T, Wichmann C, Jing Z, Neef A, Revelo NH, et al. Disruption of adaptor protein 2μ (AP -2μ) in Cochlear hair cells impairs vesicle reloading of synaptic release sites and hearing. The EMBO Journal. 2015;**34**:2686-2702

[25] Pangšrič T, Lasarow L, Reuter K, Takago H, Schwander M, Riedel D, et al. Hearing requires Otoferlin-dependent efficient replenishment of synaptic vesicles in hair cells. Nature Neuroscience. 2010;**13**:869-876

[26] Starr A, Sininger Y, Nguyen T, Michalewski H. Cochlear receptor and Auditory pathway activity in Auditory neuropathy. Ear and Hearing. 2001;**22**:91-99

[27] Roux I, Safieddine S, Nouvian R, Grati M, Simmler MC, Bahloul A, et al. Otoferlin, defective in a human deafness form, is essential for exocytosis at the Auditory ribbon synapse. Cell. 2006;**127**:277-289

[28] Johnson CP, Chapman ER. Otoferlin is a calcium sensor that directly regulates SNARE-mediated membrane fusion. The Journal of Cell Biology. 2010;**191**:187-197

[29] Varga R, Avenarius MR, Kelley PM, Keats BJ, Berlin CI, Hood LJ, et al. OTOF mutations revealed by genetic analysis of hearing loss families including a potential temperature sensitive auditory neuropathy allele. Journal of Medical Genetics. 2006;**43**(7):576-581

[30] Brandt A, Striessnig J, Moser T. Cav 1.3 channels are essential for development and presynaptic activity of cochlear inner ear hair cells. Journal of Neurosscience. 2003;**23**(34):10832-10840

[31] Qi F, Zhang R, Chen J, Zhao F, Sun Y, Du Z, et al. Down-regulation of Cav 1.3.in auditory pathway promotes age-related hearing loss by enhancing

calcium-mediated oxidative stress in male mice. Aging. 2019;**11**:6490-6502

[32] Schrauwen I, Helfmann S, Inagaki A, Predoehl F, Tabatabaiefar MA, Picher MM, et al. A mutation in CABP2, expressed in Cochlear hair cells, causes autosomal-recessive hearing impairment. American Journal of Human Genetics. 2012;**91**:636-645

[33] Seal RP, Akil O, Yi E, Weber CM, Grant L, Yoo J, et al. Sensorineural deafness and seizures in mice lacking vesicular glutamate transporter 3. Neuron. 2008;**57**:263-275

[34] Ryu N, Sagong B, Park HJ, Kim MA, Lee KY, Choi JY, et al. Screening of the SLC17A8 gene as a causative factor for autosomal dominant non-syndromic hearing loss in Koreans. BMC Medical Genetics. 2016;**17**:6

[35] Ryu N, Lee S, Park HJ, Lee B, Kwon TJ, Bok J, et al. Identification of a novel splicing mutation within SLC17A8 in a Korean family with hearing loss by whole-exome sequencing. Gene. 2017;**627**:233-238

[36] Shearer AE, Eppsteiner RW, Frees K, Tejani V, Sloan-Heggen CM, Brown C, et al. Genetic variants in the peripheral Auditory system significantly affect adult Cochlear implant performance. Hearing Research. 2017;**348**:138-142

[37] Ranieri M, Del Bo R, Bordoni A, Ronchi D, Colombo I, Riboldi G, et al. Optic atrophy plus phenotype due to mutations in the OPA1 gene: Two more Italian families. Journal of the Neurological Sciences. 2012;**15**:146-149

[38] Amati-Bonneau P, Valentino ML, Reynier P, Gallardo ME, Bornstein B, Boissière A, et al. OPA1 mutations induce mitochondrial DNA instability and optic atrophy 'plus' phenotypes. Brain. 2008;**131**:338-351

[39] Hudson G, Amati-Bonneau P, Blakely EL, Stewart JD, He L, Schaefer AM, et al. Mutation of OPA1 causes dominant optic atrophy with external ophthalmoplegia, ataxia, deafness, and multiple mitochondrial DNA deletions: A novel disorder of mtDNA maintenance. Brain. 2008;**131**:329-337

[40] Diaz-Horta O, Abad C, Sennaroglu L, Foster J 2nd, DeSmidt A, Bademci G, et al. ROR1 is essential for proper innervation of auditory hair cells and hearing in humans and mice. Proceedings of the National Academy of Sciences of the United States of America. 2016;**113**(21):5993-5998

[41] Tranebjærg L, Strenzke N, Lindholm S, Rendtorff ND, Poulsen H, Khandelia H, et al. Correction to: The CAPOS mutation in ATP1A3 alters Na/K-ATPase function and results in auditory neuropathy which has implications for management. Human Genetics. 2018;**137**:111-127

[42] Heimer G, Sadaka Y, Israelian L, Feiglin A, Ruggieri A, Marshall CR, et al. CAOS-episodic cerebellar ataxia, areflexia, optic atrophy, and sensorineural hearing loss: A third allelic disorder of the ATP1A3 gene. Journal of Child Neurology. 2015;**30**:1749-1756

[43] Paquay S, Wiame E, Deggouj N, Boschi A, De Siati RD, Sznajer Y, et al. Childhood hearing loss is a key feature of CAPOS syndrome: A case report. International Journal of Pediatric Otorhinolaryngology. 2018;**104**:191-194

[44] Goswamy J, Bruce IA, Green KMJ, O'Driscoll MP. Cochlear implantation in a patient with Sensori-neural deafness secondary to Charcot-Marie-tooth

disease. Cochlear Implants International. 2012;**13**:184-187

[45] Kabzińska D, Korwin-Piotrowska T, Drechsler H, Drac H, Hausmanowa-Petrusewicz I, Kochański A. Late-onset Charcot-Marie-tooth type 2 disease with hearing impairment associated with a novel Pro105Thr mutation in the MPZ gene. American Journal of Medical Genetics. 2007;**143**:2196-2199

[46] Rance G, Fava R, Baldock H, Chong A, Barker E, Corben L, et al. Speech perception ability in individuals with Friedreich ataxia. Brain. 2008;**131**:2002-2012

[47] Delmaghani S, Del Castillo FJ, Michel V, Leibovici M, Aghaie A, Ron U, et al. Mutations in the gene encoding Pejvakin, a newly identified protein of the afferent Auditory pathway, cause DFNB59 Auditory neuropathy. Nature Genetics. 2006;**38**:770-778

[48] Saphiro SM. Bilirubin toxicity in the developing nervous system. Pediatric Neurology. 2003;**29**:410-421

[49] Saphiro SM, Nakamura H. Bilirubin and the auditory system. Journal of Perinatology. 2001;**21**(Suppl. 1):S52-S55

[50] Riggs WJ, Roche JP, Giardina CK, Harris MS, Bastian ZJ, Fontenot TE, et al. Intraoperative electrocochleographic characteristics of Auditory neuropathy Spectrum disorder in Cochlear implant subjects. Frontiers in Neuroscience. 2017;**11**:416

[51] Buchman CA, Roush PA, Teagle HF, Brown CJ, Zdanski CJ, Grose JH. Auditory neuropathy characteristics in children with cochlear nerve deficiency. Ear and Hearing. 2006;**27**(4):399-408

[52] Bielecki I, Horbulewicz A, Wolan T. Prevalence and risk factors for Auditory neuropathy Spectrum disorder in a screened newborn population at risk for hearing loss. International Journal of Pediatric Otorhinolaryngology. 2012;**76**:1668-1670

[53] Chen GD. Hidden cochlear impairments. Journal of Otology. 2018;**13**:37-43

[54] Xiong B, Liu Z, Liu Q, Peng Y, Wu H, Lin Y, et al. Missed hearing loss in tinnitus patients with Normal audiograms. Hearing Research. 2019;**384**:107826

[55] Iliadou VV, Ptok M, Grech H, Pedersen ER, Brechmann AA, Deggouj NN, et al. A european perspective on auditory processing disorder-current knowledge and future research focus. Frontiers in Neurology. 2017;**8**:622

[56] Guest H, Munro KJ, Prendergast G, Millman RE, Plack CJ. Impaired speech perception in noise with a normal audiogram: No evidence for Cochlear Synaptopathy and No relation to lifetime noise exposure. Hearing Research. 2018;**364**:142-151

[57] Fontenot TE, Giardina CK, Teagle HF, Park LR, Adunka OF, Buchman CA, et al. Clinical role of electrocochleography in children with Auditory neuropathy Spectrum disorder. International Journal of Pediatric Otorhinolaryngology. 2017;**99**:120-127

[58] Chandan HS, Prabhu P. Audiological changes over time in adolescents and young adults with an auditory neuropathy spectrum disorder. European Archives of Oto-Rhino-Laryngology. 2015;**272**:1801-1807

[59] Wynne DP, Zeng FG, Bhatt S, Michalewski HJ, Dimitrijevic A, Starr A. Loudness adaptation accompanying

ribbon synapse and auditory nerve disorders. Brain. 2013;**136**:1626-1638

[60] Rance G, McKay C, Grayden D. Perceptual characterization of children with Auditory neuropathy. Ear and Hearing. 2004;**25**(1):34-46

[61] Chen W, Huang S, Huanng Y, Duan B, Xu Z, Wang Y. Short-term outcomes of infants with a hyperbilirubinemia-associated auditory neuropathy spectrum disorder in the neonatal intensive care unit. International Journal of Otorhinolaryngology and Head and Neck Surgery. 2023;**268**:189-196

[62] Psarommatis I, Florou V, Fragkos M, et al. Reversible auditory brainstem responses screening failures in high-risk neonates. European Archives of Oto-Rhino-Laryngology. 2011;**268**:189-196

[63] Uus K. Transient Auditory neuropathy in infants: How to conceptualize the recovery of Auditory brain stem response in the context of newborn hearing screening? Seminars in Hearing. 2011;**32**:123-128

[64] Kemp DT. Stimulated acoustic emissions from within the human Auditory system. The Journal of the Acoustical Society of America. 1978;**64**:1386-1391

[65] Prieve B, Fitzgerald T. Otoacoustic emissions. In: Katz J, editor. Handbook of Clinical Audiology. Philadelphia, PA, USA: Wolters Kluwer Health; 2015

[66] Glattke TJ. Otoacoustic Emissions—Clinical Applications. 2nd ed. New York, NY, USA: Thieme; 2002

[67] Pappa AK, Hutson KA, Scott WC, David WJ, Fox KE, Masood MM, et al. Hair cell and neural contributions to the Cochlear summating potential. Journal of Neurophysiology. 2019;**121**:2163-2180

[68] Dallos P, Cheatham MA. Production of cochlear potentials by inner and outer hair cells. The Journal of the Acoustical Society of America. 1976;**60**:510-512

[69] Santarelli R. Information from cochlear potentials and genetic mutations helps localize the lesion site in auditory neuropathy. Genome Medicine. 2010;**2**:91

[70] Santarelli R, Arslan E. Electrocochleography in Auditory neuropathy. Hearing Research. 2002;**170**:32-47

[71] Durrant JD, Wang J, Ding DL, Salvi RJ. Are inner or outer hair cells the source of summating potentials recorded from the round window? The Journal of the Acoustical Society of America. 1998;**104**:370-377

[72] do Amaral Soares I, de Lemos Menezes P, Carnaúba ATL, de Andrade KCL, Lins OG. Estudo do microfonismo coclear na neuropatia auditiva. Brazilian Journal of Otorhinolaryngology. 2016;**82**:722-736

[73] Snyder RL, Schreiner CE. The auditory neurophonic: Basic properties. Hearing Research. 1984;**15**:261-280

[74] Raveh E, Buller N, Badrana O, Attias J. Auditory neuropathy: Clinical characteristics and therapeutic approach. American Journal of Otolaryngology. 2007;**28**:302-308

[75] Berlin CI, Bordelon J, StJohn P, Wilensky D, Hurley A, Kluka E, et al. Reversing click polarity may uncover auditory neuropathy in infants. Ear and Hearing. 1998;**19**(1):37-47

[76] Auditory KK. Neuropathy Spectrum Disorders. In: Kaga K, editor. ABRs and

Electrically Evoked ABRs in Children. Modern Otology and Neurotology. Tokyo: Springer; 2022

[77] Meleca JB, Stillitano G, Lee MY, Lyle W, Carol Liu YC, Anne S. Outcomes of audiometric testing in children with Auditory neuropathy Spectrum disorder. International Journal of Pediatric Otorhinolaryngology. 2020;**129**:109757

[78] Walker E, McCreery R, Spratford M, Roush P. Children with auditory neuropathy spectrum disorder fitted with hearing aids applying the American Academy of Audiology Pediatric amplification guideline: Current practice and outcomes. Journal of the American Academy of Audiology. 2016;**27**:204-218

[79] Berlin CI, Hood LJ, Morlet T, Wilensky D, Li L, Mattingly KR, et al. Multi-site diagnosis and management of 260 patients with auditory neuropathy/dyssynchrony (Auditory neuropathy spectrum disorder). International Journal of Audiology. 2010;**49**:30-43

[80] Breneman AI, Gifford RH, Dejong MD. Cochlear implantation in children with auditory neuropathy spectrum disorder: Long-term outcomes. Journal of the American Academy of Audiology. 2012;**23**:5-17

[81] Shearer AE, Hansen MR. Auditory synaptopathy, auditory neuropathy, and cochlear implantation. Laryngoscope Investigative Otolaryngology. 2019;**4**:429-440

[82] Teagle HFB, Roush PA, Woodard JS, Hatch DR, Zdanski CJ, Buss E, et al. Cochlear implantation in children with auditory neuropathy spectrum disorder. Ear and Hearing. 2010;**31**:325-335

[83] Crispino G, Di Pasquale G, Scimemi P, Rodriguez L, Ramirez FG, de Siati RD, et al. BAAV mediated GJB2 gene transfer restores gap junction coupling in Cochlear organotypic cultures from deaf Cx26Sox10Cre mice. PLoS One. 2011;**6**:e23279

[84] Saidia AR, Ruel J, Bahloul A, Chaix B, Venail F, Wang J. Current advances in gene therapies of genetic auditory neuropathy spectrum disorder. Journal of Clinical Medicine. 2023;**12**(3):738

Chapter 3

Mitochondrial Hearing Loss: Diagnosis and Management

Charvi Malhotra and Peter Kullar

Abstract

Mitochondrial hearing loss (MHL) arises from mutations in mitochondrial DNA (mtDNA) or in nuclear genes coding for mitochondrial proteins, which impair inner ear function resulting in hearing loss. Diagnosis of MHL requires a comprehensive evaluation, including genetic tests, clinical assessments, and audiological examination. Treatment options for MHL are limited, with supportive measures to enhance communication and restore hearing function being the primary options. Ongoing research is investigating new therapies that target mitochondrial dysfunction and regenerative techniques to restore hearing function. It is crucial to understand the underlying mechanisms of MHL and develop effective interventions to mitigate its negative impact.

Keywords: mitochondria, hearing loss, diagnosis, treatment, neurogenetics

1. Introduction

Mitochondria, subcellular organelles found within eukaryotic cells, form a flexible network and serve various functions in addition to their well-known role in cellular energy production. These organelles have evolved to acquire multiple cellular functions over time including provision of cellular energy through ATP generation, crucial involvement in metabolic pathways, and apoptosis. Consequently, when mitochondria fail to function properly, it can negatively impact various aspects of cellular physiology and contribute to the development of different human diseases, including hearing loss.

The process of hearing relies on the conversion of sound pressure waves into neural signals by the inner hair cells of the cochlea. These signals are then transmitted to the auditory cortex through auditory neurons. Any disruption along this pathway can result in hearing loss, a complex condition influenced by multiple factors that can affect both individuals with mitochondrial disease and the general population.

Mitochondrial diseases are both genetically and phenotypically heterogeneous and can be caused by mutations in mitochondrial DNA (mtDNA) or the nuclear genes that encode mitochondrial proteins. Mitochondrial disease can involve potentially any organ at any age and involve either a single or multiple organs [1].

MHL is an important feature of many mitochondrial diseases, both in isolation (non-syndromic) and as a feature of systemic disease (syndromic). Some of the syndromes associated with mitochondrial hearing loss include Kearns-Sayre syndrome

(KSS), Mitochondrial encephalopathy, lactic acidosis and stroke-like syndrome (MELAS), and maternally inherited diabetes and deafness (MIDD) syndrome. Each of these syndromes is associated with the loss of hearing along with multiple other systemic manifestations [2–4].

Mitochondrial disease is rare, affecting approximately 1 in 5000 individuals, but it contributes significantly to the overall burden of hearing loss [2, 5]. Mitochondrial dysfunction is estimated to contribute to around 5% of non-syndromic post-lingual hearing loss and approximately 1% of pre-lingual cases [3, 5]. Additionally, studies suggest that mitochondrial mutations may also contribute to age-related hearing loss [3].

Mitochondria play a vital role in producing cellular energy through oxidative phosphorylation. In the auditory system, the inner ear contains specialized sensory hair cells that convert sound vibrations into electrical signals for the brain to interpret. Any disruption in mitochondrial function can severely impact the energy supply and cellular homeostasis of these hair cells, leading to hearing loss. Additionally, mitochondrial dysfunction can affect functionality of the stria vascularis, which is responsible for endolymph production and ion composition maintenance [1, 5]. Moreover, the spiral ganglion neurons can also be impacted by mtDNA mutations that result in loss of signal transduction from the auditory nerve to the brain.

Mitochondrial hearing loss is primarily caused by mutations in the mitochondrial DNA, which can occur in various genes responsible for mitochondrial function [1, 5, 3, 6]. These mutations are usually inherited from the mother due to the maternal inheritance pattern of mitochondrial DNA [1, 4]. However, spontaneous mutations can also occur during mitochondrial DNA replication, leading to mitochondrial hearing loss [2, 3, 6].

Mitochondrial DNA mutations can result in decreased ATP production, leading to cellular dysfunction in the inner ear [1, 7]. ATP deficiency can impair the normal functioning of hair cells, which are responsible for transmitting sound signals to the brain. Additionally, the stria vascularis can be impacted due to lack of proper ion composition of the endolymph. Mitochondria play a crucial role in generating reactive oxygen species (ROS) within cells during oxidative phosphorylation. The presence of noise has been shown to elevate the production of mitochondrial ROS, surpassing the cellular antioxidants' capacity and leading to oxidative stress. Consequently, cochlear hair cells may undergo apoptosis triggered by mitochondria, potentially resulting in their demise [1, 2, 5, 6, 8, 9].

2. Clinical presentation

Mitochondrial hearing loss presents with a diverse range of clinical manifestations, exhibiting considerable heterogeneity in terms of severity, age of onset, and progression of hearing impairment [1, 2, 4–6, 8]. The clinical features can vary among affected individuals and can include unilateral or bilateral hearing loss. The age at which hearing loss manifests can range from infancy to adulthood, and the progression of the condition can be gradual or sudden.

The degree of hearing impairment observed in individuals with mitochondrial hearing loss can vary widely, ranging from mild to profound [5, 8]. The specific frequencies of sound that are affected may also vary, resulting in different patterns of hearing loss. Some individuals may experience greater difficulty perceiving high-frequency sounds, while others may have impairments in the low-frequency range.

It is important to note that mitochondrial dysfunction can extend beyond the auditory system and affect other organ systems, leading to a wide array of associated symptoms. Neurological abnormalities, such as seizures, developmental delays, and cognitive impairments, may be observed in individuals with mitochondrial hearing loss [2, 5, 6, 8–10]. Additionally, myopathy, characterized by muscle weakness and fatigue, and visual impairment, including optic atrophy and retinitis pigmentosa, can be present in syndromic disease [2, 3, 5, 8].

There are various syndromic causes of mitochondrial hearing loss. One major cause is maternally inherited diabetes and deafness (MIDD), which is characterized by the development of both diabetes and hearing loss, typically in adulthood [4]. The severity of hearing loss can vary from mild to profound. Kearns-Sayre Syndrome is a rare mitochondrial disorder characterized by a triad of symptoms: progressive external ophthalmoplegia, heart block, and pigmentary retinopathy [3, 8, 9]. Hearing loss is a common feature of KSS, and it can be sensorineural, conductive, or mixed.

MELAS (Mitochondrial Encephalomyopathy, Lactic Acidosis, and Stroke-like episodes) syndrome is a multisystem disorder caused by mitochondrial DNA mutations [8, 9]. While it primarily affects the brain, it can also lead to hearing loss, among

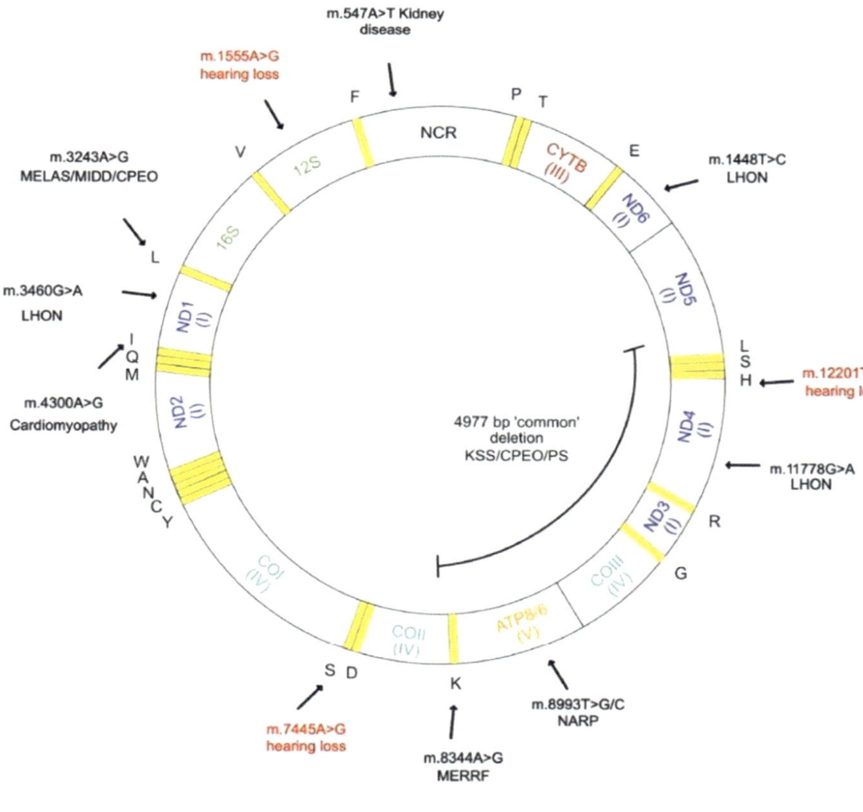

Figure 1.
Primary mtDNA mutations linked to human disease. A selection of clinically relevant primary mtDNA mutations linked to mitochondrial disease with their associated phenotypes. LHON, Leber's hereditary optic neuropathy; NARP, neurogenic weakness, ataxia and retinitis pigmentosa; KSS, Kearns-Sayre syndrome; CPEO, chronic progressive external ophthalmoplegia; MERRF, myoclonic epilepsy and ragged red fibres; MELAS, mitochondrial myopathy lactic acidosis and stroke like episodes; MDD, maternally inherited diabetes and deafness.

other symptoms such as muscle weakness, impaired exercise tolerance, stroke-like episodes, encephalopathy, and high levels of lactic acid in the blood [3, 8, 9, 11].

There are several diseases inherited from mothers have been linked to mutations in mitochondrial DNA. Specifically, the mt.1555A>G mutation (see **Figure 1**) occurring in mtDNA impacts the gene responsible for rRNA, leading to a structural alteration in the human ribosome [12]. Consequently, this renders the ribosome vulnerable to binding with the widely used antibiotic, aminoglycosides. This particular mutation has been associated with non-syndromic hearing loss and is prevalent among Asian populations as one of the most frequently observed mitochondrial DNA mutations [11, 12].

Moreover, the mt.3243A>G mutation (see **Figure 1**) is linked to patients with MELAS syndrome [13]. This variant is associated with early-onset hearing loss that typically occurs in early infancy with a gradual course. Due to the stroke-like episodes that occur in this syndrome, there are also cases of sudden onset hearing loss with this mitochondrial DNA variant [14].

Furthermore, the impact of mitochondrial hearing loss extends beyond the physical manifestations, affecting various aspects of an individual's life, including communication, social interactions, and educational attainment. Difficulties in speech understanding, particularly in noisy environments, can lead to challenges in daily communication and academic performance [1, 3]. Consequently, individuals with mitochondrial hearing loss may benefit from speech therapy, educational accommodations, and support services to optimize their communication abilities and overall quality of life.

3. Diagnosis

Accurate diagnosis of mitochondrial hearing loss relies on a comprehensive evaluation that includes clinical assessment, genetic testing, and audiological examinations [1, 2]. A thorough patient history and physical examination can provide valuable insights into the clinical features and potential risk factors associated with mitochondrial dysfunction. Healthcare providers should inquire about a family history of hearing loss, other associated symptoms, and the presence of neurologic or visual abnormalities [1, 2, 15].

Genetic testing plays a crucial role in confirming the diagnosis of mitochondrial hearing loss. It involves analyzing the mitochondrial DNA (mtDNA) for specific mutations known to be associated with hearing loss. Molecular genetic techniques are utilized to identify the presence of pathogenic mutations in mtDNA [8, 15]. It is important to note that mutations in mtDNA can be heteroplasmic, meaning they are present in varying proportions within an individual's cells. Therefore, genetic testing may require the analysis of multiple tissues, such as blood, saliva, or skin fibroblasts, to accurately assess the mutation load [5, 15].

Whole exome sequencing (WES) can be a valuable tool for investigating the genetic basis of sensorineural hearing loss (SNHL). WES allows for a comprehensive analysis of the protein-coding regions of the genome, including those genes coding for mitochondrial proteins. It enables the simultaneous screening of thousands of genes associated with various genetic disorders, including those known to be related to SNHL. This broad approach increases the likelihood of identifying the underlying genetic cause of SNHL in patients [13, 16]. WES can uncover novel genetic variants that may not have been previously associated with SNHL. This can lead to the identification of new genes or pathways involved in hearing loss, expanding our understanding of the condition and potentially leading to new therapeutic targets [13, 16]. Additionally, knowledge of the genetic cause of SNHL can have implications for personalized treatment and management strategies. It can help determine the prognosis, guide the selection of appropriate interventions, and inform decisions regarding hearing aids, cochlear implants, or other assistive devices [13, 16, 17].

Another approach that can be used to aid diagnosis is mitochondrial DNA sequencing. The mitochondrial genome is separate and contained within the mitochondria, therefore whole genome sequencing cannot provide any information about mt DNA. Mitochondrial DNA sequencing can provide valuable information regarding genetic coding of essential proteins that contribute the functionality of auditory structures [16].

Audiological testing is an integral component of the diagnostic workup for mitochondrial hearing loss. Pure-tone audiometry is performed to assess hearing thresholds across different frequencies, providing information about the type, severity, and

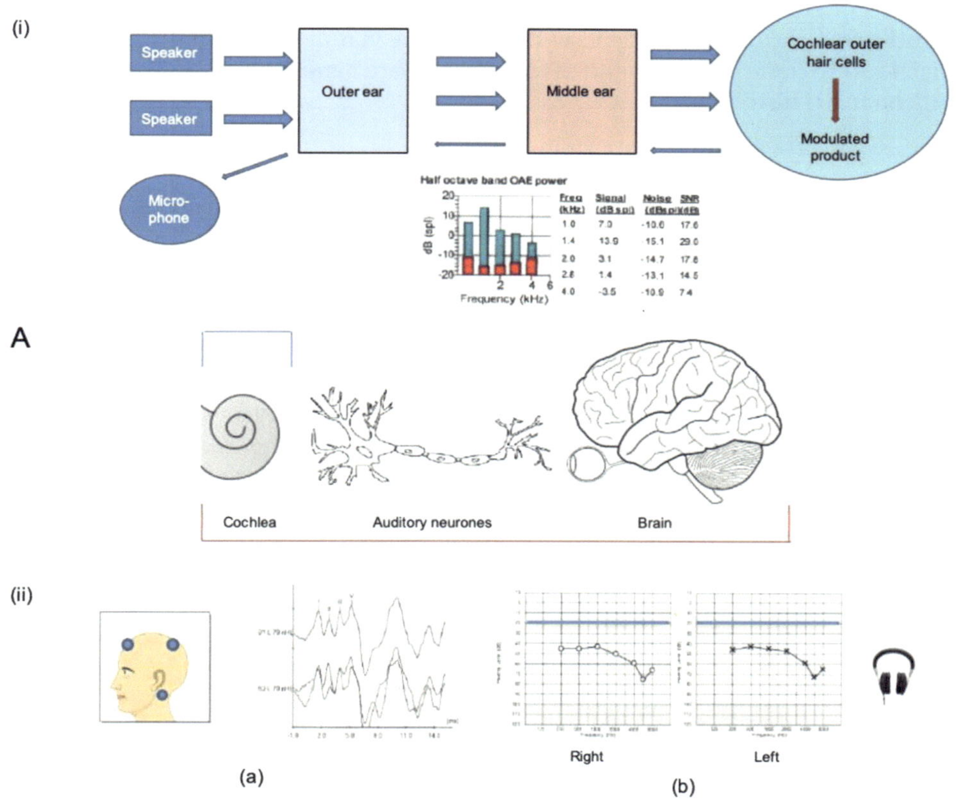

Figure 2.
Audiological assessment of diagnosos of hearing loss. (A) Schematic representation of the auditory conduction pathway from the cochlea via neuronal auditory brain structures to the auditory cortex. (i) OAFs: A speaker generated tone is delivered to the ear by an indwelling ear probe which also measures the modulated product (in the case of DPOAEs) generated by the stimulated cochlear outer hair cells. Cochlea function is specifically measured (represented by blue diagrammatic brackets in Panel A). (ii) (a) Auditory brainstem response (ABR): position of skull electrodes and representation of elecrophysilogical response of auditory pathway (waves I–V marked). (ii) (b) PTA: Audioframs of the right and left ears showing pan-frequency hearing loss with raised thresholds (lower limit of normal hearing marked with horizontal blue line). Subject responds to different frequency tones presented by headphones. (ii) Both ABR and PTA measure response of the entire auditory pathway (represented by red diagrammatic bracketsin Panel A).

configuration of hearing loss [10]. Speech audiometry evaluates an individual's ability to understand speech and discriminate between different speech sounds. Otoacoustic emissions (OAEs) and auditory brainstem response (ABR) testing can help assess the function of the inner ear and the auditory nerve pathways (see **Figure 2**). These audiological examinations aid in confirming the presence of hearing loss, characterizing its nature and extent, and ruling out other potential causes of hearing impairment [10, 17].

In cases where the clinical suspicion for mitochondrial hearing loss is high but genetic testing results are inconclusive or unavailable, other diagnostic modalities may be considered. Biochemical analyses, such as measuring the activity of respiratory chain complexes in muscle biopsies or assessing lactate and pyruvate levels in blood or cerebrospinal fluid, can provide indirect evidence of mitochondrial dysfunction [5, 7]. Neuroimaging techniques, including magnetic resonance imaging (MRI), can help identify structural abnormalities or functional changes in the brain or inner ear that may be associated with mitochondrial dysfunction [7].

Moreover, the diagnosis of mitochondrial hearing loss requires specialized expertise and a multidisciplinary approach. Audiologists, geneticists, otolaryngologists, and other healthcare professionals with experience in mitochondrial disorders play a crucial role in the accurate diagnosis and appropriate management of individuals with mitochondrial hearing loss.

4. Management

The management of mitochondrial hearing loss involves a multidisciplinary approach aimed at optimizing communication abilities and addressing the specific needs of affected individuals. While currently there is no cure for mitochondrial hearing loss, various strategies can be employed to improve functional outcomes and enhance quality of life.

As previously discussed, there are various syndromes that are associated with mitochondrial hearing loss. As a result, it is important to acknowledge the management required for the complex systemic manifestations associated with these syndromes. It's important for individuals with such syndromes to receive regular medical follow-ups to monitor their condition, manage symptoms, and address any new developments. The management approach may vary depending on the specific needs and symptoms of each individual, so it's essential to work closely with a healthcare team experienced in mitochondrial disorders [1, 8]. For example, symptomatic treatment is provided for other manifestations of MELAS syndrome, such as cardiac abnormalities, hearing loss, muscle weakness, and gastrointestinal issues [1, 3, 15]. Medications, therapies, and lifestyle modifications may be employed based on the specific symptoms and their severity. Additionally, in the case of KSS, it is essential to consider the ophthalmic symptoms including regular eye exams, corrective lenses, cardiologic interventions and close monitoring [1, 3, 8].

Audiological rehabilitation plays a central role in managing mitochondrial hearing loss. Hearing aids are commonly prescribed to individuals with residual hearing to amplify sound and enhance audibility. These devices can improve speech understanding and facilitate communication in daily activities. Regular audiological assessments and adjustments are important to ensure that hearing aids are appropriately fitted and calibrated to individual needs [8, 17].

In cases of very severe hearing loss, another therapy option is the use of cochlear implants. As another form of sensorineural hearing loss, mitochondrial hearing loss in theory should have the same efficacy in improving auditory symptoms. Some studies have cited improvement of hearing in patients with Kearns-Sayre and MNGIE syndromes [15]. A recent systematic review identified 9 of 11 studies showing favorable audiometric outcomes with CI in patients with MHL [17]. Karkos et al. conducted a 12-month review of MELAS patients with CI indicating positive results are preserved for at least 12 months [18]. However, larger studies with longer follow up are needed to determine whether hearing results are preserved long term.

In addition to hearing aids, assistive listening devices (ALDs) can further enhance communication abilities for individuals with mitochondrial hearing loss. ALDs include devices such as personal FM systems, induction loop systems, and Bluetooth-enabled devices. These technologies improve sound transmission and reduce background noise, particularly in challenging listening environments, such as classrooms, public venues, or workplaces [6, 8, 9, 17]. Audiologists can provide guidance on selecting and using ALDs effectively.

Communication strategies and education are vital for individuals with mitochondrial hearing loss and their families. Techniques such as lip-reading, sign language, and speech therapy can supplement auditory input and facilitate effective communication. Speech therapy can help improve speech production, language skills, and overall communication abilities. Additionally, educating family members, friends, and educators about mitochondrial hearing loss and its impact can foster understanding and support in various social settings [1, 17].

Living with hearing loss can have a significant psychological and emotional impact on individuals. Psychosocial support and counseling services can provide a supportive environment for individuals with mitochondrial hearing loss and their families. These services can help individuals cope with the challenges associated with hearing loss, manage stress, and promote overall mental well-being. Support groups and online communities can also offer a platform for sharing experiences, seeking advice, and finding a sense of belonging [8, 6].

Genetic counseling is an important aspect of the management of mitochondrial hearing loss. Genetic counselors can provide information about the inheritance patterns, recurrence risks, and available genetic testing options. They can guide individuals and families in making informed decisions regarding family planning and reproductive options. Genetic counseling also facilitates the identification of at-risk family members who may benefit from early detection and intervention [6–8, 17, 19].

Finally, regular monitoring and consistent follow-up are crucial for individuals with mitochondrial hearing loss. Audiological evaluations should be conducted at regular intervals to assess changes in hearing thresholds, adjust hearing aids or assistive devices, and provide ongoing support. Additionally, individuals with mitochondrial hearing loss may benefit from periodic assessments by otolaryngologists, geneticists, and other specialists to monitor overall health and address any associated systemic manifestations of mitochondrial dysfunction [2, 5, 6, 8].

5. Future directions of mitochondrial disease treatment

While significant progress has been made in understanding mitochondrial hearing loss, further research is needed to advance our knowledge and develop more effective strategies for diagnosis, treatment, and prevention of the condition. Several areas of investigation show promise for future directions in the field.

a. Genetic discoveries and personalized medicine: continued exploration of the genetic basis of mitochondrial hearing loss will contribute to the identification of novel causative genes and mutations. Whole-exome sequencing and genome-wide association studies hold potential for unraveling the complex genetic architecture underlying the condition. Such discoveries will facilitate the development of personalized medicine approaches, enabling tailored interventions based on an individual's specific genetic profile [6].

b. Targeting mitochondrial dysfunction: further understanding of the molecular mechanisms involved in mitochondrial dysfunction in hearing loss is essential for the development of targeted therapies. Emerging evidence suggests that various therapeutic agents, such as antioxidants, mitochondrial biogenesis enhancers, and modulators of mitochondrial dynamics, may hold promise for preserving or improving mitochondrial function in the auditory system [2]. Preclinical studies and clinical trials investigating the efficacy and safety of these interventions are warranted.

c. Regenerative medicine: regenerative approaches aimed at restoring damaged or lost auditory structures offer a potential avenue for treating mitochondrial hearing loss. Stem cell-based therapies, including the use of pluripotent stem cells and induced pluripotent stem cells, hold promise for generating functional hair cells and auditory neurons in vitro and in vivo [19]. The integration of tissue engineering and gene editing technologies further enhances the prospects of regenerating damaged auditory tissues, paving the way for potential curative interventions.

d. Novel drug therapies: the identification of small molecules and pharmacological agents that can specifically target the underlying molecular pathways involved in mitochondrial dysfunction may offer new avenues for therapeutic intervention. High-throughput screening techniques can aid in the discovery of potential drug candidates that enhance mitochondrial function, reduce oxidative stress, and mitigate cellular damage in the auditory system [2]. An example of mitochondrial disease enzyme replacement therapy is the use of fusion propionyl co-A carboxylase (PCC) for the fatal metabolic disorder propionic acidemia [20].

e. Non-invasive monitoring techniques: the development of non-invasive methods for monitoring mitochondrial function and assessing disease progression in individuals with mitochondrial hearing loss is an area of ongoing research. Imaging techniques, such as functional magnetic resonance imaging (fMRI) and positron emission tomography (PET), hold potential for evaluating mitochondrial metabolism and bioenergetics in vivo [7]. These non-invasive monitoring tools can provide valuable insights into the efficacy of therapeutic interventions and aid in the assessment of treatment outcomes.

f. Preventive strategies: identifying individuals at risk for mitochondrial hearing loss and implementing preventive measures are crucial for minimizing the impact of the condition. Genetic counseling and carrier screening programs can help identify individuals who are at risk of passing on mitochondrial mutations to their offspring. Early detection and intervention, such as newborn hearing screening programs and regular audiological assessments, may enable timely intervention and support for affected individuals, leading to improved outcomes.

6. Conclusion

Mitochondrial hearing loss is an umbrella terms that describes a range of conditions affecting mitochondrial function in pertinent structures of the auditory pathway. These conditions can be caused by mutations to mitochondrial DNA, as well as nuclear genes that cause dysfunction of inner ear hair cells, the stria vascularis, and even the auditory neurons as well. Although its pathogenesis remains poorly understood, current research points toward factors like ATP deficiency and oxidative damage being crucial factors. Diagnosing mitochondrial hearing loss requires comprehensive evaluation including clinical assessment, genetic testing and audiological tests - unfortunately there is currently no cure available and treatment focuses mainly on improving communication abilities and supporting quality-of-life improvements.

Additional research initiatives are required to increase our understanding of the pathogenesis of mitochondrial hearing loss and develop effective treatments. The development of mitochondrial-targeted therapies, such as antioxidants and gene therapy, holds promise for the treatment of mitochondrial hearing loss [2]. Additionally, research into stem cell-based regenerative therapies for the repair and regeneration of hair cells in the inner ear is being explored as a potential treatment strategy [5]. These treatment modalities will be tailored to the unique biophysical profile of each patient and provides the potential for a greater and more specific clinical response.

In conclusion, mitochondrial hearing loss is a complex condition that requires further research and understanding. While there are currently limited treatment options, ongoing research holds promise for the development of effective therapies to mitigate the impact of mitochondrial hearing loss and improve the lives of affected individuals. Continued efforts in research, diagnosis, and treatment of mitochondrial hearing loss are essential to improve upon our knowledge base and provide better management strategies for individuals with this condition.

Conflict of interest

The authors declare no conflict of interest.

Author details

Charvi Malhotra and Peter Kullar*
Department of Otolaryngology, Head and Neck Surgery, Stanford University School of Medicine, Stanford, CA, USA

*Address all correspondence to: pk234@stanford.edu

References

[1] Fancello V, Fancello G, Palma S, Monzani D, Genovese E, Bianchini C, et al. The Role of Primary Mitochondrial Disorders in Hearing Impairment: An Overview. Medicina (Kaunas). 19 Mar 2023;**59**(3):608. DOI: 10.3390/medicina59030608. PMID: 36984609; PMCID: PMC10058207

[2] Kang J, Wang C, Lu Y. Mitochondrial-targeted therapies for hearing loss: A mini-review. Frontiers in Cellular Neuroscience. 2021;**15**:674768

[3] Liu Y, Xue J, Zhao D, Chen L, Yuan Y, Wang Z. Audiological evaluation in Chinese patients with mitochondrial encephalomyopathies. Chinese Medical Journal. 2014;**127**(12):2304-2309

[4] Smith RJ, Bale JF Jr, White KR. Sensorineural hearing loss in children. Lancet. 2005;**365**(9462):879-890. DOI: 10.1016/S0140-6736(05)71047-3

[5] Fernandez-Vizarra E, Enriquez JA, Perez-Martos A, Montoya J, Fernandez-Silva P. Tissue-specific differences in mitochondrial activity and biogenesis. Mitochondrion. 2011;**11**(1):207-213. DOI: 10.1016/j.mito.2010.09.011

[6] Lieberman AP, Shakkottai VG, Albin RL, Anderson KE, Ard MC, Ashizawa T, et al. Patient-centered outcome measures as decision-making tools for the management of neurodegenerative diseases: A multi-stakeholder perspective. Journal of Personalized Medicine. 2020;**10**(3):103

[7] Muller BA, Kamerer AM, Epperson CN. Positron emission tomography (PET) neuroimaging biomarkers for preclinical detection of Alzheimer's disease. Neurobiology of Disease. 2020;**134**:104699

[8] Kullar PJ, Quail J, Lindsey P, et al. Both mitochondrial DNA and mitonuclear gene mutations cause hearing loss through cochlear dysfunction. Brain. 2016;**139**(Pt 6):e33. DOI: 10.1093/brain/aww051

[9] Li JN, Han DY, Ji F, et al. Successful cochlear implantation in a patient with MNGIE syndrome. Acta Oto-Laryngologica. 2011;**131**(9):1012-1016. DOI: 10.3109/00016489.2011.579623

[10] Doosti A, Lotfi Y, Moosavi A, Bakhshi E, Talasaz AH. Distortion product otoacoustic emission (DPOAE) as an appropriate tool in assessment of otoprotective effects of antioxidants in noise-induced hearing loss (NIHL). Indian Journal of Otolaryngology Head and Neck Surgery. 2014;**66**(3):325-329. DOI: 10.1007/s12070-014-0721-7

[11] Li P, Li S, Wang L, et al. Mitochondrial dysfunction in hearing loss: Oxidative stress, autophagy and NLRP3 inflammasome. Frontiers in Cell and Development Biology. 2023;**11**:1119773. DOI: 10.3389/fcell.2023.1119773

[12] Ou YH, Chen AW, Fan JY, et al. Aminoglycoside-associated nonsyndromic deafness and speech disorder in mitochondrial A1555G mutation in a family: A case report. Medicine (Baltimore). 2018;**97**(42):e12878. DOI: 10.1097/MD.0000000000012878

[13] Sun C, Wu S, Chen R, et al. Whole exome sequencing is an alternative method in the diagnosis of mitochondrial DNA diseases. Molecular Genetics &

Genomic Medicine. 2022;**10**(6):e1943. DOI: 10.1002/mgg3.1943

[14] Uimonen S, Moilanen JS, Sorri M, Hassinen IE, Majamaa K. Hearing impairment in patients with 3243A-->G mtDNA mutation: Phenotype and rate of progression. Human Genetics. 2001;**108**(4):284-289. DOI: 10.1007/s004390100475

[15] Scarpelli M, Zappini F, Filosto M, Russignan A, Tonin P, Tomelleri G. Mitochondrial sensorineural hearing loss: A retrospective study and a description of cochlear implantation in a MELAS patient. Genetic Research International. 2012;**2012**:287432. DOI: 10.1155/2012/287432

[16] Ye F, Samuels DC, Clark T, Guo Y. High-throughput sequencing in mitochondrial DNA research. Mitochondrion. 2014;**17**:157-163. DOI: 10.1016/j.mito.2014.05.004

[17] Zia N, Nikookam Y, Muzaffar J, Kullar P, Monksfield P, Bance M. Cochlear implantation outcomes in patients with mitochondrial hearing loss: A systematic review and narrative synthesis. Journal of International Advanced Otology. 2021;**17**(1):72-80. DOI: 10.5152/iao.2020.9226

[18] Karkos P, Anari S, Johnson I. Cochlear implantation in patients with MELAS syndrome. European Archives of Oto-Rhino-Laryngology. 2004;**262**:322-324

[19] Roccio M, Edge AS, Perny M. Regenerative medicine for the treatment of hearing loss. Clinical Pharmacology & Therapeutics. 2020;**107**(3):572-579

[20] Darvish-Damavandi M, Ho HK, Kang TS. Towards the development of an enzyme replacement therapy for the metabolic disorder propionic acidemia. Molecular Genetics in Metabolism Report. 2016;**8**:51-60. DOI: 10.1016/j.ymgmr.2016.06.009

Chapter 4

Potential Mechanisms of Hearing Loss Due to Impaired Potassium Circulation in the Organ of Corti

Guillermo Spitzmaul, Ezequiel Rías and Leonardo Dionisio

Abstract

Hearing loss (HL) is a common condition that significantly affects an individual's quality of life. Impaired potassium circulation in the organ of Corti (OC), including the movement of potassium into hair cells (HCs) and from hair cells to supporting cells (SCs), can contribute to hearing loss. This chapter aims to provide a better understanding of cochlear potassium ion homeostasis and its dysfunction in this context. Sensorineural hearing loss (SNHL) is caused by damage to the inner ear or the auditory nerve. Various factors contribute to it, including aging, exposure to loud noise, genetics, medications, and infections. In all of them, some level of potassium circulation alteration is present. Potassium plays a crucial role in hearing function as it is the moving charge that depolarizes hair cells in response to sound perception. It generates the endocochlear potential (EP) which provides the driving force for potassium movement. Disruptions in potassium circulation due to molecular alterations in ion channels and transporters can lead to hair cells dysfunction and cell death. Moreover, drugs that affect potassium circulation can also cause hearing loss. Understanding the molecular and tissue changes resulting from potassium circulation deficits is essential for developing targeted treatments and preventive measures for potassium-related hearing disorders.

Keywords: hearing loss, potassium homeostasis, hair cells, ion channels, KCNQ4, supporting cells

1. Introduction

Hearing loss (HL) is a common condition nowadays that reduces hearing capacity. HL can be caused by a variety of factors, and it can have a significant impact on a person's quality of life [1, 2]. In this chapter, we will explain the importance of potassium (K^+) circulation for proper hearing function and how it can cause HL, primarily focusing on K^+ movement from hair cells (HCs) to supporting cells (SCs). By the end of this chapter, we aim to have a better understanding on cochlear K^+ ion homeostasis and how its dysfunction contributes to very common HL processes.

Sensorineural hearing loss (SNHL) is the most common type of HL, affecting millions of people worldwide [2–4]. SNHL occurs when there is damage to the inner ear

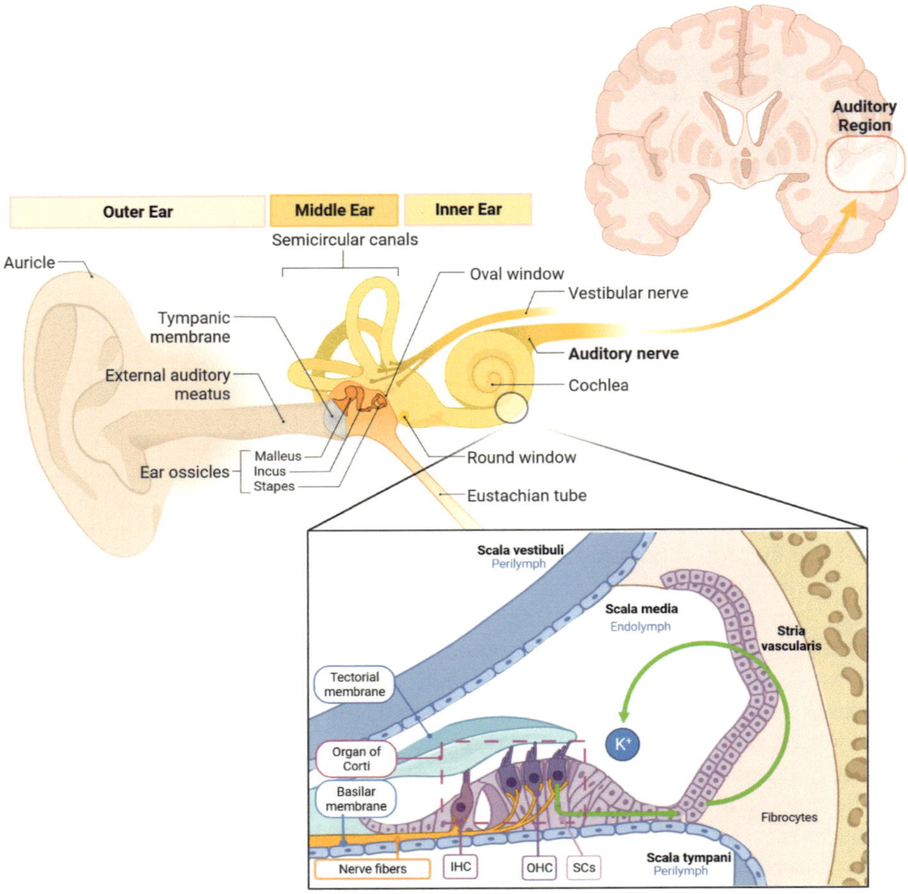

Figure 1.
Auditory pathway and potassium circulation in cochlea. Schematic representation of the auditory system, composed by: The outer, the middle, and the inner ear; and scheme of the auditory pathway to auditory cortex in the brain. Inset of the cochlea's cross section depicts the scala vestibuli and scala tympani (both filled with perilymph) and the scala media filled with endolymph, containing the OC: IHCs, OHCs, and SCs. Schematic representation of the K^+ recirculation from the OHCs to the endolymph through SCs and Stria vascularis (green arrows). This figure is original for this work.

or the auditory nerve [5]. Unlike conductive HL, which occurs when sound is blocked from reaching the inner ear, SNHL occurs when sound is not effectively transmitted to the brain (**Figure 1**) [2, 6]. This type of HL can be caused by a variety of factors, including aging, exposure to loud noise, genetics, some drugs, and certain medical conditions [7–10]. Age-related hearing loss (ARHL), also known as presbycusis, is a common sensory disorder among the elderly. It is characterized by a decline in hearing sensitivity and speech discrimination, delayed central processing of acoustic information, and impaired localization of sound sources. Multiple mechanisms have been proposed for age-related cochlear degeneration, and it appears that both genetic and environmental factors play a role. Noise-induced hearing loss (NIHL) is a significant occupational health risk in developed countries. NIHL can also result from unsafe recreational, social, and residential noise exposures. People with excessive exposure to noise are frequently the population with a lifestyle which may affect auditory function. Exposure to loud noises, such as explosions or prolonged exposure to high sound levels, can cause damage to the delicate structures within the inner ear. This can lead to temporary or permanent HL, depending on the severity and duration of the exposure. Genetic factors play a significant role in the development of SNHL. Mutations in genes such as those coding for calcium (Ca^{2+}) channel and K^+ channels in sensory HCs of the cochlea can cause hereditary deafness, but many others have been elucidated [6, 11–13]. Also certain medications, such as aminoglycoside antibiotics and some drugs for cancer treatment, can be toxic to the inner ear, causing damage to the HCs and auditory neurons. This damage can be temporary or permanent, depending on the drug and the dosage. Lastly on the causes of HL, infections, such as prenatal toxoplasmosis, rubella, meningitis or cytomegalovirus, can cause inflammation and damage to the inner ear, leading to SNHL [6].

K^+ is essential for the proper functioning of hearing. This ion is found in high concentration in the endolymph contained in the scala media of the cochlea. This high concentration of K^+ generates the endocochlear potential (EP), which, in conjunction with the HCs resting membrane potential, creates a strong driving force for the entry of this ion when sound causes bending of the stereocilia bundle [14]. After sound perception, K^+ leaves the HCs and returns to the stria vascularis through gap junctions (GJs) and transporters present in the surrounding SCs. The flow and recycling of K^+ ions play a vital role in the conversion of sound vibrations into electrical signals that can be transmitted to the brain for auditory perception [14–22].

Molecular alterations in channels and transporters involved in the process of K^+ circulation lead to HCs dysfunction and, ultimately, cell death. Moreover, drugs that alter K^+ circulation can result in HL [23–28]. Most of these changes impacts primarily on outer hair cells (OHCs) function and survival [29]. For these reasons, we focus on this sensory cell type in this chapter. Understanding the molecular, tissue, and innervation changes that occur in HCs due to deficits in K^+ circulation is crucial for advancing our knowledge of hearing loss mechanisms, developing targeted treatments, identifying preventive measures, and enabling personalized interventions. Such understanding has the potential to improve the diagnosis, management, and overall quality of life for individuals affected by K^+-related hearing disorders.

2. Anatomy and physiology of the organ of Corti

The organ of Corti (OC) is a complex structure located in the spiral-shaped cochlea of the inner ear, playing a crucial role in the process of hearing by converting sound vibrations into interpretable electrical signals. The OC rests on the basilar membrane, a thin and flexible membrane spanning the length of the cochlea. It separates the scala media from the scala tympani. Within the OC, there are specialized sensory cells known as HCs, specifically the inner hair cells (IHCs) and outer hair cells (OHCs), responsible for the conversion of sound vibrations into electrical signals. Above the OC lies the tectorial membrane, a gelatinous structure that extends over the HCs, playing a pivotal role in the mechanotransduction process (see further). SCs encompass the OC, providing structural support, and safeguarding the HCs, while also regulating the ionic composition of the perilymph to maintain proper HC function [15]. Furthermore, the neuronal connection to the central nervous system is facilitated by the spiral ganglion (SG), a cluster of neurons situated within the cochlea. The fibers of the SG neurons establish connections with the HCs, transmitting the electrical signals generated by the HCs to the auditory nerve (**Figure 1**).

Collectively, these components work harmoniously to convert sound vibrations into electrical signals, facilitating their transmission to the brain and enabling the perception and interpretation of sounds [30].

2.1 Structure and function of hair cells

As mentioned above, there are two types of sensory HCs in the cochlea that detect sound vibrations: IHCs and OHCs. These cells possess small, finger-like projections called stereocilia on their apical surface, facing endolymph, the high-K^+ fluid that filled the scala media (**Figure 2**). When stimulated by sound vibrations, the stereocilia of the HCs move, opening mechanoreceptor channels and initiating the generation of electrical signals. While both types of HCs depolarize in response to K^+ entrance, their specific functions and contributions to auditory processing differ. IHCs primarily serve the role of transmitting auditory information to the brain, whereas OHCs play a role in amplifying sound signals and fine-tuning the sensitivity of the cochlea [31, 32]. The depolarization caused by the entrance of K^+ is a unique feature among mammals and allows ion movement following its electrochemical gradient from endolymph to cytosol at the apical membrane and exit at the basal membrane to the extracellular fluid between HCs and SCs. The depolarization of the HCs leads to their activation upon reaching the receptor potential (RP), which represents the membrane voltage threshold that triggers the opening of CaV1.3 voltage-dependent calcium channels in IHCs [33] and initiate the process of electromotility in OHCs (see further) [32].

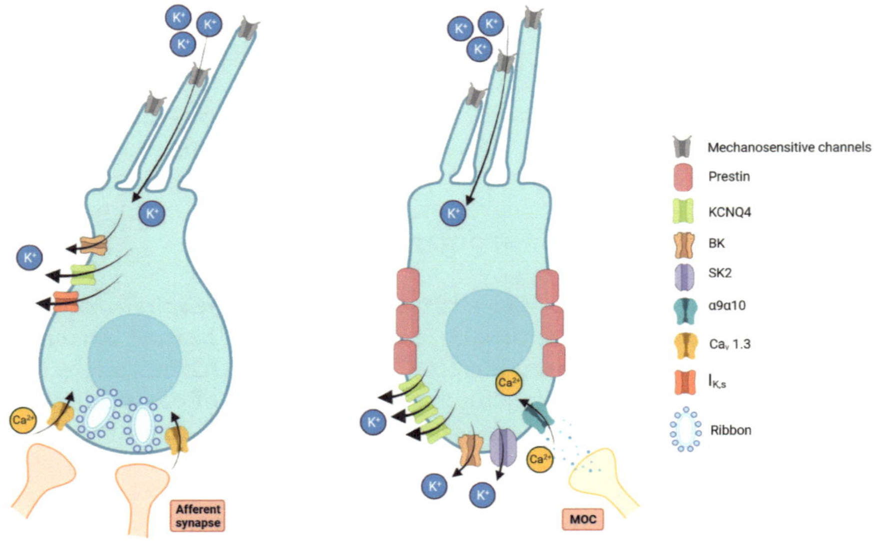

Figure 2.
Potassium movement in hair cells. Illustration depicting the IHC (left), with the influx of K^+ through the mechanosensitive channels, and the efflux of this ion mediated by the channels responsible of the $I_{K,n}$, $I_{K,s}$, an $I_{K,f}$ currents. Also, the Ca^{2+} channels which are responsible for the neurotransmitter release from the ribbon and the afferent synapses are depicted. On the right, schematic representation of the OHC, with the influx of K^+, also through mechanosensitive channels, and its efflux mediated by different K^+ channels, mainly KCNQ4. Efferent synapse through MOC terminals is also depicted, and the α9α10 nAChR is responsible for the modulation of hearing sensitivity. This figure is original for this work.

2.2 Dieter's cells structure and function

The sensory cells in the OC are surrounded by a heterogeneous group of cells denominated SCs. Among them, there is a subgroup constituted by the Dieter's cells (DCs), disposed across the OC in three rows under the OHCs. The DCs play an important role keeping the structure of the organ, acting mainly as a support, but also in homeostasis of ions and other molecules, and modulation of extracellular matrices **(Figure 3)** [34, 35].

DCs are characterized for presenting an elongated body, extending from the reticular lamina to the basilar membrane [36]. Structurally, these cells have an apical region, consisting on an extension projecting from their medial region to the reticular lamina, denominated "phalangeal process" which forms tight junctions with the OHCs at the level of the reticular lamina [37], a medial region cup-shaped, which contains and binds through tight and adherents junctions to the base of the OHCs, and a basal region holding the nucleus and most of organelles [38–40]. The medial region of the DCs envelopes nerves contacting them and the basal pole of OHCs [41]. The cytoskeleton of these cells is commonly called "Dieter's stalk" [36] and consists of microtubules, intermediate filaments and actin, and extends from the basilar membrane to the reticular lamina through the phalangeal process. The cytoskeletal structure has a conical shape thickening in the site contacting the basilar membrane called "basal cone" (**Figure 3**) [42].

2.3 Sound transduction in the organ of Corti

When sound waves enter the cochlea, their vibrations are transmitted through the perilymph of the scala tympani to the basilar membrane, causing the HCs to bend their stereocilia against the tectorial membrane. As explained previously, this

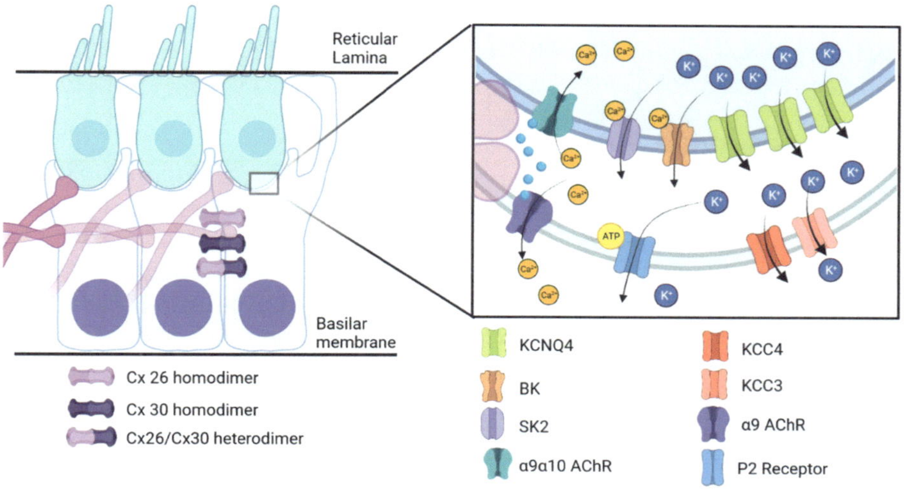

Figure 3.
Draining of potassium by the Dieter's cells. Illustration of the OHC location and DC in the OC, depicting the efferent innervation that contacts both cells. Gap junctions, composed by connexin monomers (Cx26 and Cx30), between DCs are also showed in the figure. Inset depicts the small space between the OHC and DC, showing the main channels involved in the K^+ circulation, and the efferent modulation in the hearing process. This figure is original for this work.

movement opens the mechanosensitive channels located on the stereocilia of the HCs, activating K^+ influx [6, 16]. The RPs trigger the release of the neurotransmitter glutamate by the IHCs, while activating the amplification process in the OHCs [43].

Vesicle release in IHCs occurs in the basolateral membrane, which contains the active zones characterized by the presence of synaptic ribbons that supply ultrafast and precise synaptic vesicles for exocytosis, to release glutamate into the synaptic cleft (**Figure 2**, left) [43, 44]. The released neurotransmitters then stimulate postsynaptic afferent nerve fibers from the SG neurons, sending electrical signals to the brain for sound interpretation through the auditory pathway [16, 45]. The primary function of OHCs is to amplify and fine-tune the sound signals before they reach the IHCs. The physiology of OHCs involves several key mechanisms that contribute to their capabilities [46]. It includes three main features:

a. Electromotility: one of the defining properties of OHCs is their ability to change shape in response to RPs. It is enabled by the presence of a protein called prestin in the lateral membrane of OHCs (**Figure 2**, right). When a sound stimulus is detected, a RP is generated across the cell membrane, leading to a contraction or elongation of the OHCs. This mechanical movement enhances the sensitivity and selectivity of the cochlea to different sound frequencies.

b. Basilar membrane motility: electromotility of OHCs has a direct effect on the mechanics of the basilar membrane. The movement of OHCs alters the tension and stiffness of the basilar membrane, increasing vibration intensity of IHCs in the OC. This process is known as the cochlear amplifier or the OHC amplifier.

c. Olivocochlear feedback: it involves neural connections from the brainstem to the cochlea that serve as a feedback mechanism. This efferent innervation modulates HCs excitability (**Figure 2**, right).

These mechanisms, collectively named "the active process," are crucial for our ability to detect and perceive sounds accurately, and it can be disrupted by factors such as noise exposure or genetic mutations.

2.4 Efferent innervation of the organ of Corti

The auditory system has two efferent neuronal components originated in the lateral and medial nuclei of superior olivary complex (LOC and MOC, respectively) [47]. LOC fibers make synaptic contacts with afferent fibers that contact IHCs in adult, while MOC fibers make synaptic contacts with the OHCs [48]. LOC function is still not fully understood. The main effect of MOC efferent innervation is to inhibit the cochlear response by reducing the amplification gain of the OHCs. This effect is observed as a reduction in the motility of the basilar membrane and as a transient loss of sensitivity of the auditory nerve to sound [49]. The efferent fibers directly contact the OHCs, producing inhibitory synaptic currents once activated [50]. Paradoxically, this inhibition is mediated by an excitatory current generated by the nicotinic acetylcholine receptor (nAChR) composed by the $\alpha9$ and $\alpha10$ subunits [51, 52]. The $\alpha9\alpha10$ nAChR is a cationic channel with high Ca^{2+} permeability [53, 54]. In the OHCs, the entry of Ca^{2+} through this channel leads to the activation of Ca^{2+}-dependent K^+ channels, SK2 and BK, resulting in hyperpolarization of the cell membrane through the efflux of K^+ ions through these channels [55, 56]. It is believed that Ca^{2+} entry through α9α10 nAChR triggers the release of cytoplasmic Ca^{2+} from cisterns located near the efferent synapses, and this ion would activate the SK2 channels [57]. The release of cytoplasmic Ca^{2+} from these cisterns is modulated by the ryanodine family of channels [58]. In this way, the efferent system modulates the activity of the OHCs, preventing excessive depolarization, for example, during prolonged exposure to a sound stimulus [47]. It has been demonstrated that an exacerbation of efferent system activity protects against acoustic damage [59]. In a model of over activation of nicotinic channels, generated by a mutation in the α9 subunit of the α9α10 receptor, increased sensitivity to acetylcholine and decreased channel desensitization were observed. Animals with this mutation had a higher acoustic threshold, showing greater protection against acoustic damage [59]. Conversely, it has also been shown that auditory overstimulation causes synaptopathy in young mice, resulting in a decrease in synaptic contacts of the OHCs [60, 61].

Besides the innervation of the sensory cell, nerve fibers making contact with DCs and other SCs were identified more than 40 years ago [62] and have since been confirmed through the labeling of synaptic terminals in the DCs of both cats and humans, using specific markers [63, 64]. Further investigations have revealed that these fibers originate from the MOC efferent system [65]. Recent findings have shown that the synapses formed by these fibers are functional and cholinergic in nature. DCs express the same type of nAChR as OHCs, specifically the α9 nAChR was identified so far [66]. The efferent innervation influences the activity of gap junction channels, thereby modulating the movement of K^+ ions through DCs. Consequently, the available evidence suggests that the MOC system may indirectly regulate the activity of OHCs by potentially exerting control over the membrane potential of DCs.

2.5 Potassium circulation in the organ of Corti

K^+ circulation plays a crucial role in hearing as it is closely linked to the proper function of the auditory system. As mentioned above, the scala media contains endolymph, a high K^+ fluid, bathing the apical membrane of both HCs. [14, 67, 68]. The influx of K^+ into HCs depolarizes them resulting in either the release of glutamate by IHCs or electromotility in OHCs, as the RP is reached. K^+ enters through a mechanoelectrical transduction complex located at the tip of stereocilia bundle [16, 30, 69]. This complex, still not fully resolved, forms a nonselective cation channel where K^+ and Ca^{2+} enter [30, 69]. After the entry of K^+ ions into the HCs, their removal becomes necessary for the hearing perception to continue. This is where K^+ circulation plays a crucial role, to repolarize the resting membrane potential. Specialized channels and transporters are responsible for pumping the K^+ ions out of the HCs and back into the endolymphatic fluid of the cochlea (**Figure 1**, inset) [14, 15, 22].

One of the channels responsible for these functions is the KCNQ4 voltage-gated K^+ channel. KCNQ4 is primarily responsible for generating the main K^+ conductance current in OHCs known as $I_{K,n}$. It is predominantly expressed at the basal pole of OHCs, where it plays a crucial role facilitating K^+ efflux (**Figure 2**) [70–75]. Although to a lesser extent, KCNQ4 is also expressed in IHCs, as determined by gene and protein expression and functional properties of the IHCs (**Figure 2**) [71, 73, 76–82]. In this cell, it generates the K^+ current $I_{K,n}$, one of the three main K^+ currents in IHCs [16]. Impaired surface expression or reduced activity of the KCNQ4 channel leads to functional deterioration of the OC and has been associated with different types of HL: age-related hearing loss [23, 83–86], noise-induced hearing loss [87–89], and genetic hearing loss [71, 85, 86, 90, 91].

Other K^+ channels involved in the K^+ efflux are the Ca^{2+}-activated K^+ channels BK and SK2 (**Figure 2**). They differ from each other in their affinity to Ca^{2+}, single-channel conductance, and voltage sensitivity [55]. In IHCs, they are responsible for generating the $I_{K,f}$ current that contribute to cell repolarization [92]. Both channels are involved in the efferent regulation of OHCs. BK channels show tonotopic gradients of progressively increasing expression from low-frequency (apical zone) to high-frequency (basal zone) cochlear regions [55, 92–96]. On the contrary, SK2 channels increase their expression from basal to apical cochlear turns [97]. In the mature OC, BK channels are found in the neck of IHCs and in the basal pole of OHCs, in the same area where the efferent terminals are located [56]. Similar localization was observed for SK2 channels in OHCs [56, 94]. These channels are functionally coupled to ligand-gated ion channels to cause rapid postsynaptic inhibition [55, 97]. The efferent synapse activates BK and/or SK2 channels, depending on cochlear region, through α9α10 nAChR opening and Ca^{2+} entry [51, 52] hyperpolarizing the HCs [97, 98].

Once K^+ ions leave the HCs, they diffuse through the extracellular space. One appealing hypothesis for K^+ circulation suggests that these ions are reabsorbed by SCs located in the epithelial lining of the cochlea and actively transport them back into the endolymph (**Figures 1** and **3**) [14]. The closest cells to OHCs are DCs. The membrane of the DCs on the contacting surface with OHCs expresses the K-Cl cotransporters, KCC3 and KCC4 (**Figure 3**). These cotransporters belong to a protein family that plays a role in regulating cytoplasmic ion concentration, cell volume, and salt transport through the epithelia [99]. It has been hypothesized both cotransporters play the same role: capture K^+ extruded from OHCs for them to hyperpolarize. In addition of these cotransporters, it has been observed the presence of another K^+ channel expressed in the body of DCs and especially in the cup region, Kir4.1. It has been suggested this channel would be involved in the regulation of cellular physiology and presumably affect K^+ uptake [15, 100]. K^+ intake in DCs also relies on ATP-dependent channels, purinergic P2 receptors (**Figure 3**). In the extracellular space, ATP acts as a signaling molecule which allows these channels activation at the resting membrane potential for ions entrance, mainly of K^+ [101].

Dieter's cells form a syncytium, meaning that their cytoplasm is electrically connected through GJ, allowing the initiation of potassium recycling toward the stria vascularis in favor of its electrochemical gradient. There are different isoforms of CONNEXINs (Cx) in the inner ear, although only two are expressed in DCs: Cx26 and Cx30 [102]. Their expression levels differ along the cochlea, as in SCs [103], and both are considered indispensable for hearing [20, 102]. Cx26 and 30 are capable of assemble as homomeric GJ channels (Cx26/Cx26 or Cx30/Cx30) and also as heteromeric ones (Cx26/Cx30); GJs are important for ion circulation through SCs, as well as other molecules, such as miRNA [20, 104, 105].

3. Potassium circulation deficits and molecular changes in the organ of Corti

As we mentioned before, the circulation of K^+ is crucial for maintaining the proper functioning of the HC and the overall auditory system. Disruptions in K^+ circulation can lead to hearing problems and disorders [22]. For example, impairment in the transporters responsible for removing K^+ can lead to its accumulation in the HCs, disrupting the electrical signaling process and resulting in HL. Furthermore, certain medications, such as aminoglycosides or some diuretics, can interfere with K^+ circulation and affect hearing function as a side effect [24, 26, 27, 106].

3.1 KCNQ4 channel alterations leads to hearing loss

The major pathway for K^+ exit from OHCs is the KCNQ4 channel [71]. Mutations in the gene encoding this channel subunit underlie a slowly progressive dominant form of human deafness, named DFNA2. Patients carry dominant negative (dn) mutations that lead to HL over years [86, 107–109]. Mouse models with alterations in the *Kcnq4* gene or in the channel function by pharmacological agents, such as salicylate or aminoglycosides, have been helpful in studying the pathophysiological mechanisms underlying KCNQ4 channel dysfunction [26, 28, 71, 110, 111]. The loss of KCNQ4 function in OHCs can result in sustain depolarization due to intracellular K^+ accumulation, which consequently leads to their degeneration due to chronic cellular stress [71]. When KCNQ4 is absent, cochlear OHCs degenerate first at the basal turn of the cochlea, which mediates high-frequency hearing, and progress to the apical turn with time, affecting IHCs and SG neurons [71, 110]. At this moment, three transgenic mouse models carrying dn *Kcnq4* gene mutations found in DFNA2 patients have been analyzed [71, 112, 113]. Two of them are located in the pore region, W276S and G286S [71, 112], while the other, G228D, was in the intracellular S4–S5 linker region [113]. In heterozygosity, the KCNQ4 mutant subunits in each case assemble with either wild-type, mutant, or combination of both subunits, forming homo- or heteromeric channels, which drastically reduce their conductance and in consequence, the $I_{K,n}$ current of OHCs. Similar to KCNQ4 knock-out (KO) model, these mouse models exhibit HL with OHCs loss over time, starting in the basal turn and progressing over time to middle and apical turn albeit with a slower time course than KO. The first two models exhibit a relatively fast loss of OHCs with the preservation of IHCs. For the last model, IHCs loss was also observed starting four to eight weeks later than in OHCs [113]. The absence or mutations of the KCNQ4 channel subunit impact in the membrane potential, being differently reduced in OHCs and IHCs [71]. This depolarization would increase Ca^{2+} influx through voltage-gated Ca^{2+} channels into these cells and may thereby underlie the degeneration processes. Notably, in these models, hearing impairment tend to be uniform across all frequencies, implying dysfunction along the entire cochlea. However, the loss of OHCs invariably begins at the basal turn and gradually progresses over time. These results indicate an uncoupling between cellular functionality and survival, highlighting our incomplete understanding of the cellular and molecular mechanisms involved in this process.

Same results were obtained when KCNQ4 channels function was diminished. For example, pharmacological inhibition of KCNQ4 by linopirdine in an adult guinea pig model has been shown to cause acute HL through compromised function and severe OHCs degeneration in the basal turn, which corresponds to the high-frequency range of the cochlea [28]. Given its important role in K^+ circulation and the pathological consequences of impaired KCNQ4 channel activity, activation of the KCNQ4 channel has been proposed as a treatment for HL [23]. In this regard, the KCNQ4 channel opener retigabine has been useful in reversing salicylate-induced cytotoxicity [25]. Furthermore, channel openers have been used to mitigate HL in an ARHL mouse model [23, 114]. These findings lead to the hypothesis that pharmacological activation of KCNQ4 channels may preserve hearing function and prevent OHCs loss in ARHL and other forms of HL [23, 114]. In addition, gene therapy to correct a dn *Kcnq4* mutation in a mouse model partially succeed to correct HL degeneration that develops in this condition [112].

3.2 BK and SK2 channels malfunction affects the hearing process

Regarding BK channels, pharmacological blockade of them has minimal effect on OHC functionality [115], and genetic deletion of the channel has little effect on cochlear sensitivity [92]. However, as BK channels contribute to the inhibitory signaling on OHCs through the MOC efferent pathway [97], mice lacking BK channels have reduced MOC inhibition with smaller efferent synapses. However, they remain functional [56, 116]. These data are in line with previous reports of mice lacking the BK channel pore-forming α-subunit that do not exhibit a congenital HL but rather develop mild progressive high-frequency HL. In contrast, mice lacking the auxiliary BK channel β1 gene do not exhibit any hearing deficits and have a normal cochlear phenotype [96].

Deletion of SK2 channels in mice showed that action potential activity was abolished in these animals [117]. In addition, efferent innervation of OHCs was severely reduced in young KO mice. OHCs from this model were completely insensitive to exogenous ACh, implying absent or otherwise dysfunctional nAChR [95]. Another animal model lacking SK2 channel showed that they are necessary for long-term survival of olivocochlear fibers and synapses. Loss of the SK2 gene also results in loss of electrically driven olivocochlear effects *in vivo*, and down-regulation of ryanodine receptors involved in Ca^{2+}-induced Ca^{2+} release, the main inducer of nAChR evoked SK2 activity [94].

In conclusion, BK and SK2 channels are necessary for proper function of the OC and seem to have some degree of overlapping function in controlling OHC excitability. However, as efferent inhibition is impaired, dysfunction of these channels would lead to HL as well.

3.3 Dieter's cells channels malfunction in potassium circulation

Mouse models have played a crucial role in unraveling the function of the DCs in the OC function. Models lacking the expression of KCC3 and KCC4 ($Kcc3^{-/-}$ and $Kcc4^{-/-}$, respectively) showed the same phenotype, degeneration of HCs, probably due to osmotic stress or membrane depolarization [99, 118]. In $Kcc3^{-/-}$ mouse model, cell degeneration occurred slowly compared with $Kcc4^{-/-}$ mice; it is not known if it is due to more expression of KCC4 or different properties in the isoforms. In addition, KCC3 is expressed in type I and III fibrocytes in the stria vascularis, and both also degenerate in the absence of the protein [118].

As previously mentioned, K^+ moves between DCs using GJ channels (**Figure 3**) [14, 119, 120]. Mouse models have also been extremely useful to decipher the role of Cx in DCs. It has been reported that $Cx30^{-/-}$ mice develop profound HL and exert a negative modulation of Cx26 expression. On the other hand, $Cx26^{-/-}$ mice develop a cell degeneration that leads to HL, despite the remaining GJ remain permeable to ion flux probably due to Cx30 presence [121, 122]. It is worth noting that mutations in connexin 26 are the most common mutations found in genetically inherited HL. [123]

In addition to their role in ion and molecules flux among SCs, it has been reported that GJs in DCs could modulate OHCs electromotility: changes in gap junction permeability modify membrane potential, leading to DCs depolarization which reduces OHCs electromotility associated with nonlinear capacitance and otoacustic emissions [124]. The mechanism by which this occurs is not only related to K^+ accumulation in the extracellular space between OHCs and DCs but also to their mechanical connection. Structural cytoskeleton modifications in DCs, by its destruction, or Ca^{2+} influx which alters phalangeal process stiffness [125] alters OHCs electromotility. Also, uncoupling of the mechanical junctions described in Section 2.2 between DCs and OHCs generates the same effect [101, 124].

In conclusion, it has been demonstrated that DCs are not merely passive transporters of K^+ ions during the cochlear circulation process, but they also actively participate in modulating the electromotility of OHCs [121].

4. Conclusions

Impaired K^+ circulation in the organ of Corti can lead to HL by disrupting essential processes involved in sound transduction and cochlear function. K^+ homeostasis plays a critical role in the proper function of HCs and the conversion of sound vibrations into electrical signals. K^+ is the main electric charge that, contrary to what happens in all other excitable cells in our body, directly depolarizes sensory cells. Molecular alterations in ion channels and transporters responsible for K^+ movement can result in HCs dysfunction and cell death. In this chapter, we detailed the main channels and transporters involved in the movement of K^+ from the endolymph to the network of SCs that facilitate its return to the endolymph. In OHCs, K^+ entry from the endolymph is mediated by mechanotransduction channels in the apical region, while its extrusion is mediated by KCNQ4 channel in the basal region, facing the extracellular space. The efferent system also plays a role in modulating K^+ movement to finely tune hearing. It activates additional K^+ currents mediated by either SK2 or BK channels. K^+ is cleared from the extracellular space by DCs whose membrane contain the K^+-Cl^- cotransporter KCC3 and KCC4, the K^+ channel Kir4.1, and the purinergic P2 receptors. Once taken by DCs, K^+ moves through GJ composed of Cx26 and Cx30 back to the stria vascularis, where it is pumped back into the endolymph. Mouse models bearing alterations in these channels have helped to determine their importance in the K^+ circulation process, which generally leads to progressive HL due to OHC dysfunction and death. Overall, a comprehensive understanding of the mechanisms underlying K^+ circulation and its disruption in the OC is essential for advancing our understanding of HL, improving diagnosis and management, and ultimately enhancing the quality of life for individuals affected by K^+-related hearing disorders.

Acknowledgements

This work was supported by the grant PIP 0091 from CONICET and the grant PGI 24/B333 from UNS to G.S. and the grant PIBAA from CONICET to L.D. E.R. is a postdoctoral fellow from CONICET.

Conflict of interest

The authors declare no conflict of interest.

Appendices and nomenclature

HL: hearing loss, HCs: hair cells, IHCs: inner hair cells, OHCs: outer hair cells, MOC: medial olivochochlear complex, LOC: lateral olivochochlear complex, OC: organ of Corti, K^+: Ppotassium, Ca^{2+}: calcium, nAChR: nicotinic acetylcholine receptor, DC: Dieter's cells, SCs: supporting cells, KO: knock-out, GJ: gap junction. RP: receptor potential. SNHL: sensorineural hearing loss, ARHL: age-related hearing loss, NIHL: noise-induced hearing loss, EP: endocochlear potential, Cx: connexin, dn: dominant negative.

Author details

Guillermo Spitzmaul[1,2]*, Ezequiel Rías[1,2] and Leonardo Dionisio[1,2]

1 Institute of Biochemical Research of Bahía Blanca (INIBIBB), National Scientific and Technical Research Council (CONICET)/National University of the South (UNS), Bahía Blanca, Argentina

2 Department of Biology, Biochemistry and Pharmacy, National University of the South (UNS), Bahía Blanca, Argentina

*Address all correspondence to: gspitz@criba.edu.ar

References

[1] World Health O. World Report on Hearing. Geneva: World Health Organization; 2021

[2] Cunningham LL, Tucci DL. Hearing loss in adults. New England Journal of Medicine. 2017;**377**(25):2465-2473

[3] Haile LM, Kamenov K, Briant PS, Orji AU, Steinmetz JD, Abdoli A, et al. Hearing loss prevalence and years lived with disability, 1990-2019: Findings from the global burden of disease study 2019. The Lancet. 2021;**397**(10278):996-1009

[4] Olusanya BO, Neumann KJ, Saunders JE. The global burden of disabling hearing impairment: A call to action. Bulletin of the World Health Organization. 2014;**92**(5):367-373

[5] Vlajkovic SM, Thorne PR. Molecular mechanisms of sensorineural hearing loss and development of inner ear therapeutics. International Journal of Molecular Sciences. 2021;**22**(11):5647

[6] Petit C, Bonnet C, Safieddine S. Deafness: From genetic architecture to gene therapy. Nature Reviews Genetics. 12 May 2023. DOI: 10.1038/s41576-023-00597-7. Online ahead of print

[7] Zhang L, Chen S, Sun Y. Mechanism and prevention of spiral ganglion neuron degeneration in the cochlea. Frontiers in Cellular Neuroscience. 2022;**15**:814891

[8] Foster AC, Jacques BE, Piu F. Hearing loss: The final frontier of pharmacology. Pharmacology Research & Perspectives. 2022;**10**:e00970

[9] Raviv D, Dror AA, Avraham KB. Hearing loss: A common disorder caused by many rare alleles. Annals of the New York Academy of Sciences. 2010;**1214**(1):168-179

[10] Bayazit YA, Yilmaz M. An overview of hereditary hearing loss. ORL; Journal for Oto-Rhino-Laryngology and Its Related Specialties. 2006;**68**(2):57-63

[11] Del Castillo I, Morín M, Domínguez-Ruiz M, Moreno-Pelayo MA. Genetic etiology of non-syndromic hearing loss in Europe. Human Genetics. 2022;**141**(3-4):683-696

[12] Willems PJ. Genetic causes of hearing loss. The New England Journal of Medicine. 2000;**342**(15):1101-1109

[13] Shearer AE, Hildebrand MS, Schaefer AM, Smith RJH. Genetic Hearing Loss Overview. GeneReviews® [Internet]. Seattle (WA)1999-Upd; 2023 Available from: https://www.ncbi.nlm.nih.gov/pubmed/20301607

[14] Zdebik AA, Wangemann P, Jentsch TJ. Potassium ion movement in the inner ear: Insights from genetic disease and mouse models. Physiology. 2009;**24**:307-316

[15] Jang MW, Lim J, Park MG, Lee JH, Lee CJ. Active role of glia-like supporting cells in the organ of Corti: Membrane proteins and their roles in hearing. Glia. 2022;**70**(10):1799-1825

[16] Effertz T, Moser T, Oliver D. Recent advances in cochlear hair cell nanophysiology: Subcellular compartmentalization of electrical signaling in compact sensory cells. Faculty Reviews. 2020;**9**:24

[17] Mittal R, Aranke M, Debs LH, Nguyen D, Patel AP, Grati M, et al. Indispensable role of ion channels and

transporters in the auditory system. Journal of Cellular Physiology. 2017;**232**(4):743-758

[18] Liu W, Schrott-Fischer A, Glueckert R, Benav H, Rask-Andersen H. The human "Cochlear Battery"-Claudin-11 barrier and ion transport proteins in the lateral wall of the cochlea. Frontiers in Molecular Neuroscience. 2017;**10**:239

[19] Mistrik P, Ashmore J. The role of potassium recirculation in cochlear amplification. Current Opinion in Otolaryngology & Head and Neck Surgery. 2009;**17**(5):394-399

[20] Martinez AD, Acuna R, Figueroa V, Maripillan J, Nicholson B. Gap-junction channels dysfunction in deafness and hearing loss. Antioxidants & Redox Signaling. 2009;**11**(2):309-322

[21] Jin Z, Liang GH, Cooper EC, Jarlebark L. Expression and localization of K channels KCNQ2 and KCNQ3 in the mammalian cochlea. Audiology & Neuro-Otology. 2009;**14**(2):98-105

[22] Hibino H, Kurachi Y. Molecular and physiological bases of the K^+ circulation in the mammalian inner ear. Physiology. 2006;**21**:336-345

[23] Rim JH, Choi JY, Jung J, Gee HY. Activation of KCNQ4 as a therapeutic strategy to treat hearing loss. International Journal of Molecular Sciences. 2021;**22**(5):2510

[24] Sun W, Liu J, Zhang C, Zhou N, Manohar S, Winchester W, et al. Potassium channel activator attenuates salicylate-induced cochlear hearing loss potentially ameliorating tinnitus. Frontiers in Neurology. 2015;**6**:77

[25] Sheppard AM, Chen GD, Salvi R. Potassium ion channel openers, maxipost and retigabine, protect against peripheral salicylate ototoxicity in rats. Hearing Research. 2015;**327**:1-8

[26] Leitner MG, Halaszovich CR, Oliver D. Aminoglycosides inhibit KCNQ4 channels in Cochlear outer hair cells via depletion of phosphatidylinositol(4,5) bisphosphate. Molecular Pharmacology. 2011;**79**(1):51-60

[27] Gradogna A, Pusch M. Molecular pharmacology of kidney and inner ear CLC-K chloride channels. Frontiers in Pharmacology. 2010;**1**:130

[28] Nouvian R, Ruel J, Wang J, Guitton MJ, Pujol R, Puel JL. Degeneration of sensory outer hair cells following pharmacological blockade of cochlear KCNQ channels in the adult guinea pig. The European Journal of Neuroscience. 2003;**17**(12):2553-2562

[29] Furness DN. Molecular basis of hair cell loss. Cell and Tissue Research. 2015;**361**(1):387-399

[30] Goutman JD, Elgoyhen AB, Gomez-Casati ME. Cochlear hair cells: The sound-sensing machines. FEBS Letters. 2015;**589**(22):3354-3361

[31] Hudspeth AJ. Sensory transduction in the ear. In: Kandel ER, Schwartz JH, Jessell TM, editors. Principles of Neural Science. 4th ed. New York: bMcGraw-Hill; 2000. pp. 614-624

[32] McPherson DR. Sensory hair cells: An introduction to structure and physiology. Integrative and Comparative Biology. 2018;**58**(2):282-300

[33] Pangrsic T, Singer JH, Koschak A. Voltage-gated calcium channels: Key players in sensory coding in the retina and the inner ear. Physiological Reviews. 2018;**98**(4):2063-2096

[34] Wan G, Corfas G, Stone JS. Inner ear supporting cells: Rethinking the silent majority. Seminars in Cell & Developmental Biology. 2013;**24**(5):448-459

[35] Ramirez-Camacho R, Garcia-Berrocal JR, Trinidad A, Gonzalez-Garcia JA, Verdaguer JM, Ibanez A, et al. Central role of supporting cells in cochlear homeostasis and pathology. Medical Hypotheses. 2006;**67**(3):550-555

[36] Slepecky NB. Structure of the mammalian cochlea. In: Dallos P, Popper AN, Fay RR, editors. The Cochlea. New York, NY: Springer New York; 1996. pp. 44-129

[37] Li–dong Z, Jun L, Yin–yan H, Jian–he S, Shi–ming Y. Supporting cells–a new area in cochlear physiology study. Journal of Otology. 2008;**3**(1):9-17

[38] Vater M, Lenoir M. Ultrastructure of the horseshoe bat's organ of Corti. I. Scanning electron microscopy. The Journal of Comparative Neurology. 1992;**318**(4):367-379

[39] Engström H, Wersäll J. Structure and innervation of the inner ear sensory epithelia. In: Bourne GH, Danielli JF, editors. International Review of Cytology. 7. Cambridge, Massachusetts: Academic Press; 1958

[40] Engstrom H, Wersall J. The ultrastructural organization of the organ of Corti and of the vestibular sensory epithelia. Experimental Cell Research. 1958;**14**(Suppl 5):460-492

[41] Parsa A, Webster P, Kalinec F. Deiters cells tread a narrow path--the Deiters cells-basilar membrane junction. Hearing Research. 2012;**290**(1-2):13-20

[42] Engstrom H, Wersall J. Structure of the organ of Corti. II. Supporting structures and their relations to sensory cells and nerve endings. Acta Oto-Laryngologica. 1953;**43**(4-5):323-334

[43] Rutherford MA, von Gersdorff H, Goutman JD. Encoding sound in the cochlea: From receptor potential to afferent discharge. The Journal of Physiology. 2021;**599**(10):2527-2557

[44] Moser T. 2.23-Presynaptic physiology of Cochlear inner hair cells. In: Fritzsch B, editor. The Senses: A Comprehensive Reference. 2nd ed. Oxford: Elsevier; 2020. pp. 441-467

[45] Oliver DL, Cant NB, Fay RR, Popper AN. The Mammalian Auditory Pathways: Synaptic Organization and Microcircuits. Cham, Switzerland: Springer; 2018

[46] Ashmore J. Cochlear outer hair cell motility. Physiological Reviews. 2008;**88**(1):173-210

[47] Guinan JJ Jr. Olivocochlear efferents: Their action, effects, measurement and uses, and the impact of the new conception of cochlear mechanical responses. Hearing Research. 2018;**362**:38-47

[48] Fuchs PA. Synaptic transmission at vertebrate hair cells. Current Opinion in Neurobiology. 1996;**6**(4):514-519

[49] Guinan JJ Jr. Olivocochlear efferents: Anatomy, physiology, function, and the measurement of efferent effects in humans. Ear and Hearing. 2006;**27**(6):589-607

[50] Glowatzki E, Fuchs PA. Cholinergic synaptic inhibition of inner hair cells in the neonatal mammalian cochlea. Science. 2000;**288**(5475):2366-2368

[51] Elgoyhen AB, Vetter DE, Katz E, Rothlin CV, Heinemann SF, Boulter J. Alpha10: A determinant of nicotinic cholinergic receptor function in mammalian vestibular and cochlear mechanosensory hair cells. Proceedings of the National Academy of Sciences of the United States of America. 2001;**98**(6):3501-3506

[52] Elgoyhen AB, Johnson DS, Boulter J, Vetter DE, Heinemann S. Alpha 9: An acetylcholine receptor with novel pharmacological properties expressed in rat cochlear hair cells. Cell. 1994;**79**(4):705-715

[53] Gomez-Casati ME, Fuchs PA, Elgoyhen AB, Katz E. Biophysical and pharmacological characterization of nicotinic cholinergic receptors in rat cochlear inner hair cells. The Journal of Physiology. 2005;**566**(Pt 1):103-118

[54] Weisstaub N, Vetter DE, Elgoyhen AB, Katz E. The alpha9alpha10 nicotinic acetylcholine receptor is permeable to and is modulated by divalent cations. Hearing Research. 2002;**167**(1-2):122-135

[55] Rohmann KN, Wersinger E, Braude JP, Pyott SJ, Fuchs PA. Activation of BK and SK channels by efferent synapses on outer hair cells in high-frequency regions of the rodent cochlea. The Journal of Neuroscience. 2015;**35**(5):1821-1830

[56] Maison SF, Pyott SJ, Meredith AL, Liberman MC. Olivocochlear suppression of outer hair cells in vivo: Evidence for combined action of BK and SK2 channels throughout the cochlea. Journal of Neurophysiology. 2013;**109**(6):1525-1534

[57] Fuchs PA. A 'calcium capacitor' shapes cholinergic inhibition of cochlear hair cells. The Journal of Physiology. 2014;**592**(16):3393-3401

[58] Narita K, Akita T, Hachisuka J, Huang S, Ochi K, Kuba K. Functional coupling of Ca(2+) channels to ryanodine receptors at presynaptic terminals. Amplification of exocytosis and plasticity. The Journal of General Physiology. 2000;**115**(4):519-532

[59] Taranda J, Maison SF, Ballestero JA, Katz E, Savino J, Vetter DE, et al. A point mutation in the hair cell nicotinic cholinergic receptor prolongs cochlear inhibition and enhances noise protection. PLoS biology. 2009;**7**(1):e18

[60] Boero LE, Castagna VC, Di Guilmi MN, Goutman JD, Belen Elgoyhen A, Gomez-Casati ME. Enhancement of the medial olivocochlear system prevents hidden hearing loss. The Journal of Neuroscience. 2018;**38**(34):7440-7451

[61] Jensen JB, Lysaght AC, Liberman MC, Qvortrup K, Stankovic KM. Immediate and delayed cochlear neuropathy after noise exposure in pubescent mice. PLoS One. 2015;**10**(5):e0125160

[62] Wright CG, Preston RE. Efferent nerve fibers associated with the outermost supporting cells of the organ of Corti in the guinea pig. Acta Oto-Laryngologica. 1976;**82**(1-2):41-47

[63] Liberman MC, Dodds LW, Pierce S. Afferent and efferent innervation of the cat cochlea: Quantitative analysis with light and electron microscopy. The Journal of Comparative Neurology. 1990;**301**(3):443-460

[64] Nadol JB Jr, Burgess BJ. Supranuclear efferent synapses on outer hair cells and Deiters' cells in the human organ of Corti. Hearing Research. 1994;**81**(1-2):49-56

[65] Burgess BJ, Adams JC, Nadol JB Jr. Morphologic evidence for innervation of Deiters' and Hensen's cells in the guinea pig. Hearing Research. 1997;**108**(1-2):74-82

[66] Zhao H-B, Liu L-M, Yu N, Zhu Y, Mei L, Chen J, et al. Efferent neurons control hearing sensitivity and protect hearing from noise through the regulation of gap junctions between cochlear supporting cells. Journal of Neurophysiology. 2022;**127**(1):313-327

[67] Hibino H, Nin F, Tsuzuki C, Kurachi Y. How is the highly positive endocochlear potential formed? The specific architecture of the stria vascularis and the roles of the ion-transport apparatus. Pflügers Archiv. 2010;**459**(4):521-533

[68] Bazard P, Frisina RD, Acosta AA, Dasgupta S, Bauer MA, Zhu X, et al. Roles of key ion channels and transport proteins in age-related hearing loss. International Journal of Molecular Sciences. 2021;**22**(5):6158

[69] Fettiplace R, Kim KX. The physiology of mechanoelectrical transduction channels in hearing. Physiological Reviews. 2014;**94**(3):951-986

[70] Holt JR, Stauffer EA, Abraham D, Géléoc GS. Dominant-negative inhibition of M-like potassium conductances in hair cells of the mouse inner ear. The Journal of Neuroscience. 2007;**27**(33):8940-8951

[71] Kharkovets T, Dedek K, Maier H, Schweizer M, Khimich D, Nouvian R, et al. Mice with altered KCNQ4 K^+ channels implicate sensory outer hair cells in human progressive deafness. The EMBO Journal. 2006;**25**(3):642-652

[72] Kharkovets T, Hardelin JP, Safieddine S, Schweizer M, El-Amraoui A, Petit C, et al. KCNQ4, a K^+-channel mutated in a form of dominant deafness, is expressed in the inner ear and the central auditory pathway. Proceedings of the National Academy of Sciences of the United States of America. 2000;**97**(8):4333-4338

[73] Marcotti W, Johnson SL, Holley MC, Kros CJ. Developmental changes in the expression of potassium currents of embryonic, neonatal and mature mouse inner hair cells. The Journal of Physiology. 2003;**548**(Pt 2):383-400

[74] Housley GD, Ashmore JF. Ionic currents of outer hair cells isolated from the guinea-pig cochlea. The Journal of Physiology. 1992;**448**:73-98

[75] Marcotti W, Kros CJ. Developmental expression of the potassium current IK,n contributes to maturation of mouse outer hair cells. The Journal of Physiology. 1999;**520**(Pt 3):653-660

[76] Oliver D, Knipper M, Derst C, Fakler B. Resting potential and submembrane calcium concentration of inner hair cells in the isolated mouse cochlea are set by KCNQ-type potassium channels. The Journal of Neuroscience. 2003;**23**(6):2141-2149

[77] Beisel KW, Rocha-Sanchez SM, Morris KA, Nie L, Feng F, Kachar B, et al. Differential expression of KCNQ4 in inner hair cells and sensory neurons is the basis of progressive high-frequency hearing loss. The Journal of Neuroscience. 2005;**25**(40):9285-9293

[78] Beisel KW, Nelson NC, Delimont DC, Fritzsch B. Longitudinal gradients of KCNQ4 expression in spiral ganglion and cochlear hair cells correlate with progressive hearing loss in DFNA2. Brain

Research. Molecular Brain Research. 2000;**82**(1-2):137-149

[79] Kimitsuki T, Komune N, Noda T, Takaiwa K, Ohashi M, Komune S. Property of I(K,)(n) in inner hair cells isolated from guinea-pig cochlea. Hearing Research. 2010;**261**(1-2):57-62

[80] Dierich M, Altoe A, Koppelmann J, Evers S, Renigunta V, Schafer MK, et al. Optimized tuning of auditory inner hair cells to encode complex sound through synergistic activity of six independent K(+) current entities. Cell Reports. 2020;**32**(1):107869

[81] Winter H, Braig C, Zimmermann U, Geisler HS, Franzer JT, Weber T, et al. Thyroid hormone receptors TRalpha1 and TRbeta differentially regulate gene expression of Kcnq4 and prestin during final differentiation of outer hair cells. Journal of Cell Science. 2006;**119**(Pt 14):2975-2984

[82] Jeng JY, Carlton AJ, Johnson SL, Brown SDM, Holley MC, Bowl MR, et al. Biophysical and morphological changes in inner hair cells and their efferent innervation in the ageing mouse cochlea. The Journal of Physiology. 2021;**599**(1):269-287

[83] Peixoto Pinheiro B, Vona B, Lowenheim H, Ruttiger L, Knipper M, Adel Y. Age-related hearing loss pertaining to potassium ion channels in the cochlea and auditory pathway. Pflügers Archiv. 2021;**473**(5):823-840

[84] Van Eyken E, Van Laer L, Fransen E, Topsakal V, Lemkens N, Laureys W, et al. KCNQ4: A gene for age-related hearing impairment? Human Mutation. 2006;**27**(10):1007-1016

[85] Homma K. The pathological mechanisms of hearing loss caused by KCNQ1 and KCNQ4 variants. Biomedicine. 2022;**10**(9):2254

[86] Zhang X, Wang H, Wang Q. Progression of KCNQ4 related genetic hearing loss: A narrative review. Journal of Bio-X Research. 2021;**4**(4):151-157

[87] Wang Q, Li W, Cai C, Hu P, Lai R. miR-153/KCNQ4 axis contributes to noise-induced hearing loss in a mouse model. The Journal of Physiological Sciences: JPS. 2021;**71**(1):28

[88] Jaumann M, Dettling J, Gubelt M, Zimmermann U, Gerling A, Paquet-Durand F, et al. cGMP-Prkg1 signaling and Pde5 inhibition shelter cochlear hair cells and hearing function. Nature Medicine. 2012;**18**(2):252-259

[89] Van Laer L, Carlsson PI, Ottschytsch N, Bondeson ML, Konings A, Vandevelde A, et al. The contribution of genes involved in potassium-recycling in the inner ear to noise-induced hearing loss. Human Mutation. 2006;**27**(8):786-795

[90] Kubisch C, Schroeder BC, Friedrich T, Lütjohann B, El-Amraoui A, Marlin S, et al. KCNQ4, a novel potassium channel expressed in sensory outer hair cells, is mutated in dominant deafness. Cell. 1999;**96**(3):437-446

[91] Jung J, Lin H, Koh YI, Ryu K, Lee JS, Rim JH, et al. Rare KCNQ4 variants found in public databases underlie impaired channel activity that may contribute to hearing impairment. Experimental & Molecular Medicine. 2019;**51**(8):1-12

[92] Pyott SJ, Meredith AL, Fodor AA, Vazquez AE, Yamoah EN, Aldrich RW. Cochlear function in mice lacking the BK channel alpha, beta1, or beta4 subunits.

The Journal of Biological Chemistry. 2007;**282**(5):3312-3324

[93] Pyott SJ, Duncan RK. BK channels in the vertebrate inner ear. International Review of Neurobiology. 2016;**128**:369-399

[94] Murthy V, Maison SF, Taranda J, Haque N, Bond CT, Elgoyhen AB, et al. SK2 channels are required for function and long-term survival of efferent synapses on mammalian outer hair cells. Molecular and Cellular Neurosciences. 2009;**40**(1):39-49

[95] Kong JH, Adelman JP, Fuchs PA. Expression of the SK2 calcium-activated potassium channel is required for cholinergic function in mouse cochlear hair cells. The Journal of Physiology. 2008;**586**(22):5471-5485

[96] Ruttiger L, Sausbier M, Zimmermann U, Winter H, Braig C, Engel J, et al. Deletion of the Ca^{2+}-activated potassium (BK) a-subunit but not the BKb1-subunit leads to progressive hearing loss. Proceedings of the National Academy of Sciences of the United States of America. 2004;**101**(35):12922-12927

[97] Wersinger E, McLean WJ, Fuchs PA, Pyott SJ. BK channels mediate cholinergic inhibition of high frequency cochlear hair cells. PLoS One. 2010;**5**(11):e13836

[98] Evans MG. Acetylcholine activates two currents in guinea-pig outer hair cells. The Journal of Physiology. 1996;**491**(2):563-578

[99] Boettger T, Hübner CA, Maier H, Rust MB, Beck FX, Jentsch TJ. Deafness and renal tubular acidosis in mice lacking the K-Cl co-transporter Kcc4. Nature. 2002;**416**(6883):874-878

[100] Taylor RR, Jagger DJ, Forge A. Defining the cellular environment in the organ of Corti following extensive hair cell loss: A basis for future sensory cell replacement in the cochlea. PLoS One. 2012;7(1):e30577

[101] Zhu Y, Liang C, Chen J, Zong L, Chen GD, Zhao HB. Active cochlear amplification is dependent on supporting cell gap junctions. Nature Communications. 2013;**4**:1786

[102] Forge A, Becker D, Casalotti S, Edwards J, Marziano N, Nevill G. Gap junctions in the inner ear: Comparison of distribution patterns in different vertebrates and assessement of connexin composition in mammals. The Journal of Comparative Neurology. 2003;**467**(2):207-231

[103] Zhao HB, Yu N. Distinct and gradient distributions of connexin26 and connexin30 in the cochlear sensory epithelium of guinea pigs. The Journal of Comparative Neurology. 2006;**499**(3):506-518

[104] Zhu Y, Zong L, Mei L, Zhao HB. Connexin26 gap junction mediates miRNA intercellular genetic communication in the cochlea and is required for inner ear development. Scientific Reports. 2015;**5**:15647

[105] Boulay AC, del Castillo FJ, Giraudet F, Hamard G, Giaume C, Petit C, et al. Hearing is normal without connexin30. The Journal of Neuroscience. 2013;**33**(2):430-434

[106] Ding D, Liu H, Qi W, Jiang H, Li Y, Wu X, et al. Ototoxic effects and mechanisms of loop diuretics. Journal of Otology. 2016;**11**(4):145-156

[107] Dominguez LM, Dodson KM. Genetics of hearing loss: Focus on

DFNA2. The Application of Clinical Genetics. 2012;**5**:97-104

[108] Nie L. KCNQ4 mutations associated with nonsyndromic progressive sensorineural hearing loss. Current Opinion in Otolaryngology & Head and Neck Surgery. 2008;**16**(5):441-444

[109] De Leenheer EM, Ensink RJ, Kunst HP, Marres HA, Talebizadeh Z, Declau F, et al. DFNA2/KCNQ4 and its manifestations. Advances in Oto-Rhino-Laryngology. 2002;**61**:41-46

[110] Carignano C, Barila EP, Rias EI, Dionisio L, Aztiria E, Spitzmaul G. Inner hair cell and neuron degeneration contribute to hearing loss in a DFNA2-like mouse model. Neuroscience. 2019;**410**:202-216

[111] Wu T, Lv P, Kim HJ, Yamoah EN, Nuttall AL. Effect of salicylate on KCNQ4 of the guinea pig outer hair cell. Journal of Neurophysiology. 2010;**103**(4):1969-1977

[112] Noh B, Rim JH, Gopalappa R, Lin H, Kim KM, Kang MJ, et al. In vivo outer hair cell gene editing ameliorates progressive hearing loss in dominant-negative Kcnq4 murine model. Theranostics. 2022;**12**(5):2465-2482

[113] Cui C, Zhang L, Qian F, Chen Y, Huang B, Wang F, et al. A humanized murine model, demonstrating dominant progressive hearing loss caused by a novel KCNQ4 mutation (p.G228D) from a large Chinese family. Clinical Genetics. 2022;**102**(2):149-154

[114] Peixoto Pinheiro B, Muller M, Bos M, Guezguez J, Burnet M, Tornincasa M, et al. A potassium channel agonist protects hearing function and promotes outer hair cell survival in a mouse model for age-related hearing loss. Cell Death & Disease. 2022;**13**(7):595

[115] Skinner LJ, Enée V, Beurg M, Jung HH, Ryan AF, Hafidi A, et al. Contribution of BK Ca2+-activated K+ channels to auditory neurotransmission in the guinea pig cochlea. Journal of Neurophysiology. 2003;**90**(1):320-332

[116] Roux I, Wersinger E, McIntosh JM, Fuchs PA, Glowatzki E. Onset of cholinergic efferent synaptic function in sensory hair cells of the rat cochlea. The Journal of Neuroscience. 2011;**31**(42):15092-15101

[117] Johnson SL, Adelman JP, Marcotti W. Genetic deletion of SK2 channels in mouse inner hair cells prevents the developmental linearization in the Ca2+dependence of exocytosis. The Journal of Physiology. 2007;**583**(2):631-646

[118] Boettger T. Loss of K-Cl co-transporter KCC3 causes deafness, neurodegeneration and reduced seizure threshold. The EMBO Journal. 2003;**22**(20):5422-5434

[119] Kikuchi T, Kimura RS, Paul DL, Adams JC. Gap junctions in the rat cochlea: Immunohistochemical and ultrastructural analysis. Anatomy and embryology (Berl). 1995;**191**(2):101-118

[120] Santos-Sacchi J, Dallos P. Intercellular communication in the supporting cells of the organ of Corti. Hearing Research. 1983;**9**(3):317-326

[121] Zhao HB. Hypothesis of K(+)-recycling defect is not a primary deafness mechanism for Cx26 (GJB2) deficiency. Frontiers in Molecular Neuroscience. 2017;**10**:162

[122] Zhu Y, Chen J, Liang C, Zong L, Jones RO, Zhao HB. Connexin26 (GJB2) deficiency reduces active cochlear amplification leading to late-onset hearing loss. Neuroscience. 2015;**284**:719-729

[123] Chan DK, Chang KW. GJB2-associated hearing loss: Systematic review of worldwide prevalence, genotype, and auditory phenotype. The Laryngoscope. 2014;**124**(2):E34-E53

[124] Yu N, Zhao HB. Modulation of outer hair cell electromotility by cochlear supporting cells and gap junctions. PLoS One. 2009;**4**(11):e7923

[125] Dulon D, Blanchet C, Laffon E. Photoreleased intracellular Ca2+ evokes reversible mechanical responses in supporting cells of the guinea-pig organ of Corti. Biochemical and Biophysical Research Communications. 1994;**201**(3):1263-1269

Chapter 5

Comparison of Information and Communication Technology Provision in Higher Education for Students with Hearing Disabilities across Different Countries

Manal Alkharji

Abstract

The purpose of this chapter is to investigate the most important information and communication technologies (ICT) that should be provided to students with hearing disabilities in higher education institutions by reviewing the most important research, studies, and recent literature in several countries at the present time and comparing them. The primary goal is to communicate the importance of ICT and highlight how they benefit students with hearing disabilities in colleges and universities. This chapter gives examples of ICT being offered across several countries. The result of the present review shows that there are a few successful experiences regarding the provision of ICT in higher education. Showcasing the significance and usefulness of ICT use for students with hearing disabilities in obtaining information and communicating in the classroom. Additionally, ICT availability in higher education institutions differs from country to country. ICT in higher education should be prioritized by governments since they enable students with hearing disabilities to overcome barriers present in conventional higher education programs.

Keywords: C-print, deaf, hard of hearing, hearing disabilities, higher education, ICT, real-time captioning

1. Introduction

Technology made great strides throughout the last decade of the twentieth century and the beginning of the twenty-first century, especially in the areas of Information and Communication Technologies (ICT), which had an impact on educational systems. The students with disabilities have benefited from this advancement, among other groups. Many laws have emphasized the rights of individuals with disabilities by enabling them to use technology and communication methods that foster the greatest possible intellectual and social development [1]. Article 9 of the Convention on the Rights of Persons with Disabilities (CRPD) specifically emphasizes the duty of Member States to ensure access to ICT. Thus recognizing the importance of ICT application in the modern age [2].

The modern educational trends emphasize the need to find the best technologies and the most effective means concerned with providing an interactive educational environment. That is suitable for attracting the interest of students with hearing disabilities and urging them to learn as well as improving the outcomes [3]. According to Zirzow, education is a field greatly impacted by technology for the purposes of instruction and communication [4]. Therefore, the influence of ICT is extended to the field of higher education for students with hearing disabilities in all its specializations. This means improving classrooms through the provision of technological devices, such as computers, real-time captioning, C-Print, and whiteboard [5, 6].

2. ICT for students with hearing disabilities in higher education

ICT in education refers to the adoption of generic information technologies in the teaching and learning process [7]. Computer and network hardware, as well as associated communication software, are all parts of ICT. In other words, ICT includes information technology in addition to devices and tools represented in the computer and its applications, and all other electronic and digital means of assistance [8, 9]. Modified or specialized instructional technologies are used with students with disabilities to improve their performance and capabilities [1].

There should be as many avenues as possible for students with hearing disabilities to access information. Therefore, the inclusion of technology for these students in teaching is very important. According to United Nations, ICT should be used to promote greater inclusiveness and involvement. ICT has a higher role in this regard to educate students with hearing disabilities at the same pace as their peers [8]. ICT makes it easier for them to participate in the educational process and academic development [10]. Therefore, students with hearing disabilities in higher education institutions should be equipped with the requisite technological know-how to use the technology that is made available to them. This is done to guarantee that technological services are used effectively because developing these abilities boosts students' academic performance [11]. According to Peng and Daud, the integration of ICT into the classroom of students with hearing disabilities is more complicated because they are generally classified as visual learners [12]. Therefore, technology in education is crucial for these students because their nature of learning to access the information is visually orientated [13].

As ICT is a visual medium, it allows students with hearing disabilities to expand both their general knowledge and language use without being reliant on spoken word. This is done by displaying pictures, signs, or writings on a screen [8]. It is one of the primary methods used to transmit information to these pupils since it fosters their ability to learn and process information [14]. Therefore, technology should be made available to all teachers and students with hearing disabilities and adapting it to make it applicable in the learning environment. It is an essential aspect when providing educational services in the classrooms that include students with hearing disabilities because the visual display plays a key role in understanding a task [5, 13].

The benefits of using ICT in teaching and learning are based on the opportunities it provides for alternate forms of communication, offering access to educational resources in a more convenient way [15]. The use of ICT in teaching process at higher education institutions helps students with hearing disabilities to access educational resources and enhances motivation by enabling them to actively participate in learning experiences. Moreover, the use of ICT in teaching helps these students learn effectively, promotes access to the general curriculum, develops independent work skills, as well as improves access to education and enhances educational and employment opportunities for students with hearing disabilities [16]. In addition, the use of ICT can help them improve their language skills.

Both Students with hearing disability rehabilitated by hearing aids or cochlear implants and students with hearing disability non-rehabilitated could benefit from ICT. According to Peng and Daud, whatever the degree of hearing loss for students, it is possible to compensate this loss through the use of ICT services that help them obtain information within the classroom [12].

Despite the importance of ICT in the education of students with hearing disabilities in higher education, many of them today lack access to the most up-to-date ICT tools and technologies [13]. Effective technological integration in education is hampered by significant barriers. ICT integration in students with hearing disabilities' classrooms is more complex and difficult to learn in some ways. This is because the students have different levels of hearing loss which either directly or indirectly affect them [12]. Secondly, there is not a single, obvious way to incorporate technology into educational environments [17]. Thirdly, barriers that were identified by Lartz et al. included the interactions between sign language interpreters and the technology at the same time during the lectures, and difficulties in coordinating information from the faculty members, the interpreter, and the technology [18]. According to Chong and Shaffe, without the ICT, the students with hearing disabilities are unable to fully participate in the classroom discussions [19]. Furthermore, researchers mentioned that the use of technologies in the learning process of students with hearing disabilities is not often addressed in secondary schools, and this has ramifications when they attend higher education [20].

To overcome these obstacles, previous researchers have recommended involving faculty members and students with hearing disabilities in the planning processes of using the assistive technology. Faculty members need to be willing to use ICT in their classes and have access to resources when needed [8]. Also, Lartz et al. recommended that the technology planning for a classroom should be done by all the stakeholders, such as faculty members, students with hearing disabilities, and interpreters [18]. Moreover, Al-Rayes recommended that modern technology must be employed in the teaching of students with hearing disabilities, as well as training faculty members on designing websites and electronic tests for these students [21]. Furthermore, students with hearing disabilities should be able to read subtitles and use wireless devices in the classroom to listen to higher education instructors.

Many studies indicated that students with hearing disabilities in higher education institutions used a group of technologies, such as the internet, e-mail, messaging, real-time captioning, C-Print, and whiteboard [5, 6, 18, 22]. The use was justified by the fact that a few of the faculty members who instructed students with hearing disabilities in universities were fluent sign language communicators. Thus, technology was the primary means of communication with students with hearing disabilities during the lectures [18]. Obviously, faculty members should choose the best technological devices and tools to support their students' learning processes while considering their individual peculiarities and special requirements [17]. A detailed explanation of each technology is stated below:

2.1 Real-time captioning

One of the devices that is used by students with hearing disabilities in higher education institutions is real-time captioning [11]. Real-time captioning, known as speech-to-text, is one method of providing communication access [23]. It is a technological device that transforms audio content into a text display to facilitate information access and improve communication opportunities [5]. Real-time captioning, often referred to as live transcription or speech-to-text, is a service that provides students with hearing disabilities with immediate access to spoken communication in lectures and conversations [24]. The text message is displayed on the screen and includes conversations and audios [12]. Also, caption is a visual tool that assists the learning process of students with hearing disabilities and overcomes the hurdles they face in classrooms and enhances reading skills [5].

Captioning is the most valuable element to the students with hearing disabilities in a higher education level. It appears to be a useful tool for supporting hearing disabilities college students in accessing information and communicating [24]. This service is suitable for those students who do not benefit from hearing assistive devices, and students who have difficulty following lessons [11]. Offline captions are created by playing a video and the online captions in real-time are transferred into written texts. Therefore, using captions facilitates access to discussions and lectures by students with hearing disabilities [5]. According to Stinson and Stevenson, students with hearing disabilities perform better academically after receiving captioning services because it facilitates their learning [11].

Previously, research suggested that students with hearing disabilities prefer notes created in real-time systems rather than handwritten notes. This is because they provided a permanent record that a student can review after class to remember relevant information [22, 25]. Moreover, handwritten notes have limitations. They can be messy or disorganized since note-takers could not write nearly as rapidly as faculty members can talk [26]. As an illustration, explanatory publications that are published in real time retain the most information from faculty members, even though the notes taken may differ from those of note-takers. Nevertheless, the availability of such notes may lead to increased workload rate of students with hearing disabilities, requiring time and a lot of extra effort to identify the important points [24]. According to Kawas, Karalis, Wen, and Ladner, there are several problems related to the use of real-time captioning in university, such as limited control, and complex settings [27].

2.2 C-print

One of the first technological devices that students with hearing disabilities used in colleges and universities was Computer-Aided Transcription System (C-print) [28]. The C-Print service was first provided in 1996. In 2015, more than 2000 students were trained to provide this service. In recent years, the use of C-Print service has grown significantly. C-Print is a computer-related system which is used in lectures to help students with hearing disabilities to transcribe and print speech [22]. It is a system of real-time transcription and conversion of speech into written text. It is considered a printed literal version of what was said in lectures. By saving texts created during lessons and saving them in electronic form, it gives students with hearing disabilities a reference method to remember lectures [22]. Additionally, the computer-saved text file is used by being edited, printed, and then distributed to tutors and students with hearing disabilities [28].

Stinson et al. presented different benefits of C-Print services. First, the display remains on the screen long enough to allow students with hearing disabilities to fill in information they might have missed from the interpreter or faculty members. Second, a hard copy of the lecture transcript is available after class in the computer's memory [22]. Third, it can be useful for students with hearing disabilities in writing their assignments or improving their written language [29]. According to Elliot, Stinson, McKee, Everhart, & Francis, C-Print usage and academic performance were positively correlated because it improves students' educational opportunities [30]. Furthermore, the results of Stinson et al. indicated that the students with hearing disabilities preferred the use of the C-Print service because it was much more detailed than the handwritten notes [22].

More so, there are many technological devices that help students with hearing disabilities benefit from hearing remnants and improve learning outcomes, such as interactive whiteboard and e-textbooks [3, 6]. Interactive whiteboard is one of the various methods which is used to deliver helpful learning experiences. It has become popular in the last ten years because it facilitates and improves the learning of these students [6]. Students with hearing disabilities benefit from interactive whiteboards because they can see what is going on and what they need to do without having to listen to the teachers. Written instructions combined with demonstrations enable for hearing student involvement without the requirement for listening or speaking [8]. Additionally, in educational settings, e-textbooks are becoming more common. Collaboration and interaction are made easier with the material, other students, and the teacher through interactive features including surveys, quizzes, note-exchange, and instructor remarks. Also, the usage of digital recorders by students who have mild to moderate hearing loss is frequently beneficial. The technology allows students with hearing disabilities to record lectures, which may then be played back later. This can be especially helpful in settings without additional listening devices [10].

3. ICT provision for students with hearing disabilities in higher education in different countries

3.1 United States of America (USA)

In the USA, there are many public and private higher education institutions that provide services to students with hearing disabilities such as Gallaudet University and the National Technical Institute for the Deaf (NTID). According to Stinson et al. approximately 75% of students with hearing disabilities receive their education alongside hearing classmates [22]. More and more of these students enroll in normal colleges alongside peers who can hear. More than 23,000 of the 25,000 students with hearing disabilities participating in postsecondary education in the USA are doing so in programs with a hearing student majority [31]. According to Hyde et al., students with hearing disabilities frequently struggle to understand speakers and other participants when they attend classes with hearing students [23]. Therefore, ICT helps these students to understand the speakers.

According to Braun et al., there are centers in the US providing ICT for students with hearing disabilities, such as the NTID, which provides global teaching and learning resources to better support these students in higher education [29]. The NTID, a college of Rochester Institute of Technology (RIT), was founded in 1965 to offer technical and professional education programs to students with hearing disabilities, along with arts and sciences curriculum, to better prepare them for life and work [23]. At the NTID, real-time captioning and systems such as C-Print are provided which is a speech-to-text system that helps students with hearing disabilities access information in the educational environment. Computer and Internet technologies have also been utilized to their advantage [16].

Hyde et al. examined a significant communication tool created at NTID, the C-Print real-time captioning service, which is utilized to improve students' communication access at RIT and other colleges and universities [23]. Captioning is a commonly used system in many US higher education institutions. Also, C-Print, TypeWell, and Communication Access Real-Time Translation (CART) are the main systems used in US higher education institutions to provide real-time captions. Therefore, the C-Print real-time captioning system has been in development by a team of academics and developers at NTID for the past 25 years [23]. C-Print and TypeWell offer meaning captions, which means the caption translates spoken language into a simple-to-read format using a standard keyboard [24].

3.2 Kingdom of Saudi Arabia (KSA)

After King Fahad bin Abdul-Aziz's approval on March 8, 2001, students with hearing disabilities may apply to higher education institutions, ensuring they had the same access to higher education possibilities as other students [32]. Even though there are 30 public universities and 12 private universities in the KSA, the statistics showed that there are few higher education institutions that provide programs to students with hearing disabilities [33]. Based on the royal approval, departments for these students were opened at the College of Telecom and Information (CTI), the Arab Open University (AOU), and King Saud University (KSA) [32]. At the CTI, the department of special technology program is one of the first introductory programs for students with hearing disabilities in higher education. In 2005 and 2006, special classes for these students were opened at the CTI in Riyadh, Hail, and Al Qassim city. Each department has classrooms and computer labs [21].

In 2011, KSU prepared the university environment for the admission of students with hearing disabilities by equipping the halls with the necessary requirements and techniques for their education [32]. Additionally, the classrooms have been equipped with advanced and modern technological devices. To assist students with hearing disabilities with writing reports and conducting library or online searches, additional services are offered. In a higher education program for students with hearing disabilities at KSU, Al-Hawi conducted a study with the intention of determining the reality of ICT use among faculty members and support staff. The researcher used a questionnaire-based survey using descriptive methodology. The sample consisted of 26 faculty members and support staff who were in the program. The findings showed that the internet, computers, smart boards, and electronic mail systems were the most common and widely utilized technology among KSU faculty members and support staff. However, the challenges that prevented them from using the ICT were the result of poor awareness of its importance in teaching students with hearing disabilities [3].

Within the same context, a study by Salem identified the reality and the obstacles of using educational technologies among students with hearing disabilities at the same university. The study sample consisted of 40 students. The results showed that the use of technology in learning was moderate, and the poor level of Arabic language in reading and writing among the students with hearing disabilities was the most important obstacle which limits the use of technology. The results indicated that the amount of technology use in education was moderate and that the main barrier limiting the use of technology among students with hearing disabilities was their low proficiency in reading and writing Arabic [34]. There was empirical evidence that students with hearing disabilities did not gain skills above the level of third-to-fourth grade in reading and writing [35].

According to Al-Kharji and Cheong, students with hearing disabilities do better academically if technology is used more effectively in Saudi universities because it significantly aided these students in gaining access to and remembering lecture material [32]. Despite this, some universities face challenges in the effective use of these devices [34]. Al-Hawi and Al-Rayes recommended that the Saudi universities must increase the availability of hardware, software, educational devices, and applications necessary for the uses of ICT directed specifically at serving the students with hearing disabilities, including computers, digital speakers, and headphones [3, 21].

3.3 United Arab Emirates (UAE)

In the UAE, each student with disabilities is integrated and educated by the Ministry of Education. Students with hearing disabilities are included in all educational levels up to the undergraduate level. Also, they get special education along with other hearing students to take advantage of educational possibilities when they become available [36]. In UAE higher education institutions, students with hearing disabilities utilize computers to sharpen their writing and linguistic abilities. These students can learn how to use ICT tools and resources for education. Through their visual memories, they use digital information resources for reading, writing, and social engagement [37]. Moreover, there are several reports on the use of the Internet for educational purposes whether for self-learning or teaching, accessing information, enhancing thinking abilities, or increasing knowledge. The outcomes of these reports highlight how crucial the Internet is for students with hearing disabilities. This is since having access to and using the Internet is now a requirement for these students to be successful in their academic endeavors [1].

Al Ain University (AAU) was one of the first universities in Al Ain and Abu Dhabi that started a program for students with hearing disabilities to obtain a bachelor's degree in Applied Sociology and Special Education in 2015. The programs began with 30 and 38 students [1]. As a foundation for innovation and to better prepare students with hearing disabilities for the job market, AAU has been motivated to incorporate contemporary technologies into the educational process in its curricula and instructional goals. As a result, the institution has given the usage of ICT a lot of consideration. The AAU supplies a variety of materials and technological equipment for the courses and has high-speed Internet connections. Furthermore, the university website includes learning tools like Microsoft Team, Moodle, and Egate, electronic courses are also offered [1]. Kaba and Ellala presented several recommendations to the UAE higher education institutions. First, academic programs should make sure that students with hearing disabilities have access to computers and the Internet on campus. Second, institutions must arrange training sessions and workshops on how to successfully use computers and the Internet for academic purposes for these students [1].

3.4 Russia

In Russia, since 1934, Bauman Moscow State Technical University (BMSTU) is one of the most important universities that has provided students with hearing disabilities with an opportunity for education. Subsequently, in 1994 a Deafness Center was established within BMSTU, with greater focus on the needs of students. This center provides many technological devices, the most important of which are smart boards, computers, projectors equipped with classrooms, as well as PowerPoint presentations and MS Word materials [16].

In BMSTU, the C-Print system is not available, but the "in-class notes" approach has been used. In this approach, faculty members are responsible for taking notes and all conversations by typing on their computer to be displayed on a screen. This method is quite effective but very time-consuming. Kirsanova et al. mentioned that although there are various programs for students with hearing disabilities in Russia, there is a need for improvement regarding the use of ICTs in teaching students with hearing disabilities. It also recommended to organize training courses in the use of ICT for faculty members who work with these students. In addition to experimenting with new technologies and methods [16].

3.5 Europe

The European Union (EU) has established directives that would provide ICT accessibility by 2023, such as audiovisual media services, electronic communications, and websites. Its objective is ICT accessibility for students with disabilities. The most of member states have regulating bodies in place and regulations to support and encourage the accessibility of ICT services as well as websites and mobile applications. However, availability varies from country to another [38].

Most EU countries, including the United Kingdom, Norway, Germany, France, Denmark, Slovakia, Sweden, Ireland, Switzerland, and Netherlands have policies in place to make it easier for students with hearing disabilities to access information, communication, and education as well as ICT services. A growing number of accessible communication tools are being developed for these students, such as offline and closed captions, text and video relay services, video remote interpreting services that may be accessed through an application or as a web service, and communication access real-time translation (CART), and other augmentation and alternative communication methods [38].

Also, in these countries, there has been a growing interest in employing teachers for students with hearing disabilities, educating professionals and staff about the ICT accessibility issues, as well as digital accessibility, such as web and electronic document accessibility, and real-time captioning. Moreover, accessibility has been implemented to websites and mobile applications of higher education institutions based on the Royal Decree 1112/2018 in Spain [38]. They gave them the chance to learn, connect with others, and use the same services in a way that was efficient and fair in universities and colleges. In contrast, many countries still do not have closed captioning, and sign languages do not consistently provide comprehensive information [39].

3.5.1 Slovenia

In Slovenia, very few students with disabilities effectively completed their studies in higher education [10]. According to the Deaf and Hard of Hearing Clubs Association of Slovenia, the students with hearing disabilities are most affected by this issue, and they are also the least educated group in Slovenia [40]. The educational process in Slovenian higher education institutions can be made easier for the students with hearing disabilities so that they can follow lectures. Since these students must rely more on their vision owing to hearing loss, supportive visual media aids like graphs, tables, and spreadsheets are frequently employed for computer education [41]. In Slovenia, various pieces of technology and software are presently used in classrooms and institutions to assist students with hearing disabilities [10].

3.6 Australia

Few universities in Australia offer specialist help for students with hearing disabilities; Instead, it offers general disability support departments in 39 institutions. When needed, it hires tutors and interpreters. Griffith University is one of the few universities in Australia with a specialist curriculum for these students, which enrolls more than 32,000 students over five sites in Southeast Queensland [23]. Students with hearing disabilities have a long history at Griffith; the university's Deaf Student Support Program (DSSP), which was founded in 1985, is still active today. This program provides some ICT services such as captioned videos and professional tutorial assistance. Almost ten years ago, the majority of other Australian universities have created a variety of support services for these students [23].

A retrospective analysis of students with hearing disabilities' experiences at Griffith during a 20-year period, as well as the experiences of graduates in employment and further education, was conducted by the Center for Deaf Studies and Research. The study's goals were to determine which academic, social opportunities, and support services helped graduates with hearing disabilities transition successfully into the workforce and how much their university experiences contributed to that achievement. There were 72 participants, including present and former Griffith University students. The bulk (70%) had attended the institution between 2000 and 2005 and were enrolled or recent graduates [23]. The study asked respondents about communication technologies used. Participants clearly said that the availability of their selected academic program was the main factor in their decision to attend the university (76%). Furthermore, 21% of respondents said that knowing about Griffith University's support services played a significant role in their decision. Peer note-taking was most frequently used (65%), followed by laptop computer note-taking (19%). 35% of the students with hearing disabilities reported using technology and communication aids, such as hearing aids, Frequency Modulation (FM) devices, web services, e-mail, and short message service, while 36% of these students used interpreters. Overall, the students with hearing disabilities enrolling at this university demonstrated significant and successful engagement in their academic, social, and professional endeavors [23].

3.7 New Zealand

According to Hyde et al., the transition process for students with hearing disabilities in New Zealand has only ever been investigated in the study of Powell, which was carried out in (2011). According to the study's findings on transition, New Zealand students' learning and participation experiences when they started postsecondary study were significantly influenced by their level of understanding of their own learning needs, and familiarity with the variety of resources available, including ICT [23, 42]. Moreover, the problems it revealed are still relevant today. Since the study, neither the delivery of support services nor the use of and expertise with various technological aids has changed. For students with hearing disabilities in New Zealand, there is still no planning available for the transition of these students to higher education [23]. Consequently, any progress toward inclusive education at the postsecondary level for students with hearing disabilities must be on par with hearing students. Additionally, there must be a greater understanding of the academic and technology needs of students with hearing disabilities before they move from compulsory education to higher education. Also, there must be decisions about providing supportive technology services to these students before enrolling in higher education [23].

3.8 South Africa

In South Africa, there are some higher education institutions which accept students with hearing disabilities but do not offer necessary academic support or inclusive curriculum. According to Bell and Swart, students with hearing disabilities are getting more access to higher education, but they are still underrepresented and receive inadequate support, which frequently leads to subpar academic results. Both in established and developing countries, including South Africa, students with hearing disabilities are still underrepresented in higher education [43]. In addition, very little study has been done in South Africa on the teaching and learning requirements of these students in higher education or on the services and techniques they need to succeed academically. Consequently, universities are under increasing pressure to enhance the overall teaching and learning support offered to these students in order to have a beneficial impact on these students' overall academic experience and economic independence [43].

4. Discussion

In many countries, ICTs have the potential to be an effective instrument for increasing educational possibilities for students with disabilities. ICTs have generally lowered the entrance requirements for higher education. Therefore, ICT should be made available and systematically used in countries since it also improves research, teaching, and learning [44]. In order to use ICT effectively, policies must be clearly stated, operationalize specific plans for targets, and guarantee the availability of necessary resources. For instance, increases in the number of faculty members who use online reporting, and increases in the percentage of courses that incorporate ICT technologies in their design and delivery [45]. As asynchronous learning is made feasible by ICTs through online course materials, students no longer have to rely entirely on printed books and other materials for their educational needs. The Internet has made it possible for a limitless number of students to have access to a multitude of educational resources in practically every subject and across a range of media [44].

Students with hearing disabilities around the world have had the opportunity to benefit from the changes that occurred when technology was provided and used in higher education institutions [32]. Prior studies investigated how students with hearing disabilities from various parts of the world used ICT tools and resources in higher education institutions [1]. Bell and Swart, stated that although more and more students are being admitted to universities in both developed and developing countries, they are still under supported in some countries, which frequently leads to subpar academic performance [43]. Furthermore, most of the research on the academic inclusion of students with hearing disabilities in higher education has been conducted in settings with specialized support services, as the kind and scope of support services vary considerably between countries [23].

The use of facilities that are related with computers such as e-mail and the Internet is nothing new in many developed countries [16]. In contrast, there are some countries that do not provide the necessary support for students with hearing disabilities in higher education [23]. The current review of previous studies that examined the provision of ICT to students with hearing disabilities in higher education in several countries found that countries such as the US and Australia provide real-time captioning which is a speech-to-text system to help these students access information in the educational classrooms. Students with hearing disabilities use real-time captioning at universities and colleges such as NTID and Griffith University to help them get over communication obstacles caused by learning in hearing-predominant settings [24]. They also took advantage of computer and Internet technologies, web services, e-mail, and SMS to improve their achievement [16]. Another factor in improving the performance of these students in the US is the provision of C-Print system in higher education institutions for many years. Results from several previous studies showed that undergraduate students with hearing disabilities who received C-print services in their classes have benefited from these services because they got the important details of the lessons and there were also printable computer-saved copies. In contrast, the C-Print system is not available at BMSTU in Russia, but note-taking and in-class conversations have been utilized by faculty members by typing on their computers then displaying on the screen [28].

In other countries such as KSA, UAE, and Russia, ICT has been given a lot of attention. According to Al-Kharji and Cheong, the academic success of students with hearing disabilities in higher education institutions is greatly influenced by the technology because it has the potential to improve their ability to learn and raise their participation rate and performance [32]. In these countries, many technologies have been made available, the most important of which are computers, the internet, projectors, smart boards, PowerPoint, MS Word, Microsoft Team, and electronic mail systems. Classrooms are also equipped with advanced and modern technological devices in several universities such as BMSTU, KSU, and AAU [1, 16, 32]. This review also showed that in higher education institutions in Slovenia, computer graphs and spreadsheets are used in the classroom to help students with hearing disabilities, in addition to various technological devices [10, 41]. However, other countries such as New Zealand do not yet have any existing planning for student programs in higher education [23]. Although some higher education institutions in South Africa accepted students with hearing disabilities, they do not provide adequate services [43].

5. Conclusion and recommendations

Although many countries have programs for students with hearing disabilities in higher education, there are many obstacles related to the provision or use of ICT [46], which makes initiatives and studies related to the provision of ICT to these students in higher education institutions an urgent issue. Considering the previous literature review, a number of recommendations and suggestions were proposed that may help policymakers and decision-makers in educational practices to develop higher education programs for students with hearing disabilities more effectively. These recommendations are related to plans and guidelines that must be implemented to ensure availability, quality, and effectiveness of ICT. Considering the critical role of ICT in higher education programs for students with hearing disabilities, there is a need to pay more attention to providing communication and technology systems with focus on visual learning processes in higher education institutions in several countries. This is necessary to develop the programs to cover the needs of these students and for equitable access to higher education.

In different countries, the Ministry of Education should work side by side with stakeholders specialized in higher education programs for students with hearing disabilities in order to provide ICT that is commensurate with the abilities and needs of these students. Also, the Ministry of Education should give the higher education sector the authority to develop existing programs and open more programs for these students, while making sure to provide various ICT tools that are commensurate with the needs and capabilities of these students. Moreover, a mechanism must be put in place to evaluate the performance of higher education institutions to achieve quality and efficiency regarding the provision of ICT and training in its use [32].

In addition, institutions that have programs for students with hearing disabilities must establish a support service office to provide and evaluate the ICT. The support office shall provide ICT both in lectures such as computers, Internet, real-time captioning, C-Print system, and smart boards. According to Al-Hawi, the physical environment and the halls in higher education institutions should be equipped with the latest projectors suitable for students with hearing disabilities understanding of lectures [3].

Lastly, the current review recommends the necessity of simulating international experiences in providing ICT services to these students in higher education, by making use of successful models. It is hoped that this review will inspire future researchers to look more deeply into the readiness and use of different technologies in different higher education institutions globally. In conclusion, there are similar areas that future researchers can explore and review. Also, comparative studies are needed to compare the use of assistive technology in higher education programs for students with hearing disabilities in different countries.

Author details

Manal Alkharji
Princess Nourah Bint Abdulrahman University, Riyadh, Saudi Arabia

*Address all correspondence to: manal-alkharji@hotmail.com

References

[1] Kaba A, Ellala Z. Exploring the use of educational technology among deaf students in the United Arab Emirates. Universal Journal of Educational Research. 2020;**10**:4845-4852. DOI: 10.13189/ujer.2020.081056

[2] United Nations. Information and Communication Technology (ICT) and Disability: Toolkit on Disability for AFRICA [Internet]. 2016. Available from: https://www.un.org/development/desa/dspd/2016/11/toolkit-on-disability-for-africa-2/

[3] Al-Hawi M. The reality of using information and communication technology by teaching staff members and support staff in higher education program for deaf and hard of hearing-impaired persons at King Saud University. The Arabian Gulf Message. 2015;**37**:75-97. DOI: 10.35270/0011-037-139-004

[4] Zirzow N. Technology use by teachers of deaf and hard-of-hearing students [dissertation]. USA: West Virginia University; 2019

[5] Al-Salamah A. Using captioning services with deaf and hard of hearing students in higher education: A systematic review. American Annals of the Deaf. 2020;**165**:114-127. DOI: 10.1353/aad.2020.0012

[6] Taiwo S, Taiwo O. The effects of interactive whiteboard on the academic performance of deaf students in Federal College of Education (special), Oyo, Nigeria. EPiC Series in Education Science. 2020;**3**:234-240. DOI: 10.29007/q8fm

[7] Puspawati I, Juharoh R. Motivations and challenges on the use of ICT for teaching special needs students. In: 4th International Conference on Sustainable Innovation 2020–Social, Humanity, and Education. Indonesia: Atlantis Press; 2021. pp. 239-246

[8] Adebayo L. The Importance of ICT on the Academic Performance of Students with Hearing Impaired [Internet]. 2020. Available from: https://www.academia.edu/17606563/the_importance_of_ict_on_the_academic_performance_of_students_with_hearing_impaired

[9] Sallai G. Defining info communications and related terms. Acta Polytechnical Hungarian. 2012;**9**:5-15. DOI: 10.12700/APH.9.6.2012.6.1

[10] Kožuh I, Časar T, Zakošek A, Voglar T, Pučko M, Katarina N, et al. Smart Solutions for the Inclusion of Students with Disabilities in Higher Education. Slovenia: SSSD-HE; 2021

[11] Stinson M, Stevenson S. Effects of expanded and standard captions on deaf college students' comprehension of educational videos. American Annals of the Deaf. 2013;**158**:455-467. DOI: 10.1353/aad.2013.0033

[12] Peng C, Daud S. TPACK: A missing piece of the technology puzzle among special education (hearing impairment) teachers. In: Conference: Graduate Research in Education Seminar-GREDuc. Malaysia: University Putra Malaysia; 2015. pp. 54-62

[13] Nordin N, Yunis M, Zaharudin R, Salehi H, Mohd Yasin M, Embi M. Identifying the challenges and barriers hearing-impaired learners face with using ICT education courses. Journal of Theoretical & Applied Information Technology. 2015;**78**:327-335. DOI: 10.5901/mjss.2015.v6n4s1p248

[14] Nikolaraizi M, Vekiri I, Easterbrooks S. Investigating deaf students' use of visual multimedia resources in reading comprehension. American Annals of the Deaf. 2013;**157**:458-474. DOI: 10.1353/aad.2013.0007

[15] Watkins A, Tokareva N, Turner M. ICTs in Education for People with Disabilities. Moscow: UNESCO Institute for Information Technologies in Education; 2012

[16] Kirsanova G, Troufanova N, Inozemtseva K. A case study of using information technology teaching English to deaf and hard-of-hearing students at Bauman Moscow State Technical University (BMSTU). In: ICERI2018 Proceedings. Russia: IATED; 2018. pp. 6608-6613. DOI: 10.21125/iceri.2018.2547

[17] Altan T. The quest of TPACK in special education: The many faces of TPACK/special education teacher education. Wikibooks, The Free Textbook Project. 2013;**36**:90-98

[18] Lartz M, Stoner J, Stout L. Perspectives of assistive technology from deaf students at a hearing University. Assistive Technology Outcomes and Benefits. 2008;**5**:72-91. Available from: Eric.ed.gov/?id=EJ884369

[19] Chong A, Shaffe M. Exploring elementary special education (hearing impairment) teachers' technological pedagogical content knowledge (TPACK). In: 1st International Conference on Special Education. Thailand: SEAMEO; 2015. pp. 566-577

[20] Marinagi C, Skourlas C, Tsolakidis A. Information technology literacy for deaf and hard of hearing students in higher education. In: Strategic Innovative Marketing. Cham: Springer; 2017. pp. 697-703. DOI: 10.1007/978-3-319-33865-1_85

[21] Al-Rayes T. Rehabilitation of deaf and hard of hearing students for higher education: Why? How? The Sixth International Conference—Rehabilitation of People with Special Needs: Monitoring Reality and Sharing the Future. 2008;**2**:1126-1137. Available from: http://search.shamaa.org/FullRecord?ID=43968

[22] Stinson M, Elliot L, Kelly R. Deaf and hard-of-hearing high school and college students' perceptions of speech-to-text and interpreting/note taking services and motivation. Journal of Developmental and Physical Disabilities. 2017;**29**:131-152. DOI: 10.1007/s10882-017-9534-4

[23] Hyde M, Nikolaraizi M, Powell D, Stinson M. Critical factors toward the inclusion of deaf and hard-of hearing students in higher education. In: Marschark M, Lampropoulou V, Skordilis E, editors. Diversity in Deaf Education. USA: Oxford University Press; 2016. pp. 441-471. DOI: 10.1093/acprof: oso/9780190493073.003.0016

[24] Jolly A, Macfarlane C, Barker B. Deaf/hard of hearing students' experiences with higher education's real-time captioning services [dissertation]. USA: Utah State University; 2023. DOI: 10.31219/osf.io/8e74p

[25] Stinson M, Stinson S, Elliot L, Kelly R. Relationships between benefit and use of a speech-to-text service, perceptions of courses, and course performance. In: Annual Meeting of the American Educational Research Association; 2004; San Diego. CA. pp. 1-23

[26] Hastings D, Brecklein K, Cermak S, Reynolds R, Rosen H, Wilson J. Notetaking for Deaf and Hard of Hearing

Students. A Report of the National Task Force on Quality of Services in the Postsecondary Education of Deaf and Hard of Hearing Students. NY: Northeast Technical Assistance Center; 1997

[27] Kawas S, Karalis G, Wen T, Ladner R. Improving real-time captioning experiences for deaf and hard of hearing students. In: Proceedings of the 18th International ACM Sgaccess Conference on Computers and Accessibility. Nevada, USA: ACM; 2016. pp. 15-A23. DOI: 10.1145/2982142.2982164

[28] Everhart V, Stinson M, Mckee B, Giles P. Evaluation of a speech-to-print transcription system as a resource for mainstreamed deaf students. In: The Annual Meeting of the American Educational Research Association. 1996. pp. 1-24. Available from: Eric.ed.gov/?id=ED395407

[29] Braun D, Clark M, Marchut A, Solomon C, Majocha M, Davenport Z, et al. Welcoming deaf students into STEM: Recommendations for university science education. CBE—Life Sciences Education. 2018;**17**:1-8. DOI: 10.1187/cbe.17-05-0081

[30] Elliot L, Stinson M, McKee B, Everhart V, Francis P. College student's perceptions of the C-print speech-to-text transcription system. Journal of Deaf Studies and Deaf Education. 2001;**6**:285-298. DOI: 10.1093/deafed/6.4.285

[31] Gallaudet Research Institute. Regional and National Summary Report of Data from the 2006-2007 Annual Survey of Deaf and Hard of Hearing Children and Youth. Washington, DC: GRI Gallaudet University; 2007

[32] Al-Kharji M, Cheong L. Moderating role of hearing status on the relationship between technological factors and the academic achievement of deaf and hard of hearing students in Saudi universities. Journal of Special Needs Education. 2021;**11**:51-67

[33] Ministry of Education. University Statistics: List of Public and Privet Universities. University Education in the Kingdom of Saudi Arabia [Internet]; 2019. Available from: https://www.moe.gov.sa

[34] Salem S. The reality of students with hearing impairment using educational technologies in light of some variables in the stage of higher education. Journal of Special Education and Rehabilitation. 2017;**5**:66-113. DOI: 10.12816/0040297

[35] Al-Asim K. Reading development of students who are deaf and hard of hearing in inclusive education classrooms. Education Science. 2019;**9**:1-14. DOI: 10.3390/educsci9030201

[36] Al-Ghawi M. Gifted education in the United Arab Emirates. Cogent Education. 2017;**4**:1-18. DOI: 10.1080/2331186X.2017.1368891

[37] Wauters L, Dirks E. Interactive reading with young deaf and hardof-hearing children in ebooks versus print books. Journal of Deaf Studies and Deaf Education. 2017;**22**:243-252. DOI: 10.1093/deafed/enw097

[38] International Telecommunication Union. ICT Accessibility Assessment for the Europe Region. ITU: Publications International Telecommunication Union Europe; 2021. Available from: https://www.itu.int/en/ITU-D/Regional-Presence/Europe/Documents/Events/2020/AE20/event/D-PHCB-ICT_ACCESS_EUR.01-2021-PDF-E.pdf [Accessed: June 18, 2023]

[39] Health Europa. Deafness: Communication and Policy in Europe.

Available from: https://www.healtheuropa.com/deafness-communication-and-policy-in-europe/106343/. [Accessed: June 20, 2023]

[40] Tabaj A, Rebernik N, Kacic M, Debevc M, Dolinšek T, Brecelj V. Information and Communication Technology for the Disabled in the Job Rehabilitation Process. Ljubljana, URI: Occupational Rehabilitation Development Center; 2011

[41] Zaharudin R, Nordin N, Yasin M, Din R, Embi M. Exploring teachers' insight on ICT education via e-learning for the deaf learners. In: Proc. of the 10th WSEAS Int. Conf. on E-Activities. 2011. pp. 52-58

[42] Powell D. Floating in the mainstream: New Zealand deaf students learning and social participation experiences in tertiary education [dissertation]. Australia: Griffith University; 2011

[43] Bell D, Swart E. Learning experiences of students who are hard of hearing in higher education: Case study of a south African university. Social Inclusion. 2018;**6**:137-148. DOI: 10.17645/si.v6i4.1643

[44] Sarkar S. The role of information and communication technology (ICT) in higher education for the 21st century. Science. 2012;**1**:30-41

[45] Sarvi J, Pillay H. Integrated Information and Communication Technology Strategies for Competitive Higher Education in Asia and the Pacific. Mandaluyong City, Philippines: Asian Development Bank; 2015

[46] Abdulrahman S. Obstacles to higher education for deaf and hard of hearing students: Diagnosis, suggested, solutions, and recommendations. Education Technology. Studies and Research 2017;**34**:241-258. Available from: Search.mandumah.com/Record/876017

Chapter 6

When Hearing Loss Co-Occurs with Dementia: Challenges and Opportunities in Diagnosis and Management

Emma Broome, Clare Burgon, Eithne Heffernan, Tom Dening, Sian Calvert, Saima Rajasingam and Helen Henshaw

Abstract

Both dementia and hearing loss are highly prevalent in older adults and often co-exist, increasing the complexity of diagnosis and management of both conditions. As the population ages, an increasing number of people will experience both long-term conditions. The cause of the association is unclear, although there are several commonly proposed mechanisms. Within this chapter, we explore current challenges that exist in discriminating between symptoms and complications of hearing and cognitive difficulties, and how these factors can impact the identification and management of both conditions. Management options, including the role of audiology services and care, will be presented, and explored in context. As hearing loss has been identified as a potentially modifiable risk factor for dementia, contemporary research evidence will be highlighted, including the challenges associated with research study design and interpretation. We conclude by exploring opportunities in care, research, and knowledge exchange, offering new approaches to improve the quality of life of those living with both dementia and hearing loss and those who care for them. Throughout this chapter, we provide the perspectives of individuals who have personally dealt with these conditions, as well as the viewpoints of their caregivers. This helps us connect concepts and evidence with real-life experiences.

Keywords: dementia, hearing loss, multimorbidity, audiology, interprofessional care

1. Introduction

1.1 Overview of dementia

Dementia is a clinical syndrome caused by a range of diseases of the brain. It is characterised by cognitive impairments, most typically affecting memory, and functional limitations, such that a person starts to have difficulty managing their everyday life. The most common cause of dementia is Alzheimer's disease, which accounts for

60–70% of cases; other important causes are vascular dementia, dementia with Lewy bodies and frontotemporal dementia. Dementia may also be associated with a variety of neurological disorders (e.g., Parkinson's disease) [1, 2].

Dementia is strongly associated with increasing age, and the prevalence rate of dementia rises exponentially from mid-life to above the age of 80. Nonetheless, dementia is not caused by ageing per se, as it requires some form of brain pathology before it occurs. As a result of the growing ageing global population, numbers of people with dementia are increasing and will continue to do so, especially in low- and middle-income countries. For example, the current estimated number of people with dementia in the United Kingdom (UK) is over 900,000, increasing to 1.6 million by 2050 [3], whereas globally these figures will rise from 50 million to 150 million in the same period [4].

Dementia most typically presents with memory problems, noticed either by the person themselves or by those around them, but other early symptoms may include word-finding difficulties or problems with day-to-day functioning (e.g., getting lost, inability to maintain activities, such as hobbies or attending to email). A person may become socially withdrawn or may experience changes in their mood (e.g., anxiety or depression). As dementia progresses, functional impairment may become more severe, so that help is required with personal care tasks. There may also be changes in perception and behaviour, such as hallucinations, agitation, aggression, or apathy [5]. Eventually, dementia may lead to death, often through pneumonia if the person's swallowing reflex is impaired. In the UK, most people with dementia continue to live at home, however some individuals who require additional support may transition into residential or nursing home care.

Dementia is usually diagnosed in specialist memory clinics, with a combination of clinical, cognitive, and radiological assessment (CT or MRI scans). More specialised investigations may be undertaken, e.g., other scans or tests for Alzheimer's biochemical markers in blood or cerebrospinal fluid. These are likely to become more widely used in future. There are no curative treatments for disorders like Alzheimer's disease, though recently anti-amyloid monoclonal antibodies (aducanumab and lecanemab) [6, 7] have been shown to be of some benefit. However, these treatments require hospital administration and intensive follow-up, so are unlikely to be in general use, without massive increases in resources. Otherwise, treatment and care is supportive, including cholinesterase inhibitors (e.g. donepezil), treatment of other symptoms like depression, and provision of supportive social care, including activities and carer support.

Where cognitive decline is present but not sufficient to impact everyday life, this is referred to as 'mild cognitive impairment (MCI)', which can be a precursor to dementia, but does not always lead to dementia. The focus of this chapter is dementia, though some of the literature cited and recommendations provided may also apply to MCI.

1.2 Overview of hearing loss, cognitive impairment, and dementia

Hearing loss increases in both prevalence and severity with age. However, it is not necessarily an inevitable accompaniment of ageing, with many lifestyle factors contributing to its' development [8]. There is a greater prevalence of cognitive impairment, such as dementia and cognitive decline, in people with hearing loss, compared to those without hearing loss [9, 10], with one study finding the majority of people attending a memory clinic for concerns related to dementia were experiencing hearing loss [11].

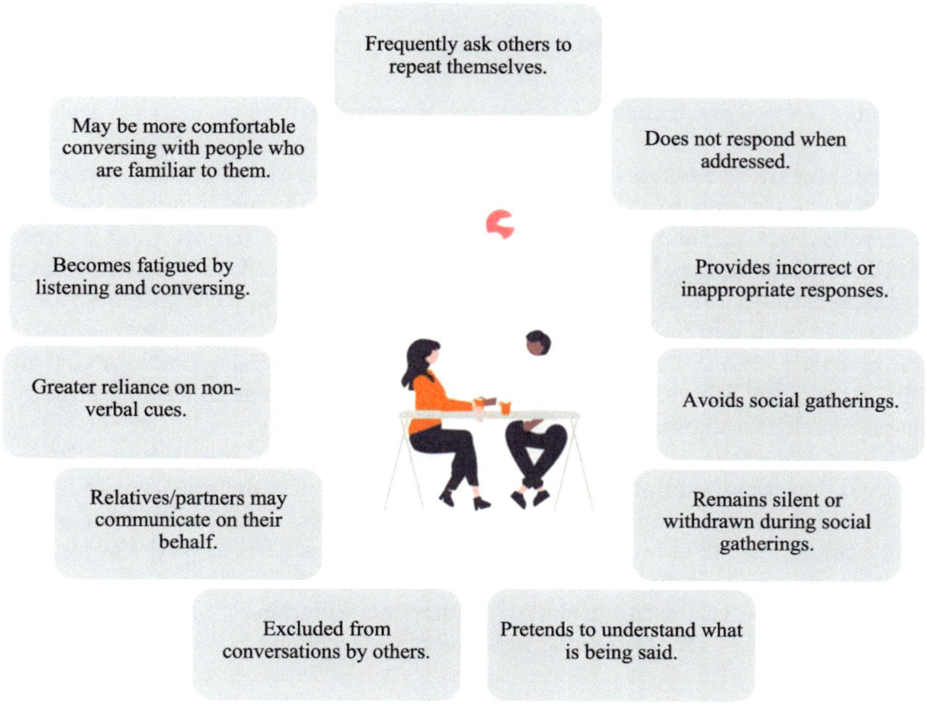

Figure 1.
Social interaction difficulties common to hearing loss and dementia.

Although a key symptom, and perhaps the most recognisable one of dementia, is memory loss, some symptoms of dementia may also be indicative of hearing loss. For example, in dementia, difficulty following conversations and needing others to repeat information is common; understanding speech may be impaired over and above any difficulties in understanding written words [12]. Similarly, key features of gradual hearing loss include difficulty following conversation in noisy environments and asking people to repeat what they said [13]. Difficulties with social interaction are common across both dementia and hearing loss (See **Figure 1**) [14–16]. In people with dementia, family members and carers may misinterpret these difficulties, attributing them solely to dementia rather than a potentially correctable hearing problem [17, 18]. Therefore, people living with hearing loss and people living with dementia may experience similar challenges, making it difficult to tell which is the cause, especially in those who live with both conditions.

Both hearing loss and dementia are associated with increased risks of the same negative outcomes or symptoms and have shared risk factors [16]. For example, they are both associated with increased frailty [19, 20]; falls [21, 22]; depression [23, 24]; social withdrawal [25, 26]; and a reduction in quality of life [27, 28]. Dementia and hearing loss can both lead to third party disability, in which the individuals' relatives or carers are also negatively affected, for example, through having to take time to support the individual, repeat things, and experience difficulties dealing with their loved ones' denial, resulting in greater burden, and reduced socialising and quality of life [29, 30]. Hearing loss may also exacerbate the behavioural and psychological symptoms associated with dementia [12], such as depression, agitation, confusion, and withdrawal. There is a risk of missing the impact of hearing loss on these factors, which may be erroneously attributed entirely to cognitive impairment [31, 32].

1.3 What mechanisms link hearing loss and dementia?

It is important to ask *how* hearing conditions contribute to cognitive impairment and dementia, not only to allow better understanding of the mechanisms at work but also to consider what therapeutic means may be useful. It is also important to consider the intimate linkage between the ear at the periphery and the central auditory processing activities of the brain. As ear and brain are linked by complex auditory pathways, they should be regarded as a whole system and not as separate entities [33]. It is noteworthy that the medial temporal lobe is a crucial meeting place for central auditory processes but also an area of the brain vulnerable to neurodegenerative processes such as Alzheimer's disease [34].

There are several hypotheses linking hearing and cognitive impairment. The first of these is that impaired hearing leads to increased cognitive demand, which is the degree of brain activity required to process cognitive tasks, such as following other people's voices [35]. In short, if you cannot hear, your brain has to work harder all the time. The effort to hear diverts processing power from other areas of activity, such as memory [36]. Eventually, this leads to a permanent depletion of cognitive reserves, though the hypothesis is perhaps vague on what the brain mechanisms underlying this may be.

The second hypothesis is that cognitive impairment results from sensory deprivation. A person with hearing loss may fail to detect auditory stimuli or else receive them in degraded form (if you cannot hear, you miss much information in your environment). This idea emphasises the impoverished auditory input rather than the increased auditory effort in the first hypothesis. It is suggested that this leads to permanent changes in brain structure and function in the auditory cortex and related brain areas, such as the hippocampus [34].

The third hypothesis suggests that there may be common cause of neurodegeneration in brain and auditory pathways. This may be the result of an underlying pathological process, for example vascular or Alzheimer's disease [37], that can affect brain areas involved in cognition and auditory processing as well as peripheral structures such as the cochlea.

The fourth hypothesis emphasises the importance of central auditory function. Central auditory dysfunction, or central auditory processing disorder, is the result of changes in the auditory processing network, which in turn lead to impaired auditory perception and speech communication [38]. It may affect around 15% of older people with acquitted hearing loss [39] and affected individuals show markedly poor perception of speech-in-noise relative to their performance on pure tone audiometry. Central auditory dysfunction may result from brain pathology, such as amyloid and tau, typical of Alzheimer's disease. People with Alzheimer's disease show evidence of central auditory dysfunction, and this may be present for several years before diagnosis [40].

The fifth hypothesis relates to social isolation and withdrawal (which can result from either hearing loss or cognitive changes but is exacerbated by the two occurring together). Social isolation is in itself a risk factor for dementia [4], which may result from the effects of decreased cognition activity and/or the effects of physical problems associated with isolation, such as heart disease and depression.

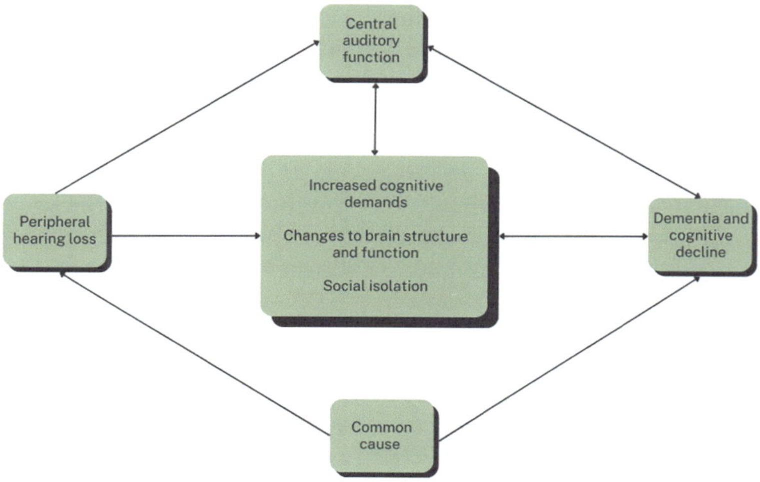

Figure 2.
Proposed framework: How hearing loss relates to dementia and cognitive decline. Adapted from [41]. This diagram offers a potential framework for understanding the connections between peripheral hearing loss and dementia/cognitive decline. The central box shows hypothesised causal pathways. A common cause (e.g., systemic vascular disease or genetic factors) may also lead to both peripheral hearing loss and dementia/cognitive decline. In addition, central auditory function may feature as a result of direct and indirect effects from the causal pathways and could serve as a marker of dementia/cognitive decline. One or more of the pathways shown may explain the association between peripheral hearing loss and dementia/cognitive decline.

It is of course conceivable that more than one mechanism may operate, or different individuals will be affected in diverse ways. These hypotheses are relevant to how hearing interventions might work. For example, it might be expected that hearing loss intervention (hearing aids or cochlear implants) would be effective against cognitive load or social withdrawal, but not against central auditory dysfunction (**Figure 2**).

2. Diagnosis

2.1 Identification of dementia and hearing loss

2.1.1 Timely diagnosis of dementia and hearing loss

Timely diagnosis of dementia and of hearing loss is important, as this enables access to information and support at the right time so that the affected individual can access suitable treatments as early as possible [42, 43]. This is particularly important as some treatments may be more effective at earlier stages, for example, non-pharmacological therapies such as cognitive stimulation therapy for dementia [44]. Hearing loss in mid-life is associated with increased risk of dementia, accounting for ~8% of all cases [4]. Whilst people with unaddressed hearing loss are at greater risk of dementia (estimated at 2x, 3x and 5x the risk for those with untreated mild, moderate, and severe hearing loss respectively) [45], those who use hearing devices may not be. Providing hearing aids or cochlear implants as early as possible could potentially help delay or reduce dementia risk [46] and might even lead to improved cognitive performance in the short-term [47]. Additionally, diagnosis enables both the individual and their family and friends to gain an explanation and understanding of what is happening, resulting in emotional and social benefits, which could result in cost savings for individuals and governments [48, 49].

Without routine screening for dementia and hearing loss in the populations at risk, timely diagnosis relies on individuals identifying symptoms and then accessing healthcare services for support. However, evidence shows that people delay seeking diagnosis or support for both dementia and hearing loss. One longitudinal study found that there was an average delay of almost nine years between an individual becoming eligible for a hearing aid (as confirmed via audiometric testing) and adopting hearing aids [50]. Delays in help-seeking are also present in people with dementia, with one in four people in the UK waiting over two years since symptoms were first experienced to seek a diagnosis from a healthcare professional [51]. This finding is consistent across Europe, where there is, on average, a gap of over a two-years between symptoms first being noticed and receiving a formal diagnosis, with almost half of carers wishing this diagnosis had been made sooner [52]. Help-seeking inequalities exist across people with dementia and hearing loss. For example, people from minority ethnic backgrounds are at greater risk of delay in seeking diagnosis for cognitive impairment [53] and treatment for hearing loss [50].

2.1.2 Seeking diagnosis

Potential reasons why individuals delay seeking a diagnosis of hearing loss and dementia are multifaceted. As age-related hearing loss occurs gradually, individuals may not initially realise that it is affecting them. People with dementia may lack insight into their own cognitive difficulties. In both cases, diagnosis may rely others to point out the problem, and require the individual to have the willingness and ability to respond to this concern [54, 55]. Furthermore, both hearing loss and dementia continue to carry stigma, which may affect help-seeking [49, 56]. For people seeking help for memory problems, there may be concerns about how a diagnosis might change their relationships and cause others to worry or treat them differently [56]. Perceptions about inaccessibility or unaffordability of services (particularly in countries without free healthcare) can significantly contribute to delayed help-seeking [57]. Having a rarer type of dementia is associated with an increased delay in help-seeking. A lack of awareness and misconceptions, such as a belief that symptoms are a normal part of ageing and that there is nothing to be done, are commonly cited reasons for not seeking help sooner [51, 52, 57]. Reasons for delayed help-seeking for hearing loss may overlap with that for dementia, such as beliefs around the limited benefits of intervention, though evidence is conflicting and sparse, with less research investigating reasons for delaying help-seeking itself, as the majority of studies focus on the uptake of hearing aids [58].

> *"What you've got here really is a... double whammy in that there's so much negativity around... hearing loss in general that it's... seen still as a kind of a weakness. People don't think twice about wearing glasses now, but they would think twice about wearing hearing aids... You almost [need to get] over that... negativity about hearing loss before you can even deal with... the cognitive... loss as well, so I can see why people will just kind of run away screaming from... the idea of either of them."*
>
> *59-year-old woman with hearing loss and tinnitus*
> *(Broome et al., [59], page 8)*

Fear of stigma, alternative beliefs about aetiology, lack of trust in health care systems due to discrimination and injustices, and lack of culturally appropriate care may also contribute to disproportionate reluctance to seek help in people from minority ethnic backgrounds [60, 61]. Similarly, previous research has shown that LGBTQ+ carers may avoid seeking help due to concerns about discrimination [62]. Less is known about reasons for delayed help-seeking for hearing loss in underserved groups, though one study of paediatric services similarly identified stigma and additionally identified a disparity in expectations of treatment based on experiences from their home country as barriers to help-seeking [63].

2.1.3 Public awareness of dementia and hearing loss

Both dementia and hearing loss can be 'hidden' conditions, meaning that they are not always recognised, understood, or accommodated for by communities and groups that are unaware of their presence. Given the reliance on individuals seeking help for symptoms of dementia and hearing loss, it is important to educate and raise awareness of these conditions and educate members of the public so that they are empowered to seek help [49]. For example, dispelling myths about dementia may include education around memory loss not being the only symptom, and both symptoms of dementia and hearing loss not being a normal part of ageing, but something that people can and should seek support for. Education about dementia and hearing loss should also include information about where to seek help, ensuring the recommended services are accessible. However, it may be important to additionally educate members of the public and clinicians about the link between dementia and hearing loss, how the two may mask one another, and how preventing or managing hearing loss may help reduce dementia.

> *"I never, ever... thought that hearing loss would be associated with a cognitive impairment... People should be made more aware of that rather than wait until it's too late and by the time you actually get a.. . diagnosis, you may well be in the stages where you're not aware enough to actually do anything about it."*
>
> *72-year-old man with tinnitus*
> *(Broome et al., [59], page 6)*

2.1.4 Challenges in diagnosis

In addition to being a barrier for the identification of dementia and/or hearing loss by individuals or their carers, common or overlapping symptoms can also impede the help-seeking process. For example, when individuals do decide to seek help for their symptoms, receiving a diagnosis for hearing loss and/or dementia may be more difficult when the two conditions co-occur.

Most primary care providers (such as family doctors) assess patients for cognitive impairment if the patient or family report symptoms. If the assessment indicates a problem, they will refer the patient to see a specialist. However, sometimes family doctors report choosing not to assess patients for cognitive problems due to concerns about the impact of a diagnosis on the patient, or concerns about limited treatment options [48]. Furthermore, as many as one in five people who express concerns about hearing loss to their primary care provider do not receive a referral for further assessment [64]. Sometimes, providers might have insufficient knowledge about hearing loss, which can lead to them to normalise or minimise its importance and impact, particularly when hearing loss is 'mild,' or to assume that it cannot be effectively treated [54, 64].

> *"My hearing [loss] results in a lot of information in conversations being incomplete and or inaccurate as I rebuild and guess at missing words. So poor memory can be seen as the issue where my memory is ok but the original information, I heard is inaccurate. Someone not recognizing this could make incorrect assumptions resulting in a poor and misleading diagnosis."*
>
> *67-year-old man with hearing loss*
> *(Broome et al., [59], page 8.)*

Even when referral to secondary care for further assessment is achieved, making a diagnosis of both hearing loss and dementia is further complicated by the overlap in symptoms. Hearing loss may be misdiagnosed as cognitive impairment or dementia [16, 31], and conversely cognitive impairment may first be diagnosed or dismissed as hearing loss.

Cognitive testing (both simple screening tests and more comprehensive cognitive assessments) for dementia typically relies on normal hearing, using verbal instructions and tasks. There is a growing body of literature that highlights how cognition may be underestimated if sensory impairments are not considered [65, 66]. Evidence suggests that people with hearing loss tend to perform worse than individuals with normal hearing on cognitive tests which are verbally administered [67]. Individuals with unidentified hearing loss (and even those with known hearing loss where adjustments are not made) may mis-hear key information and must work cognitively harder to understand what is required, leading to them scoring worse on cognitive assessments, and possibly being mis-diagnosed with cognitive impairment [16, 36].

Attempts have been made to adapt cognitive tests to account for sensory impairment. For example, adaptions to the Mini Mental State Examination (MMSE, a popular screening tool for cognitive impairment) include administering screening questions on written flashcards [68] or excluding three verbally administered items [69]. Data from studies evaluating these adaptations suggest that they may be acceptable for people with hearing loss, though no improvement in performance occurred. Research has also been conducted to evaluate modifications to another popular screening tool, the Montreal Cognitive Assessment (MoCA). A visual version of the MoCA, developed by Dupuis et al., [65] which removed auditory items from the standard MOCA, demonstrated a higher pass rate in comparison to the standard MoCA. Finally, Dawes et al., [70] developed a validated, sensitive, and reliable version of the MoCA-H to identify dementia in adults with hearing loss. However, whilst scoring adjustments are advised for those with lower education (12 years or less), it is not clear how it performs in those with poor literacy or dyslexia, and it is not suitable for those with dual sensory loss [70]. There remains a need for standardised diagnostic tests which are reliable and valid in these populations to detect and monitor cognitive function.

The diagnosis of hearing loss in adults with MCI/dementia can represent a significant challenge for audiology services, though some recommendations have been developed (see **Box 1**). First, audiologists are advised to consider that patients may have dementia even if it is not mentioned in their referral letter, particularly because many do not receive an 'official' diagnosis of dementia [71]. People living with dementia have varied needs, and an individualised approach to audiological assessment is recommended [71, 72]. This could entail testing in a familiar environment, such as the patient's residence, and involving carers/family in the assessment [71–73]. Whilst some people living with dementia can complete standard behavioural assessments (e.g., pure-tone audiometry, speech audiometry), others will require adaptations, such as reducing or increasing test duration, providing breaks, accepting responses other than button presses (e.g., verbal responses), and repeating the instructions throughout [71, 73]. The use of objective tests, including otoacoustic emissions or auditory evoked potentials (AEPs), is recommended in cases where behavioural tests are not possible [71]. The use of objective assessments is not without challenges; capacity to consent may be difficult to establish and the accuracy of cortical evoked potentials can be affected by level of alertness requiring observation by someone who knows the patient well and electrophysiological tests must be considered within the context of information from the patient and any other available test data [74]. If behavioural and objective testing are not possible, audiologists could review previous audiometric results, where available, and carry out a functional assessment with the patient and/or their relative carer to determine their communication abilities and needs and their potential to benefit from an audiological intervention [71].

2.2 A role for audiologists in screening cognition?

Understanding the extent of both hearing and cognitive factors is essential in developing an appropriate treatment plan [75]. Cognitive screening, through formal testing and hearing professionals asking relevant questions around cognitive status has been recommended as a useful tool in adult audiology clinics to aid in the detection of cognitive impairment, longer-term care planning and the programming of hearing aid devices [73]. This could help ensure more timely diagnosis of dementia, and also help highlight and reduce any issues with undetected cognitive impairment interfering with hearing assessment and treatment. However, consideration should also be given to the practical implementation of cognitive screening, including whether this would be acceptable to and feasible for both patients and audiologists. The need for training and appropriate questioning or use of screening tools is particularly important in this context as the provision of cognitive assessment (including history taking) currently sits outside of the scope of practice for audiology professionals.

> *"Since I was carer for my mother who had Alzheimer's, I would be only too pleased to be assessed because the earlier the treatment the better if any is needed."*
> *72-year-old woman with hearing loss*
> *(Broome et al., [59], page 6.)*
> *"Only if the audiologist had been suitably trained in dealing with a very sensitive topic."*
>
> *75-year-old woman with hearing loss*
> *(Broome et al., [59], page 8.)*

Recent qualitative research has suggested that patients perceive cognitive screening to be acceptable within adult audiology services [59]. However, the successful delivery of cognitive screening in adult audiology services relies upon audiologists being sufficiently trained and feeling comfortable enough to deliver and discuss such tests with a patient. Yet, a survey of hearing professionals in the United Kingdom on managing sensory and cognitive impairment in older adults highlighted limited awareness of cognitive screening tests and a lack of adequate training [76]. This clearly impacts practice as, in another UK survey, although 90% of audiologists reported a willingness to conduct cognitive assessments only 4% did so, due to lack of training, time and resources [77]. Furthermore, as discussed previously, despite attempts to make screening tools suitable for people with hearing loss, there is still a lack of valid and reliable tests that can reduce the impact of hearing loss on cognitive screening which can be implemented in hearing clinics [78]. Ultimately, cognitive screening tests only demonstrate a snapshot view into an individual's cognitive ability at the time of administration. Thus, the results may be unreliable, particularly in populations who live with sensory impairment. There are other attributes which may impact testing scores such as level of education, age of patient and mood which should be taken into account.

There remains a clear need for recommendations around direct referral pathways, (mentioned briefly by Littlejohn et al., [73]), particularly criteria for onward referral of patients from audiology to memory care services. Implementing cognitive screening within adult audiology services is one step towards addressing the challenge of an ageing population living with comorbid disorders. However, this application requires careful consideration into the management and training within clinical settings, and may be better addressed through building links between audiology and memory services. Guidance on facilitating early detection and access to memory services is essential to support audiology professionals and patients with suspected MCI/dementia.

2.3 A role for memory services in screening hearing?

Currently NICE [79] guidance recommends a referral to a memory clinic for suspected dementia, after an investigation of reversible causes of cognitive decline, including delirium, depression, and sensory impairment. It is unclear if hearing loss is investigated in all referrals to memory clinics, and in view of the evidence that adults with hearing loss often (i) do not acknowledge hearing loss and (ii) do not disclose hearing difficulties to their primary care provider [64], it is highly likely that many are not referred for audiological assessment. Once the patient is referred to a memory clinic, it is unlikely that they will receive a hearing assessment, as evidenced in a survey of professionals working in the UK National Health Service (NHS) memory services, in which only 4% reported performing hearing assessments within the clinic [77]. To address this gap, some NHS audiology services in England and Wales are piloting hearing assessments as a part of the memory clinic pathway. Initial findings indicate that service users who receive an audiological assessment as part of this pathway consider it a valuable part of their cognitive assessment, but also suggest that they may need additional information provision and follow-up appointments to maximise uptake and use of hearing aids [80].

3. Management of hearing loss

3.1 Improving care for people living with co-existing dementia and hearing loss

There has been much recent attention on understanding the link between hearing loss and dementia risk [4, 16]. A growing ageing population means that the prevalence of people living with chronic conditions is increasing, leading to an imbalance between conditions and care [81]. While prevention (or risk-reduction) efforts are crucial, they alone are insufficient to address the pressing needs of individuals currently living with co-existing dementia and hearing loss and who urgently require appropriate and ongoing support. There is no standard system of care for people living with these long-term co-occurring conditions, and the co-existence of these conditions presents unique challenges in terms of management in health and social care settings [16, 72, 82]. To enhance the care and support rendered to individuals currently living with both dementia and hearing loss and their caregivers, as well as those who will go on to live with these conditions in the future, it is imperative that we draw from and build on existing research knowledge. This will enable us to better understand the complex interplay between dementia and hearing loss, identify effective interventions, and develop and implement comprehensive care frameworks.

3.2 Health and care services for adults with hearing loss and dementia

3.2.1 Audiology services for adults with dementia

Despite an awareness of associations between dementia and hearing loss, and the potential for hearing interventions to reduce the risk of dementia and improve outcomes in patients living with both conditions, there is limited peer-reviewed evidence around effective audiological practice for people living with, or at risk of, dementia. Furthermore, although a range of interventions for people living with dementia have been developed, many of them are auditory in nature and little is known about their effectiveness specifically in people who also live with hearing loss, despite the high prevalence of this co-morbidity. This is especially important to establish for the numerous dementia interventions that rely on hearing, such as music therapy, dance therapy, drama therapy/storytelling, reminiscence therapy, counselling, and peer support groups [83].

Work has commenced on the development of practice recommendations and models of care for co-existing dementia and hearing loss (See **Box 1**) [71–73]. Littlejohn and colleagues [73] developed International Practice Recommendations for the Recognition and Management of Hearing and Vision Impairment in People with Dementia using consensus methods with key stakeholders (including professionals and lay experts). They outlined recommendations according to six domains: awareness and knowledge, recognition and detection, evaluation, management, support, and services and policies. Those recommendations specific to the management of hearing loss in adults with MCI/dementia included advance provision of information about the appointment, adjusting appointment lengths and allowing for breaks, offering domiciliary appointments where appropriate, and including caregivers/family members in the appointment, such as by providing them with written instructions on hearing aid care and troubleshooting [73].

Dawes and colleagues [70] applied [70] Brooker and Latham's VIPS model of person-centered dementia care to hearing healthcare for people living with co-existing dementia and hearing loss. The key components of the VIPS model are (i) *valuing* people with dementia and those who care for them (e.g., ensuring audiology services are accessible to all, provide dementia training to staff) (ii) seeing the *individuality* of people living with dementia (e.g., develop an understanding of the individual to build trust and rapport, use preferred communication methods,), (iii) viewing the world from the *perspective* of the person (e.g., understand they may find hearing assessments intimidating or confusing, observe their non-verbal

Prior to appointments

- Ensure the individual can be seen by an appropriately trained clinician.
- Consider appointments early in the day.
- Make contact after referral and ask about needs (communication/informational needs/format of information/accessibility/environment).
- Provide details about when and where the appointment will take place.
- Provide details about who the appointment will be with and what will happen.
- A recommendation that the individual is accompanied by a partner/spouse, family member or friend can be useful for both the individual and the clinician.
- Consider if there are any outcomes you can send in advance of the appointment for extended consideration (e.g., history taking).

During appointments

- Address the patient directly and assume capacity to consent, unless it has been confirmed otherwise.
- Consider whether a home visit is preferable and feasible.
- Keep the partner/spouse, family/friend visible.
- Keep instructions short and clear, check for understanding.
- Be prepared to vary the length of the appointment as necessary. Allow for breaks.
- Adapt testing – response modes – and hearing aid fitting. This may be easier with two clinicians present to support with the detection of response.
- Gather most important information first.
- Consider slowing the pace of stimuli presentation, collecting fewer thresholds and/or automated tests of hearing thresholds.
- Consider using pulsed tones rather than pure tones to assist with alertness and orientation.
- Where standard behavioural hearing assessment is unsuccessful, consider functional or objective tests.
- Involve the partner/spouse, family/friend where necessary to support effective hearing diagnosis and treatment options.
- Do not rule out hearing aid technology or features for people with dementia – Consider on an individual basis. However, hearing aids might not be suitable for all.
- Provide written instructions on hearing aid care and troubleshooting that can be shared with others.

Aftercare

- Consider whether a home visit is preferable and feasible.
- Offer regular follow-up hearing assessments as part of a long-term care plan.
- Provide scheduled rather than opt-in follow-ups, with service/maintenance of any hearing devices where possible.
- Be flexible in approach and care over time to deal with any changes in cognitive and hearing status.
- Provide flexibility in how you deal with e.g., missed appointments and lost hearing devices.

For detailed person-centered recommendations for providing hearing healthcare to people with dementia, please see Dawes et al., [71] and Littlejohn et al., [73].

Box 1.
Suggested adjustments to audiology and hearing services to benefit people with cognitive decline and dementia.

cues), and (iv) ensuring the person's *social* environment supports relationships and interactions that promote well-being (e.g., ensure they can invite a relative/carer to attend appointments, involve them in conversations even when communication is difficult) [71, 84].

The discussion of hearing services has largely been limited to evidence from high-income countries, particularly the USA and European nations, but dementia remains under-recognised, under-disclosed and undertreated in low- and middle-income countries [85], who also bear over 51% of the estimated $981 billion costs of hearing loss [86]. Addressing dementia and hearing loss jointly may require different approaches to those adopted in high income countries, and research is urgently needed to identify tailored solutions in low- and middle-income contexts.

3.2.2 Residential care for adults with hearing loss and dementia

The majority of residents in long-term care homes (LTCHs) live with hearing loss [87]. Many of these residents experience communication breakdowns with staff and fellow residents, often stemming from environmental issues (e.g., background noise, poor lighting), over which residents may have little control [88, 89]. Consequently, residents with hearing loss frequently struggle to participate in social activities and group conversations, which can lead them to become isolated through exclusion or withdrawal. These difficulties are exacerbated in residents with co-existing hearing loss and dementia [88, 90]. This is a critical concern given that most LTCH residents who live with dementia likely also live with hearing loss, particularly hearing loss that is undetected, untreated, or under-treated [91–93]. Of those who do own hearing aids, usage is often low, and the devices commonly become broken or lost [94, 95]. The impacts of hearing loss on residents living with dementia can include increased agitation and behavioural disturbances, accelerated cognitive decline, depression, greater carer burden, and reduced quality of life [16, 95, 96].

Numerous barriers impede the provision of hearing healthcare to residents in LTCHs, especially those living with dementia [88, 89]. First, residents and staff may consider hearing loss to be a normal aspect of ageing and thus do not seek to address it [89]. Staff may also mistake hearing difficulties for cognitive difficulties [17, 97]. Furthermore, hearing loss is not prioritised in many LTCHs, and its prevalence is under-estimated [89, 98]. Additionally, LTCHs tend to have poor links with audiology services and to have few on-site hearing healthcare facilities or resources (e.g., assistive listening devices, hearing-friendly rooms) [76, 88, 89]. Moreover, LTCHs rarely undertake routine hearing checks or appoint hearing healthcare champions [96, 99]. Several studies highlighted the lack of LTCH staff training in hearing device management, communication tactics, and hearing loss awareness, identification, and assessment [89, 96, 97, 99]. Finally, the provision of hearing healthcare to residents living with dementia is especially challenging and time consuming. For instance, they may not tolerate hearing aids, forget to wear them, struggle to use them, or may not understand why they should wear them [89, 96, 99].

A range of strategies for improving hearing healthcare in LTCH residents with dementia have been proposed. Staff training and behaviour change is recommended so that they can recognise hearing loss and understand its consequences, adopt tactics to enhance communication, and support the use and maintenance of hearing devices [76, 93, 97]. Environmental modification is also recommended, such as by reducing background noise, implementing quiet hours or quiet activities, and using sound-absorbing materials [88, 89, 93, 97]. In addition, shifting from task-focused to person-centred care, (e.g., personalised communication plans), and involving family members in hearing healthcare (e.g., changing hearing aid batteries, history taking, shared decisions) are advised [89, 93, 94]. Furthermore, practice guidelines for managing hearing loss in residents with dementia should be developed and implemented [76, 89]. Finally, strong leadership and institutional support are vital to improving hearing healthcare, particularly building relationships with audiology services and family physicians, implementing policy change, providing sufficient resources, and ensuring staff have the autonomy and training needed to provide empathetic, person-centred care [76, 89, 93, 97].

4. Opportunities for diagnosis and management

Delivering care to people living with dementia and hearing loss is complex. A comprehensive approach to care should therefore be adopted, encompassing timely diagnosis, appropriate treatment, and ongoing support [71, 82]. Many opportunities exist to improve the evidence-based care of those living with both dementia and hearing loss, spanning clinical practice, research, the health and care workforce, and effective sharing of knowledge.

4.1 Opportunities for health care services

Due to the high co-occurrence of hearing loss and dementia, both conditions cannot be diagnosed and managed effectively without acknowledging the potential for comorbidity [100]. Yet, clear and appropriate referral pathways between memory and audiology services are not often in place, and no standard best practice guidelines across services exist to ensure consistent care [77, 101]. Finally, clinicians often feel they do not have the right skills and knowledge to provide appropriate provision [102, 103]. Recently developed guidance supports the identification and management of hearing difficulties in people living with dementia [71, 73, 104]. However, there remain many unanswered questions about the best way to provide diagnoses and care to people living with dementia and hearing loss, both within and outside of hearing services. Additional evidence is required to inform best practice, whilst considering how interprofessional support can be adopted and streamlined to ease the burden on health and care services [103].

Because of the progressive nature of both conditions, guidelines for the management of hearing loss health and social care settings should include tailored training, flexibility to deal with the changing needs of the population over time, clear pathways for onward referral where necessary, and practical guidance for the joining-up of general, audiological, memory and geriatric services, as appropriate [37, 71, 94, 99]. In addition, it is imperative that consideration is given to the inclusion of individuals and communities typically underserved within healthcare. These can be defined as groups of individuals with lower inclusion than would be expected from population estimates, those with high healthcare burden that is not matched by the volume of healthcare resource designed for the group, and/or groups with important differences in how they respond to or engage with healthcare interventions, compared with other groups [105]. For example, the British Deaf Association (Scotland) produced a toolkit for people who use British Sign Language (BSL) and who are living with dementia, their families, and professionals who are supporting them. The primary aim of the toolkit is to help ensure that BSL users and their families have equal access to information and services for dementia and experience fair treatment [106].

4.2 Opportunities for research

Given the suggested beneficial role for hearing devices in the reduction of risk for cognitive decline and dementia in adults with hearing loss via the UK Biobank cohort [45] and meta-analysis of published studies [47], further high-quality randomised controlled trials that seek to answer the question of whether hearing loss intervention can delay, reduce, or prevent cognitive decline or dementia are of paramount importance for researchers and clinicians. In the United States, the Ageing and Cognitive Health Evaluation in Elders (ACHIEVE) study was a randomised controlled trial designed to determine whether treating hearing loss in older adults could reduce cognitive decline that can precede dementia, compared with a health education control. Initial results showed that the hearing intervention did not reduce 3-year cognitive decline in the primary analysis of the total cohort. However, a prespecified sensitivity analysis showed that the effect differed between two different study populations that comprised the cohort, and that hearing intervention might reduce cognitive change over 3 years in populations of older adults at *increased risk* for cognitive decline [107]. The study was extended to examine longer-term outcomes.

However, trials of this nature present a number of challenges for the research community. First, withholding any hearing loss intervention from individuals identified as eligible and likely to benefit from them (e.g., to create a clinical trial control group) can be unethical if not appropriately managed and addressed. Linked to this, those in the control group who decide to obtain hearing intervention during the study period may need to leave the study [107]. Third, individuals who may benefit most from the intervention (i.e., for ACHIEVE, those at greater risk of cognitive decline and dementia) may not be the same individuals who volunteer take part in health research through standard recruitment routes. Finally, although a key goal for research in the field is to understand how hearing loss relates to dementia risk and to find treatments to reduce that risk, there is a current pressing need for research that addresses the challenges faced by the vast number of people who already live with both long-term conditions.

Incorporating the perspectives of people living with hearing loss and dementia, their caregivers, and healthcare professionals, across the entire research process, from design and conduct to dissemination, is crucial to fostering comprehensive and impactful outcomes in the realm of hearing loss and dementia. These stakeholders bring invaluable insights based on real-world experiences, which can greatly enrich the relevance and applicability of research findings [108]. Research priority setting exercises involving key stakeholders are important for identifying where research would make the most difference [109]. By involving patients and their caregivers, researchers can ensure that the research questions and methodologies resonate with the challenges they face on a daily basis [110], reducing waste in research, and ultimately yielding interventions that are more practical and effective. Involving healthcare professionals provides unique clinical perspective that aid in the translation of findings into actionable recommendations, bridging the gap between research and practice, and ensuring that the outcomes are not only scientifically rigorous but also relevant to the needs of the individuals receiving care. Collaboration among researchers, patients, caregivers, and healthcare professionals enhances the credibility and validity of research outcomes whilst facilitating ownership and shared responsibility in addressing the complex interplay between hearing loss and dementia. Yet the focus of research needs to be widened from single disease models to the complex challenges associated with managing and treating individuals with multiple long-term health conditions [100].

Priority setting exercises have previously been completed for both hearing (mild-moderate hearing loss in adults) [111], and dementia [112, 113] as individual conditions, but until recently, these have not been considered in combination. In 2023, a James Lind Alliance Priority Setting Partnership in co-existing dementia and hearing conditions was launched in collaboration with key charities: RNID and Alzheimer's Research UK [114] It is the first such partnership to bring together two specific disease areas. It involves identifying and prioritising research questions about the prevention, diagnosis, and management of these co-existing conditions. The partnership emphasises the need to consider hearing conditions other than hearing loss that are potentially important for people with dementia (such as tinnitus and hyperacusis). It also promotes the representation of individuals and groups who may be typically underserved in research (e.g., LGBTQ+ communities, unpaid carers, individuals from ethnic minority groups, people with lived experience of hearing loss and dementia, including those with early onset dementia and members of the Deaf community). Emerging priority research questions can guide research funders and commissioners, investigators, campaigners, and policymakers, to achieve tangible impact.

4.3 Opportunities for developing the health and care workforce

Taking a holistic, patient-centred care approach to the management of individual living with multiple health conditions is a challenge not only for dementia and hearing loss. For individuals experiencing a range of multiple long-term conditions, evidence has shown that integrated approaches to healthcare are more effective than services that address conditions on an individual basis [115–117]. Yet, hearing healthcare is still in its' infancy when it comes to integration with other healthcare services, largely due to organisational and financial constraints [115].

In the interim, important steps can be made to nurture holistic practices in hearing care. For example, the incorporation of training into curriculums for primary care providers (e.g., family doctors) on hearing loss in isolation *and* alongside cognitive impairment and dementia would serve to increase detection and onward referral, to support early diagnosis. A good example is provided by the Royal College of General Practitioners via their Deafness and hearing loss toolkit [118]. Furthermore, greater awareness and consideration of hearing loss by family doctors about the importance and common comorbidities of hearing conditions can help ensure that treatment and referrals are harmonised [100].

With an increasing number of people living with dementia and hearing conditions, there is a need to consider how to build capacity and support the development of a skilled clinical academic research workforce [119, 120]. There should also be an emphasis on supporting the development and delivery of research within dementia and hearing services to enable the growth of research activities for patient benefit. Identifying strategies to support professionals in conducting and delivering research is crucial, enabling them to contribute to advancing knowledge and improving clinical practices in these domains. The challenge is with increasing caseloads due to an ageing population [121], how can clinicians be supported to engage in both research and upskilling practices.

4.4 Opportunities for the sharing of knowledge

Efforts are urgently required to raise public awareness of dementia, of hearing loss, and of the importance of addressing declines in hearing to promote overall brain health [122]. Rather than focusing on dementia risk reduction, emphasising the positive aspects of preserving and enhancing hearing can motivate people to take proactive measures, not only to safeguard against potential cognitive decline but to embrace a fuller and more connected life experience. Just as physical exercise is championed for its positive impact on overall health, nurturing auditory health through hearing care can be highlighted as a strategy to support lifelong cognitive vitality.

In addition to public health endeavours, the sharing of research needs, efforts and findings with patients and the public is paramount for bridging the gap between the scientific community and society. When people have access to credible and evidence-based information, they are more likely to trust medical recommendations and follow best practices [123]. Enhanced public dissemination of research fosters transparency and greater awareness of emerging health treatments, enabling individuals, and their families to make informed decisions about their ongoing healthcare.

5. Conclusions

Within this chapter, we have explored the multifaceted challenges that exist in discriminating between symptoms and complications of hearing and cognitive difficulties and how these impact patient research and care. Insights from those with lived experience of hearing loss and dementia and their carers offer important perspectives on challenges faced, as well as what we might do to address them. A collaborative approach integrating across healthcare specialties and expertise is likely to offer significant advances for diagnoses and care.

We discuss the proposed mechanisms linking hearing loss and dementia and review emerging research evidence about the role hearing rehabilitation might play in reducing the risk and progression of cognitive decline and dementia. We also highlight the many challenges associated with research addressing these issues and take a forwards look to the evidence we can expect to see in years to come. Practical suggestions, backed by health and care professionals, provide guidance for clinical adaptations that can improve quality of life for patient and their experiences of care.

As we enter a new horizon in our understanding of comorbid conditions, this chapter identifies opportunities to overcome challenges faced by clinicians and researchers alike, to improve evidence-based care and support for people living with dementia and hearing loss and the people who care for them.

Acknowledgements

EB, CB, EH, SC and HH are supported by funding from the National Institute for Health and Care Research (NIHR) Biomedical Research Centre (BRC-1215-20003) and NIHR Clinical Research Network East Midlands (UF18 and TF53). HH, EB and EH are also supported by NIHR funding award PB-PG-2018-2111-016, and EB and EH by NIHR Three Schools Dementia Career Development Awards. The views expressed in this chapter are those of the author(s) and not necessarily those of the NHS, the NIHR, or the Department of Health and Social Care.

Conflict of interest

The authors declare no conflicts of interest.

Notes/thanks/other declarations

The authors wish to thank all of the participants and patient research partners who contributed to the research cited in this chapter. We also wish to thank Ms. Sandra Smith and Ms. Izabela Popis from the NIHR Nottingham Biomedical Research Centre for their assistance.

Author details

Emma Broome[1,2], Clare Burgon[1,2], Eithne Heffernan[1,2], Tom Dening[3], Sian Calvert[1,2], Saima Rajasingam[4] and Helen Henshaw[1,2]*

1 National Institute for Health and Care Research (NIHR) Nottingham Biomedical Research Centre, Nottingham, United Kingdom

2 Hearing Sciences, Mental Health and Clinical Neurosciences, School of Medicine, University of Nottingham, Nottingham, United Kingdom

3 Mental Health and Clinical Neurosciences, School of Medicine, University of Nottingham, Nottingham, United Kingdom

4 Vision and Hearing Sciences, Anglia Ruskin University, Cambridge, United Kingdom

*Address all correspondence to: helen.henshaw@nottingham.ac.uk

References

[1] Davis L, Dening T. Diagnostic, management and nursing challenges of less common dementias: Parkinsonian dementias and Huntington's disease. British Journal of Neuroscience Nursing. 2021;**17**:68-76

[2] Davis L, Karim Z, Dening T. Diagnostic, management and nursing challenges of less common dementias: Frontotemporal dementia, alcohol-related dementia, HIV dementia and prion diseases. British Journal of Neuroscience Nursing. 2022;**18**:26-37

[3] Alzheimer's Research UK; Prevalence and Incidence. Prevalence and Incidence – Dementia Statistics Hub. 2023. Available from: https://dementiastatistics.org/about-dementia/prevalence-and-incidence/#:~:text=The%20number%20of%20people%20living%20with%20dementia%20in%20the,exceed%201.5%20million%20by%202050 [Accessed: August 29, 2023]

[4] Livingston G, Huntley J, Sommerlad A, Ames D, Ballard C, Banerjee S, et al. Dementia prevention, intervention, and care: 2020 report of the Lancet Commission. The Lancet. 2020;**396**:413-446

[5] Sandilyan MB, Dening T. Signs and symptoms of dementia. Nursing Standard. 2014;**29**:42

[6] Van Dyck CH, Swanson CJ, Aisen P, Bateman RJ, Chen C, Gee M, et al. Lecanemab in early Alzheimer's disease. New England Journal of Medicine. 2023;**388**:9-21

[7] Budd Haeberlein S, Aisen PS, Barkhof F, Chalkias S, Chen T, Cohen S, et al. Two randomized phase 3 studies of aducanumab in early Alzheimer's disease. The Journal of Prevention of Alzheimer's Disease. 2022;**9**:197-210

[8] Tsimpida D, Kontopantelis E, Ashcroft D, Panagioti M. Socioeconomic and lifestyle factors associated with hearing loss in older adults: A cross-sectional study of the English Longitudinal Study of Ageing (ELSA). BMJ Open. 2019;**9**:e031030. DOI: 10.1136/bmjopen-2019-031030

[9] Huang AR, Jiang K, Lin FR, Deal JA, Reed NS. Hearing loss and dementia prevalence in older adults in the US. JAMA. 2023;**329**:171-173

[10] Lau K, Dimitriadis PA, Mitchell C, Martyn-St-James M, Hind D, Ray J. Age-related hearing loss and mild cognitive impairment: A meta-analysis and systematic review of population-based studies. The Journal of Laryngology and Otology. 2022;**136**:103-118

[11] Nirmalasari O, Mamo SK, Nieman CL, Simpson A, Zimmerman J, Nowrangi MA, et al. Age-related hearing loss in older adults with cognitive impairment. International Psychogeriatrics. 2017;**29**:115-121

[12] Hardy CJD, Marshall CR, Golden HL, Clark CN, Mummery CJ, Griffiths TD, et al. Hearing and dementia. Journal of Neurology. 2016;**263**:2339-2354

[13] RNID. Signs of Hearing Loss. 2018. Available from: https://rnid.org.uk/information-and-support/hearing-loss/signs-of-hearing-loss/ [Accessed: August 30, 2023]

[14] Burgon C, Goldberg S, van der Wardt V, Harwood RH. Experiences and understanding of apathy in people with neurocognitive disorders and their carers: A qualitative interview study. Age and

Ageing. 2023;**52**:afad031. DOI: 10.1093/ageing/afad031

[15] Heffernan E, Withanachchi CM, Ferguson MA. 'The worse my hearing got, the less sociable I got': A qualitative study of patient and professional views of the management of social isolation and hearing loss. Age and Ageing. 2022;**51**:afac019. DOI: 10.1093/ageing/afac019

[16] Ray M, Dening T, Crosbie B. Dementia and hearing loss: A narrative review. Maturitas. 2019;**128**:64-69. DOI: 10.1016/j.maturitas.2019.08.001

[17] Slaughter SE, Hopper T, Ickert C, Erin DF. Identification of hearing loss among residents with dementia: Perceptions of health care aides. Geriatric Nursing (Minneap). 2014;**35**:434-440. DOI: 10.1016/j.gerinurse.2014.07.001

[18] Hopper T, Hinton P. Hearing loss among individuals with dementia: Barriers and facilitators to care. Canadian Journal of Speech-Language Pathology and Audiology. 2012;**36**:302-313

[19] Petermann-Rocha F, Lyall DM, Gray SR, Esteban-Cornejo I, Quinn TJ, Ho FK, et al. Associations between physical frailty and dementia incidence: A prospective study from UK Biobank. Lancet Healthy Longevity. 2020;**1**:e58-e68

[20] Tian R, Almeida OP, Jayakody DMP, Ford AH. Association between hearing loss and frailty: A systematic review and meta-analysis. BMC Geriatrics. 2021;**21**:333

[21] Jiam NT, Li C, Agrawal Y. Hearing loss and falls: A systematic review and meta-analysis. Laryngoscope. 2016;**126**:2587-2596

[22] Tinetti ME, Speechley M, Ginter SF. Risk factors for falls among elderly persons living in the community. New England Journal of Medicine. 1988;**319**:1701-1707

[23] Enache D, Winblad B, Aarsland D. Depression in dementia: Epidemiology, mechanisms, and treatment. Current Opinion in Psychiatry. 2011;**24**:461-472

[24] Lawrence BJ, Jayakody DMP, Bennett RJ, Eikelboom RH, Gasson N, Friedland PL. Hearing loss and depression in older adults: A systematic review and meta-analysis. Gerontologist. 2020;**60**:e137-e154

[25] Kuiper JS, Zuidersma M, Voshaar RCO, Zuidema SU, van den Heuvel ER, Stolk RP, et al. Social relationships and risk of dementia: A systematic review and meta-analysis of longitudinal cohort studies. Ageing Research Reviews. 2015;**22**:39-57

[26] Weinstein BE, Ventry IM. Hearing impairment and social isolation in the elderly. Journal of Speech, Language, and Hearing Research. 1982;**25**:593-599

[27] Dalton DS, Cruickshanks KJ, Klein BEK, Klein R, Wiley TL, Nondahl DM. The impact of hearing loss on quality of life in older adults. Gerontologist. 2003;**43**:661-668

[28] Keating N, Gaudet N. Quality of life of persons with dementia. The Journal of Nutrition, Health & Aging. 2012;**16**:454-456

[29] Scarinci N, Worrall L, Hickson L. Factors associated with third-party disability in spouses of older people with hearing impairment. Ear and Hearing. 2012;**33**:698-708

[30] Lind C, Meyer C, Young J. Hearing and cognitive impairment and the role of the international classification of functioning, disability and health as a

rehabilitation framework. Seminars in Hearing. 2016;**37**:200-215

[31] Kricos PB. Providing hearing rehabilitation to people with dementia presents unique challenges. Hearing Journal. 2009;**62**:39-40

[32] Mamo SK, Oh E, Lin FR. Enhancing communication in adults with dementia and age-related hearing loss. Seminars in Hearing. 2017;**38**:177-183

[33] Johnson JCS, Marshall CR, Weil RS, Bamiou D-E, Hardy CJD, Warren JD. Hearing and dementia: From ears to brain. Brain. 2021;**144**:391-401

[34] Griffiths TD, Lad M, Kumar S, Holmes E, McMurray B, Maguire EA, et al. How can hearing loss cause dementia? Neuron. 2020;**108**:401-412

[35] Martini A, Castiglione A, Bovo R, Vallesi A, Gabelli C. Aging, cognitive load, dementia and hearing loss. Audiology and Neurotology. 2015;**19**:2-5. DOI: 10.1159/000371593

[36] Uchida Y, Sugiura S, Nishita Y, Saji N, Sone M, Ueda H. Age-related hearing loss and cognitive decline—The potential mechanisms linking the two. Auris Nasus Larynx. 2019;**46**:1-9

[37] Shen Y, Ye B, Chen P, Wang Q, Fan C, Shu Y, et al. Cognitive decline, dementia, Alzheimer's disease and presbycusis: Examination of the possible molecular mechanism. Frontiers in Neuroscience. 2018;**12**:394

[38] Sardone R, Battista P, Panza F, Lozupone M, Griseta C, Castellana F, et al. The age-related central auditory processing disorder: Silent impairment of the cognitive ear. Frontiers in Neuroscience. 2019;**13**:1-9

[39] Quaranta N, Coppola F, Casulli M, Barulli O, Lanza F, Tortelli R, et al. The prevalence of peripheral and central hearing impairment and its relation to cognition in older adults. Audiology and Neurotology. 2015;**19**:10-14

[40] Tarawneh HY, Menegola HK, Peou A, Tarawneh H, Jayakody DMP. Central auditory functions of Alzheimer's disease and its preclinical stages: A systematic review and meta-analysis. Cell. 2022;**11**:1007

[41] Powell DS, Oh ES, Reed NS, Lin FR, Deal JA. Hearing loss and cognition: What we know and where we need to go. Frontiers in Aging Neuroscience. 28 Feb 2022;**13**:769405. DOI: 10.3389/fnagi.2021.769405

[42] Prince M, Bryce R, Ferri C. World Alzheimer Report 2011: The Benefits of Early Dagnosis and Intervention. 2011. Available from: https://www.alz.co.uk/research/WorldAlzheimerReport2011.pdf [Accessed: October 24, 2023]

[43] World Health Organization. Deafness and Hearing Loss. 2023. Available from: https://www.who.int/news-room/fact-sheets/detail/deafness-and-hearing-loss [Accessed: August 30, 2023]

[44] Woods B, Rai HK, Elliott E, Aguirre E, Orrell M, Spector A. Cognitive stimulation to improve cognitive functioning in people with dementia. Cochrane Database of Systematic Reviews. 2023;**1**:1-186

[45] Lin FR, Metter EJ, O'Brien RJ, Resnick SM, Zonderman AB, Ferrucci L. Hearing loss and incident dementia. Archives of Neurology. 2011;**68**:214-220

[46] Jiang F, Mishra SR, Shrestha N, Ozaki A, Virani SS, Bright T, et al. Association between hearing aid use and all-cause and cause-specific dementia: An

analysis of the UK Biobank cohort. The Lancet Public Health. 2023;**8**:e329-e338

[47] Yeo BSY, Song HJJMD, Toh EMS, Ng LS, Ho CSH, Ho R, et al. Association of hearing aids and cochlear implants with cognitive decline and dementia: A systematic review and meta-analysis. JAMA Neurology. 2023;**80**:134-141. DOI: 10.1001/jamaneurol.2022.4427

[48] Alzheimer's Association. Why get checked? Alzheimer's disease and dementia. 2023. Available from: https://www.alz.org/alzheimers-dementia/diagnosis/why-get-checked [Accessed: August 30, 2023]

[49] The Lancet Public Health. Addressing hearing loss at all ages. Lancet Public Health. 2023;**8**:e318

[50] Simpson AN, Matthews LJ, Cassarly C, Dubno JR. Time from hearing-aid candidacy to hearing-aid adoption: A longitudinal cohort study. Ear and Hearing. 2019;**40**:468

[51] Alzheimer's Society. 91% of People Affected by Dementia See Clear Benefits to Getting a Diagnosis. 2022. Available from: https://www.alzheimers.org.uk/news/2022-05-16/91-people-affected-dementia-see-clear-benefits-getting-diagnosis [Accessed: September 05, 2023]

[52] Woods B, Arosio F, Diaz A, Gove D, Holmerová I, Kinnaird L, et al. Timely diagnosis of dementia? Family carers' experiences in 5 European countries. International Journal of Geriatric Psychiatry. 2019;**34**:114-121

[53] Dodd E, Pracownik R, Popel S, Collings S, Emmens T, Cheston R. Dementia services for people from Black, Asian and Minority Ethnic and White-British communities: Does a primary care based model contribute to equality in service provision? Health & Social Care in the Community. 2022;**30**:622-630

[54] Parker M, Barlow S, Hoe J, Aitken L. Persistent barriers and facilitators to seeking help for a dementia diagnosis: A systematic review of 30 years of the perspectives of carers and people with dementia. International Psychogeriatrics. 2020;**32**:611-634

[55] Wallhagen MI, Pettengill E. Hearing impairment: Significant but underassessed in primary care settings. Journal of Gerontological Nursing. 2008;**34**:36-42

[56] Alzheimer's Society. New Research Reveals One in Three Wait Over a Month to Speak Out About Dementia Worries. Alzheimer's Society. 2023. https://www.alzheimers.org.uk/news/2023-05-15/new-research-reveals-one-three-wait-over-month-speak-out-about-dementia-worries [Accessed: August 30, 2023]

[57] Ng CKM, Leung DKY, Cai X, Wong GHY. Perceived help-seeking difficulty, barriers, delay, and burden in carers of people with suspected dementia. International Journal of Environmental Research and Public Health. 2021;**18**:2956

[58] Knoetze M, Manchaiah V, Mothemela B, Swanepoel DW. Factors influencing hearing help-seeking and hearing aid uptake in adults: A systematic review of the past decade. Trends Hearing. 2023;**27**:2331

[59] Broome EE, Tannirandorn P, Straus J, Beale P, Heffernan E, Dening T, et al. Patient perceptions of cognitive screening in adult audiology services: A qualitative exploration. Frontiers in Neurology. 2023;**14**:1143128

[60] Lillekroken D, Halvorsrud L, Gulestø R, Bjørge H. Family caregivers

experiences of providing care for family members from minority ethnic groups living with dementia: A qualitative systematic review. Journal of Clinical Nursing. 2023;**32**:1625-1641

[61] Kenning C, Daker-White G, Blakemore A, Panagioti M, Waheed W. Barriers and facilitators in accessing dementia care by ethnic minority groups: A meta-synthesis of qualitative studies. BMC Psychiatry. 2017;**17**:1-13

[62] Di Lorito C, Bosco A, Peel E, Hinchliff S, Dening T, Calasanti T, et al. Are dementia services and support organisations meeting the needs of lesbian, gay, bisexual and transgender (LGBT) caregivers of LGBT people living with dementia? A scoping review of the literature. Aging & Mental Health. 2022;**26**:1912-1921

[63] Grandpierre V, Fitzpatrick E, Thomas R, Sikora L, Potter B, Thomas O. Perspectives of parents of minority culture backgrounds on pediatric hearing loss services: A qualitative inquiry. Canadian Journal of Speech-Language Pathologists and Audiologists. 2019;**43**:203-215

[64] Tsimpida D, Rajasingam S, Panagioti M, Henshaw H. The leaky pipeline of hearing care: Primary to secondary care evidence from the English Longitudinal Study of Ageing (ELSA). International Journal of Audiology. 2023:1-9 [Ahead of Print]

[65] Dupuis K, Pichora-Fuller MK, Chasteen AL, Marchuk V, Singh G, Smith SL. Effects of hearing and vision impairments on the Montreal Cognitive Assessment. Aging, Neuropsychology, and Cognition. 2015;**22**:413-437

[66] Jorgensen LE, Palmer CV, Pratt S, Erickson KI, Moncrieff D. The effect of decreased audibility on MMSE performance: A measure commonly used for diagnosing dementia. Journal of the American Academy of Audiology. 2016;**27**:311-323

[67] Völter C, Götze L, Dazert S, Wirth R, Thomas JP. Impact of hearing loss on geriatric assessment. Clinical Interventions in Aging. 2020;**15**:2453-2467

[68] Uhlmann RF, Teri L, Rees TS, Mozlowski KJ, Larson EB. Impact of mild to moderate hearing loss on mental status testing: Comparability of standard and written Mini-Mental State Examinations. Journal of the American Geriatrics Society. 1989;**37**:223-228

[69] De Silva ML, Mclaughlin MT, Rodrigues EJ, Broadbent JC, Gray AR, Hammond-Tooke GD. A mini-mental status examination for the hearing impaired. Age and Ageing. 2008;**37**:593-595

[70] Dawes P, Reeves D, Yeung WK, Holland F, Charalambous AP, Côté M, et al. Development and validation of the Montreal Cognitive Assessment for people with hearing impairment (MoCA-H). Journal of the American Geriatrics Society. 2023;**71**:1485-1494

[71] Dawes P, Littlejohn J, Bott A, Brennan S, Burrow S, Hopper T, et al. Hearing assessment and rehabilitation for people living with dementia. Ear and Hearing. 2022;**43**:1089

[72] Langdon A, Heffernan E, Somerset S, Calvert S, Broome E, Dening T, et al. Recommendations for the assessment and management of co-existing dementia and hearing loss within UK audiology services. Age Ageing. 1615, 2023;**52**:afad104.060. DOI: 10.1093/ageing/afad104.060

[73] Littlejohn J, Bowen M, Constantinidou F, Dawes P, Dickinson C,

Heyn P, et al. International practice recommendations for the recognition and management of hearing and vision impairment in people with dementia. Gerontology. 2021;**68**:121-135. DOI: 10.1159/000515892

[74] British Society of Audiology. Audiological Assessment for Adults with Intellectual Disabilities. 2019. Available from: https://www.thebsa.org.uk/resources/practice-guidance-audiological-assessment-for-adults-with-intellectual-disabilities/ [Accessed: August 29, 2023]

[75] Füllgrabe C. On the possible overestimation of cognitive decline: The impact of age-related hearing loss on cognitive-test performance. Frontiers in Neuroscience. 2020;**14**:454

[76] Leroi I, Chauhan N, Hann M, Jones L, Prew S, Russell G, et al. Sensory health for residents with dementia in care homes in England: A knowledge, attitudes, and practice survey. Journal of the American Medical Directors Association. 2021;**22**:1518-1524.e12. DOI: 10.1016/j.jamda.2021.03.020

[77] Omar R, Kuo L, Costafreda SG, Hall A, Forbes M, O'Brien JT, et al. Managing comorbid cognitive impairment and hearing loss in older adults: A UK survey of audiology and memory services. Age and Ageing. 2023;**52**:afad080. DOI: 10.1093/ageing/afad080

[78] Ladduwahetty S, Dowell RC, Winton E. Dementia and cochlear implant outcomes: Can we screen for dementia effectively using the mini mental state examination in implant candidates? The Australian and New Zealand Journal of Audiology. 2013;**33**:88-102

[79] NICE. Dementia: Assessment, Management and Support for People Living with Dementia and Their Carers – NICE Guideline [NG97]. 2018. Available from: https://www.nice.org.uk/guidance/ng97 [Accessed August 30, 2023]

[80] McDonough A, Dookhy J, McHale C, Sharkey J, Fox S, Kennelly SP. Embedding audiological screening within memory clinic care pathway for individuals at risk of cognitive decline—patient perspectives. BMC Geriatrics. 2021;**21**:1-8

[81] World Health Organization. Ageing and Health 2022. 2022. Available from: https://www.who.int/news-room/fact-sheets/detail/ageing-and-health [Accessed: August 30, 2023]

[82] Bisogno A, Scarpa A, Di Girolamo S, De Luca P, Cassandro C, Viola P, et al. Hearing loss and cognitive impairment: Epidemiology, common pathophysiological findings, and treatment considerations. Life. 2021;**11**:1102

[83] Patel B, Perera M, Pendleton J, Richman A, Majumdar B. Psychosocial interventions for dementia: From evidence to practice. Advances in Psychiatric Treatment. 2014;**20**:340-349. DOI: 10.1192/apt.bp.113.011957

[84] Brooker D, Latham I. Person-centred Dementia Care: Making Services Better with the VIPS Framework. London, England: Jessica Kingsley Publishers; 2015

[85] Ferri CP, Jacob KS. Dementia in low-income and middle-income countries: Different realities mandate tailored solutions. PLoS Medicine. 2017;**14**:e1002271

[86] McDaid D, Park A-L, Chadha S. Estimating the global costs of hearing loss. International Journal of Audiology. 2021;**60**:162-170

[87] RNID. Supporting Older People with Hearing Loss in Care Settings. A Guide for Managers and Staff 2018. UK: RNID; 2018

[88] Ludlow K, Mumford V, Makeham M, Braithwaite J, Greenfield D. The effects of hearing loss on person-centred care in residential aged care: A narrative review. Geriatric Nursing. 2018;**39**:296-302. DOI: 10.1016/j.gerinurse.2017.10.013

[89] Andrusjak W, Barbosa A, Mountain G. Identifying and managing hearing and vision loss in older people in care homes: A scoping review of the evidence. Gerontologist. 2020;**60**:e155-e168. DOI: 10.1093/geront/gnz087

[90] Liu C, Chang P-S, Griffith CF, Hanley SI, Lu Y. The nexus of sensory loss, cognitive impairment, and functional decline in older adults: A scoping review. Gerontologist. 2022;**62**:e457-e467. DOI: 10.1093/geront/gnab082

[91] Jupiter T. Cognition and screening for hearing loss in nursing home residents. Journal of the American Medical Directors Association. 2012;**13**:744-747

[92] Mitoku K, Masaki N, Ogata Y, Okamoto K. Vision and hearing impairments, cognitive impairment and mortality among long-term care recipients: A population-based cohort study. BMC Geriatrics. 2016;**16**:112. DOI: 10.1186/s12877-016-0286-2

[93] Crosbie B, Ferguson M, Wong G, Walker D-M, Vanhegan S, Dening T. Giving permission to care for people with dementia in residential homes: Learning from a realist synthesis of hearing-related communication. BMC Medicine. 2019;**17**:54. DOI: 10.1186/s12916-019-1286-9

[94] Cross H, Dawes P, Hooper E, Armitage CJ, Leroi I, Millman RE. Effectiveness of hearing rehabilitation for care home residents with dementia: A systematic review. Journal of the American Medical Directors Association. 2022;**23**:450-460.e4. DOI: 10.1016/j.jamda.2021.11.011

[95] Punch R, Horstmanshof L. Hearing loss and its impact on residents in long term care facilities: A systematic review of literature. Geriatric Nursing (Minneap). 2019;**40**:138-147. DOI: 10.1016/j.gerinurse.2018.07.006

[96] Dawes P, Leroi I, Chauhan N, Han W, Harbishettar V, Jayakody DMP, et al. Hearing and vision health for people with dementia in residential long term care: Knowledge, attitudes and practice in England, South Korea, India, Greece, Indonesia and Australia. International Journal of Geriatric Psychiatry. 2021;**36**:1531-1540

[97] McCreedy EM, Weinstein BE, Chodosh J, Blustein J. Hearing loss: Why does it matter for nursing homes? Journal of the American Medical Directors Association. 2018;**19**:323-327. DOI: 10.1016/j.jamda.2017.12.007

[98] Bott A, Meyer C, Hickson L, Pachana NA. "It's huge, in a way." Conflicting stakeholder priorities for managing hearing impairment for people living with dementia in residential aged care facilities. Clinical Gerontologist. 2022;**45**:844-858. DOI: 10.1080/07317115.2020.1805537

[99] Cross H, Armitage CJ, Dawes P, Leroi I, Millman RE. Capabilities, opportunities and motivations of staff to provide hearing support to long-term care home residents with dementia. International Journal of Audiology. 2023:1-8. DOI: 10.1080/14992027.2023.2227764 [Ahead of Print]

[100] Henshaw H, Calvert S, Heffernan E, Broome EE, Burgon C, Dening T, et al. New horizons in hearing conditions. Age and Ageing. 2023;**52**:afad150. DOI: 10.1093/ageing/afad150

[101] Hampel H, Au R, Mattke S, van der Flier WM, Aisen P, Apostolova L, et al. Designing the next-generation clinical care pathway for Alzheimer's disease. Nature Aging. 2022;**2**:692-703

[102] Wright N, Stickley T, Mulla I, Bradshaw E, Buckley L, Archbold S. Hearing loss and dementia: An exploratory study of the views of audiologists. Quality Ageing Older Adults. 2014;**15**:220-231

[103] Leroi I, Himmelsbach I, Wolski L, Littlejohn J, Jury F, Parker A, et al. Assessing and managing concurrent hearing, vision and cognitive impairments in older people: An international perspective from healthcare professionals. Age and Ageing. 2019;**48**:580-587

[104] Leroi I, Constantinidou F, Langenbahn D, Heyn P, Yeung WK, Dawes P. Hearing and vision impairment in people with dementia: A guide for clinicians. Archives of Physical Medicine and Rehabilitation. 2020;**101**:1667-1670

[105] National Institute for Health and Care Research. Improving inclusion of under-served groups in clinical research: Guidance from the NIHR-INCLUDE project. 2020. Available from: www.nihr.ac.uk/documents/improving-inclusion-of-under-served-groups-in-clinical-research-guidance-from-include-project/25435 [Accessed: August 27, 2023]

[106] British Deaf Association (Scotland). Remember: The Deaf Dementia Experience in Scotland: A Toolkit for All. UK: British Deaf Association (Scotland); 2019

[107] Lin FR, Pike JR, Albert MS, Arnold M, Burgard S, Chisolm T, et al. Hearing intervention versus health education control to reduce cognitive decline in older adults with hearing loss in the USA (ACHIEVE): A multicentre, randomised controlled trial. The Lancet. 2023;**402**:786-797. DOI: 10.1016/S0140-6736(23)01406-X

[108] Miah J, Dawes P, Leroi I, Parsons S, Starling B. A protocol to evaluate the impact of involvement of older people with dementia and age-related hearing and/or vision impairment in a multi-site European research study. Research Involved Engagement. 2018;**4**:1-10

[109] Grill C. Involving stakeholders in research priority setting: A scoping review. Research Involved Engagement. 2021;**7**:1-18

[110] Chalmers I, Bracken MB, Djulbegovic B, Garattini S, Grant J, Gülmezoglu AM, et al. How to increase value and reduce waste when research priorities are set. The Lancet. 2014;**383**:156-165

[111] Henshaw H, Sharkey L, Crowe D, Ferguson M. Research priorities for mild-to-moderate hearing loss in adults. The Lancet. 2015;**386**:2140-2141

[112] Kelly S, Lafortune L, Hart N, Cowan K, Fenton M, Brayne C, et al. Dementia priority setting partnership with the James Lind Alliance: Using patient and public involvement and the evidence base to inform the research agenda. Age and Ageing. 2015;**44**:985-993. DOI: 10.1093/ageing/afv143

[113] Bethell J, Pringle D, Chambers LW, Cohen C, Commisso E, Cowan K, et al. Patient and public involvement

in identifying dementia research priorities. Journal of the American Geriatrics Society. 2018;**66**:1608-1612. DOI: 10.1111/jgs.15453

[114] Calvert S, Heffernan E, Henshaw H. Generating Priorities for Future Dementia and Hearing Research. BAA Magazine. UK: British Academy of Audiology; 2023

[115] Wallhagen MI, Strawbridge WJ, Tremblay K. Leveraging the age friendly healthcare system initiative to achieve comprehensive, hearing healthcare across the spectrum of healthcare settings: An interprofessional perspective. International Journal of Audiology. 2021;**60**:80-85

[116] Maidment DW, Wallhagen MI, Dowd K, Mick P, Piker E, Spankovich C, et al. New horizons in holistic, person-centred health promotion for hearing healthcare. Age and Ageing. 2023;**52**:afad020

[117] Vercammen C, Bott A, Saunders GH. Hearing health in the broader context of healthy living and well-being: Changing the narrative. International Journal of Audiology. 2021;**60**:1-3

[118] Royal College of General Practitioners. Deafness and Hearing Loss Toolkit. 2021. Available from: https://elearning.rcgp.org.uk/mod/book/view.php?id=12532 [Accessed August 30, 2023]

[119] Hibbert PD, Basedow M, Braithwaite J, Wiles LK, Clay-Williams R, Padbury R. How to sustainably build capacity in quality improvement within a healthcare organisation: A deep-dive, focused qualitative analysis. BMC Health Services Research. 2021;**21**:1-13

[120] National Health Service England. National Health Service Improvement; Demand and capacity – A comprehensive guide. 2022

[121] Nicol E. The ageing population in healthcare: A challenge to, and in, the workforce. Clinical Medicine. 2017;**17**:291

[122] RNID. Hearing loss and dementia: How are they linked? 2023. Available from: https://rnid.org.uk/hearing-research/hearing-loss-and-dementia-how-are-they-linked/#:~:text=hearing%20is%20an%20essential%20part,increases%20the%20risk%20five%20times [Accessed: August 30, 2023]

[123] Kington RS, Arnesen S, Chou W-YS, Curry SJ, Lazer D, Villarruel AM. Identifying credible sources of health information in social media: Principles and attributes. NAM Perspectives. 2021;**2021**:1-37. DOI: 10.31478/202107a

Chapter 7

Effect of Cochlear Implantation on Voice Quality in Patients with Hearing Impairment

Karol Myszel and Piotr Henryk Skarżyński

Abstract

Hearing impairment is a cause of many problems suffered by a patient. Apart from hearing problems also voice problems develop as a result. Already in deaf newborns, clear signs of voice disturbances appear soon after birth. Development of voice is delayed, babbling appears later and speech development depends on the time and kind of medical intervention. The reason of voice abnormalities in hearing impaired individuals is abnormal hearing control over voice production. Therefore, audiological intervention enabling better control, is an important factor for hearing and voice quality improvement. This chapter summarizes up-to-date knowledge on the influence of hearing aids and cochlear implants on voice quality of hearing impaired patients. Both literature studies and authors` own research show that the use of cochlear implants is the most effective tool of improving hearing and voice of people with hypoacusis. Cochlear implantation brings better results compared to hearing aids and the time of implantation plays a key role.

Keywords: hearing impairment, voice quality, voice disorders, cochlear implant, partial deafness, acoustic voice analysis

1. Introduction

In newborns, voice appears as a reflex immediately after birth. It continues to develop during further stages of life and, together with the onset of speech, voice becomes a useful tool for interpersonal communication. Numerous studies have demonstrated how voice production is strictly controlled by both the central nervous system and the auditory system. This means that a disorder in either of these control systems can lead to abnormalities in voice quality and changes in its acoustic structure.

Individuals deprived of full hearing suffer many problems in their social, professional, and personal lives. Prolonged hearing deprivation, particularly in children, results in problems such as loss of voice control, which is evident as dysphonia of different degrees.

Compared to healthy children, hearing-impaired children are no different in terms of their larynx. However, differences do become apparent in the first few years of life, with the degree depending on various factors, such as type and depth of hearing impairment and the method and success of rehabilitation. The type of voice disorder in poorly hearing or deaf children is usually classed as functional [1].

In infants with hearing impairment, changes can be seen in voice development within a matter of months. The voice is typically higher pitched, shows greater fluctuations in frequency, and is less constant in volume. In the first few months of life, intrinsic motivation is the major stimulus for vocalization (i.e., no external sound stimulus is needed), but later on there is a greater reliance on hearing [2, 3]. Analysis of the vocalizations of hearing-impaired children only a few months old brings out the differences compared to normally hearing children. In the first year of life, hearing-impaired children show a delay in canonical babbling, usually of 4–6 months, whereas children with normal hearing produce many more canonical syllables [4–6]. The delay depends on the severity of the hearing impairment [7, 8].

Apart from the quality of vocalization, hearing impairment can also affect the number of vocalization episodes, with hearing impaired or deaf children producing significantly less vocalizations than their healthy peers [9, 10]. The deleterious effect of hearing impairment depends strongly on its severity. For deaf children, the number of vocalizations is significantly less than in children with only partial hearing impairment, and in both groups the number of vocalizations is substantially lower than in normally hearing peers [11]. At later stages of development (i.e., 16–24 months), the transition from babbling to words is also delayed among hearing-impaired children. Later on, as speech develops, hearing-impaired children show delays or more limited use of syllables containing consonants, incorrect vowel articulation, and a smaller vocabulary [12].

Compared to normally hearing people, the voice of hearing-impaired individuals is, in general, marked by an increase in average fundamental frequency (F0), an increase in the variation of fundamental frequency (vF0), an increase in the variation of amplitude (vAm), and a decrease in phonation time [13–16]. These factors suggest that the hearing impaired have difficulty in controlling long-term frequency and amplitude during phonation. Perceptively, this difficulty manifests as vocal instability that can take the form of tremor, poor modulation, and elevated pitch. Those voice features fall into the category of 'audiogenic dysphonia'. In addition, the speech of hearing-impaired individuals is also marked by patterns of poor articulation, or 'audiogenic dyslalia'. Taken together, voice quality depends on the effective functioning of the auditory organs and adequate performance of the respiratory tract. With a functional level of hearing, it is possible to have correct voice range development, an ability to modulate voice intensity, and achievement of normal acoustic voice parameters. In brief, appropriate hearing allows normal speech and prosody to develop.

Among hearing-impaired individuals, changes in the acoustic structure of voice are seen at every developmental stage. The changes are primarily related to voice frequency. In particular, deaf and partially deaf individuals use a narrower range of frequencies in their voice and tend to have less control over pitch [17–21]. The voice of a hearing-impaired child is frequently dull, fluctuating, and harsh, and is accompanied by high muscle tension; it is often breathy, toneless, weak, monotonous, and devoid of melody. It appears that hearing impairments interfere with how the pitch, volume, rhythm, and timbre of the voice is regulated [22–24].

Other studies have demonstrated that individuals with hearing disorders often exhibit abnormalities of voice resonance – evident as nasalence [25–27] – so that voice and speech becomes nasal, dull, and rather dark. Most researchers consider that nasalence reflects inadequate central nervous system control of the velopharyngeal muscles due to a lack of auditory input [25, 28, 29]. Another potential factor in causing nasalence is a slower rate of speech [30–32]. Perceptive and acoustic examinations reveal elevated nasal resonance, even when electromyography (EMG) of the palatal muscles remains normal [33].

These studies suggest that a lack of auditory-derived control produces abnormal voice characteristics, evident as changes in aerodynamic parameters. The changes come about from poor coordination between the internal and external muscles of the larynx, and are seen as abnormalities the way antagonistic muscles develop and release tension. Comparisons of normal and hearing-impaired individuals have revealed statistically significant differences in the vital capacity of the lungs (VC), maximum sustained phonation time (MSPT), and fast adduction–abduction rate (FAAR). In particular, they show lower VC, shorter MSPT, and smaller FAAR compared to normally hearing individuals. There is also a somewhat smaller peak expiratory flow (PEF), although this difference does not reach statistical significance [34, 35].

Research on the mechanisms of respiration and chest mobility suggest that, among deaf and poorly hearing individuals, there may be abnormalities in the coordination of chest and abdominal movements. In particular, such people tend to initiate phonation using an incorrect volume of air in the lungs (either too large or too small). The mean volume of air (per syllable) is double that of normally hearing subjects. Deaf or hearing impaired individuals therefore tend to speak fewer syllables per breath, which leads to awkward breaks to breathe in at grammatically inappropriate moments [36].

2. Cochlear implantation and voice quality

Early intervention, either with hearing aids or cochlear implantation, is crucial to enable patients to receive appropriate hearing. Better auditory control of the voice will help improve the patient's voice quality. The option of whether to use a hearing aid or a cochlear implant depends on the degree of hearing impairment. Regardless of the choice, numerous studies have shown that the earlier the intervention is performed, the better are the results in terms of hearing and voice improvement.

In this context, one relevant study was conducted in the Institute of Physiology and Pathology of Hearing in Warsaw, Poland, on a group of 83 Polish school children aged 7–12 years [37]. The aim of the study was to compare the quality of the voice after using hearing aids or cochlear implants. Acoustic voice analysis was performed for each individual, and the linguistic material was a prolonged [a] vowel. The criterion for including a patient in the study was profound prelingual, sensorineural hypoacusis. The study group was divided into four subgroups according to their hearing and use of hearing devices: there were 20 children without any type of hearing device (HL), 20 children who used hearing aids (HA), 20 children with cochlear implants (CI), and 23 normal-hearing children, of the same age, who had no voice disorders (control group, NH). The children who used hearing aids or cochlear implants had undergone hearing rehabilitation 6 months previously.

After audiological intervention and rehabilitation, statistically important changes were observed in several acoustic voice parameters. The group of hearing-impaired children (HL) had the highest average fundamental frequency F0. In the hearing aid group (HA), testing performed 6 months after a hearing aid was fitted showed there was a slight decrease in the average F0 value. However, in the CI group, there was a much greater decrease in F0. The study also showed a significant decrease in the number of fundamental frequency periods (pitch periods, PER) in the hearing-impaired children compared to the control group. In the HA group, some improvements in PER were observed, but in the CI group the improvements occurred much faster. At the same time, slight decreases in smoothed amplitude perturbation quotient (sAPQ) were observed in the HL and HA groups, indicating that amplitude control stabilized quite quickly. The highest average peak amplitude variation (vAm) was found in the HL group, and the lowest in the control group (NH). Values of vAm in the HL group reached values almost twice those of vAm in the control group. These significantly lower vAm values after use of hearing aids and cochlear implants indicate that the patients had better auditory control of the voice. Noise-to-harmonic ratio (NHR) decreased in the HL and HA groups, whereas a significant increase was noted in the CI group. The soft phonation index (SPI) was found to be lower in the HA and CI groups, but higher in the CI group. F0 tremor intensity index (FTRI) in the HL group was almost twice that of the control group. In the HA and CI groups there was a significant decrease in FTRI, but it was even greater in the CI group. This reflected an observed decrease of voice tremor in the patients.

The conclusion of the study was that long-term hearing deprivation, whether minor or substantial, affects the acoustic structure of children's voices. Significant changes were found in fundamental frequency (F0), highest fundamental frequency (Fhi), variability of fundamental frequency (vF0), number of periods of fundamental frequency (PER), amplitude perturbation quotient (sAPQ), variability of amplitude (vAm), noise-to-harmonic ratio (NHR), soft phonation index (SPI), and frequency tremor index (FTRI). The implication is that patients with a profound level of hearing impairment develop long-term problems in the control of voice frequency and amplitude. Acoustic analysis confirms that the use of hearing rehabilitation devices significantly improves most acoustic voice parameters. The improvements reflect improved auditory control of voice frequency and amplitude, and a decrease in noise components and voice tremor. In particular, significantly better voice results have been seen in children who have received cochlear implants [37].

Similiar results were obtained by Campisi et al. [17] who conducted acoustic voice analysis of 21 children before and 6 months after cochlear implantation. Before cochlear implantation elevated levels of F0, vF0, and vAm were observed. After cochlear implantation, vF0 tended towards normal and there was a marked decrease in vAm, bringing more stability to voice.

In a study by Evans and Deliyski [14], patients before cochlear implantation presented abnormalities in F0, jitter, shimmer, NHR, VTI, SPI, vAm, and vF0. After cochlear implantation they noted a decrease in F0 for all subjects. After implantation the voice was more stable, while jitter, shimmer, and VTI were markedly less. After cochlear implantation all subjects had much lower nasality. Similar findings were noted by Fletcher et al. [29].

In another study of 31 children aged 2–3 years with prelingual deafness who received cochlear implants, Hocevar-Boltezar et al. [38] reported substantial improvements in jitter and shimmer 6 months after implantation and after 24 months there was a noticeable improvement in NHR. It was clear that cochlear implants improved the patients' ability to control the pitch and loudness of their voice. These findings were confirmed by Holler et al. [15].

Kishon-Rabin et al. [39] described the effects of cochlear implantation on voice in a group of post-lingually deaf patients. They noted a decrease of F0 after 1, 6, and 24 months from implantation. They also found that voice quality improved more if the intervention was undertaken earlier.

Szkiełkowska et al. [40] compared acoustic voice parameters before and after a CI in two groups of 40 children aged 3–7 and 7–12 years. After implantation, both groups received intensive rehabilitation and the voice parameters were then measured 6 months later. Most parameters improved and they correlated with better subjective voice quality. MPT was longer and voice range was wider. The main improvement of objective voice parameters were seen in Jitt, RAP, PPQ, SPPQ, VFo, ShdB, Shim, APQ, SAPQ, vAm, DUV, NUV, FTRI, and ATRI. In general, implantation followed by intensive rehabilitation allowed better control of voice frequency and amplitude, less tremor, and fewer voice breaks.

Kosztyła-Hojna et al. [41] examined voice and speech quality before and after cochlear implantation in two groups of patients: one with prelingual deafness and the other with post-lingual deafness. All patients had features of functional dysphonia, with a slight prevalence of hyperfunction in the prelingually deaf patients and hypo-function in the post-lingually deaf ones. After the CI, the quality of voice and speech in both groups improved. Improvements were mainly seen in parameters describing changes in amplitude and frequency.

Another study by Kosztyła-Hojna et al. [42] examined 21 adults with prelingual or post-lingual deafness. Before receiving a CI, the subjects showed a disturbed motorial function of the articulation organs and errors in articulation of vowels and consonants. After the CI, there was a substantial improvement in articulation, the voice became more stable, the scope of words was larger, and prosody improved [43].

3. Voice quality in partial deafness

Partial deafness (PD) is characterized by normal hearing thresholds at low frequencies and much poorer hearing thresholds (almost deaf) at high frequencies. In an audiogram this is seen as a hearing threshold curve that drops sharply at high frequencies. It is mainly seen in elderly patients, but may also affect individuals exposed to noise, take certain medications, or have a genetic predisposition. In contrast to other types of hearing impairment, the use of amplifying hearing aids in PD is constrained due to three physiological factors. The first factor is an abnormal loudness perception (recruitment), which makes the patient hear sounds louder than they really are. The second is poorer frequency resolution, which means that sound stimulation covers a larger group of hearing cells (there is an overlap of stimulus frequencies), and this leads to difficulty in the patient's sound discrimination. The third phenomenon is distortion caused by "dead areas" in the cochlea, where hearing cells are completely destroyed. In these areas, sounds cannot be perceived at all and so sounds have to be picked up by neighboring cells. Stimulation therefore covers broad areas and slightly different tones are perceived by the patient as the same. Together, these three factors mean that standard hearing aids giving unsatisfactory results for PD patients.

PD patients have therefore been left struggling to overcome their deficit. The use of cochlear implants in PD treatment has for many years been circumscribed due to the risk of damaging remaining hair cells, and hearing, while introducing an electrode into the cochlea. An important landmark in PD treatment was a novel type of cochlear implantation for this kind of dysfunction. This was done in an adult PD patient by Skarżyński and colleagues in 2002 [44], and 2 years later in a partially deaf child [45]. Success of the operation was possible thanks to the use of specially designed electrodes and a novel round window approach to the cochlea. In this way, electrical and acoustic stimulation were combined (so-called Electro-Acoustic-Stimulation, EAS), and offered a way for PD patients to receive improved hearing. Skarżyński's achievement began a systematic Partial Deafness Treatment Program in Poland, the first such program worldwide [44–49].

Like other hearing impairments, PD leads to voice abnormalities. However, the literature on the voice of PD patients before and after a CI is quite limited. The first study was done in the Institute of Physiology and Pathology of Hearing in Warsaw, Poland, by Myszel and Szkiełkowska [50]. They recruited 147 individuals, one group of 67 children aged 7–12 years and another of 80 adults. In one aspect, the voice of school-aged children was analyzed: 44 had prelingual partial deafness and 23 had normal hearing (a control group). As a second aspect, 80 adults were examined: 25 with bilateral post lingual partial deafness (13 females and 12 males) and 55 with normal hearing (28 females and 27 males, a control group). The average age of the partially deaf adults was 49.2 years and the average length of time they had had PD was 19.1 years. Voice parameters of both PD children and PD adults were tested 9 months after cochlear implantation.

All subjects were selected so as to exclude pre-existing conditions (palatal, alveolar, and lip clefts; inborn and acquired malformations of the larynx; paralytic dysphonia; allergy; gastro- esophageal reflux; thyroid disease; asthma; chronic obstructive pulmonary disease; mental or neurogenerative disorder; or delayed psychomotor development). Objective acoustic analysis of the voice was done with the Kay Elemetrics Multi Dimension Voice Program, and subjective analysis was done on the Hirano GRBAS scale.

Individuals were patients of the World Hearing Center of the Institute of Physiology and Pathology of Hearing in Kajetany, Warsaw, from 2014 to 2021. Every individual underwent a detailed anamnesis, otolaryngological examination, and hearing assessment. Hearing assessments included the use of pure tone audiometry, impedance audiometry, otoacoustic emissions, and brainstem evoked response audiometry, ensuring that patients fulfilled the PD criteria as described by Skarzynski [51].

Data analysis showed that, compared to normal hearing, PD in children leads to abnormalities in acoustic structure of the voice. The abnormalities involved most of the voice parameters, but the most important changes were in frequency, amplitude, noise, and voice tremor (F0, vF0, vAm, sAPQ, NHR, SPI, FTRI). In all the examined children, subjective assessment with GRBAS showed grade of hoarseness G1 or G2, roughness R1 or R2, breathy voice B1 or B2, and strain S1 or S2.

For the adults, the most statistically important changes involved the parameters describing frequency, amplitude, subharmonics, noise, voice breaks, and tremor (vF0, Jita, Jitt, APQ, sAPQ, RAP, vAm, %Shim, PPQ, sPPQ, DSH, NSH, DUV, NHR). However, no statistical changes were observed in F0, SPI, or VTI. Adults displayed grade of hoarseness G1 or G2, roughness R1 or R2, breathy voice B1, asthenic A1 or A2, and strain S1 or S2. The voice of all PD patients appeared to be slightly harsh, rough, breathy, or asthenic.

Both children and adults were examined 9 months after cochlear implantation. In children, the biggest improvement in voice parameters was observed in frequency, amplitude, noise, and tremor. Normal values were seen in F0, vF0, vAm, sAPQ, NHR, and FTRI. In adults, statistically significant improvements were observed in parameters describing frequency, amplitude, noise, voice irregularities, and subharmonics; normal parameters were seen in vF0, vAm, sAPQ, Shim, NHR, DUV, DSH, and NSH.

In subjective assessment, the voice of PD patients also improved after receiving a CI, especially in grade, roughness, and breathiness. The improvements made their voices less harsh, less breathy, and less asthenic. Apart from the perceptive improvement, strong correlations were observed between the voice quality assessed subjectively and acoustic voice parameters: G (grade) correlated with vF0 and Shim; R (roughness) correlated with DSH and NSH; B (breathiness) correlated with NSH and NHR; and A (asthenic) correlated with DUV. A weak correlation was observed between S (strain) and both DUV and NHR.

It was concluded that PD leads to voice abnormalities both in children and adults. In both groups statistically significant changes involved parameters describing frequency, amplitude, and presence of noise. The number of years of hearing deprivation was an important factor in determining changes in the voice. In adult PD patients, voice abnormalities affected a wider range of acoustic parameters.

In both children and adults, it is clear that there is a strong correlation between acoustic voice parameters and subjective features. Importantly, cochlear implantation in PD patients strongly improves the voice, normalizing its acoustic structure and subjective character.

4. Summary

Hearing impairment leads to disruption of auditory control of the voice via the central nervous system, creating voice disorders classified as dysphonia. The degree of dysphonia depends on when the hearing loss began (prelingual or post-lingual), its duration, and its severity.

Children born with hearing impairment do start to develop a voice, but its development is delayed compared to healthy children and further development into good speech requires audiological intervention.

Patients with hearing impairment develop voice disorders of a functional type, and these are evident both in perceptual assessments as well as in objective examinations (i.e. acoustic voice parameters). The changes are mostly seen in terms of amplitude, frequency, tremor, and noise. The voice of hearing-impaired patients is usually rough, breathy, asthenic, and strained. Some patients develop nasality. Apart from a different voice characteristic in hearing-impaired patients, there are also morphological changes of the larynx, articulatory organs, and changes in chest biomechanics.

Numerous studies conducted worldwide have demonstrated that, depending on the severity of the hearing loss, the use of hearing aids or cochlear implants improves hearing ability. After regaining auditory control, the voice quality improves in all types of hearing impairment, both in children and in adults. Research shows that, in general, cochlear implants are more effective and improve voice quality faster than hearing aids. The voice of children with cochlear implants is better as soon as a few months after intervention, and the improvement continues progressively. Objective parameters describing changes in amplitude and frequency steadily improve, and tremor and noise decrease or disappear. Perceptive assessment shows the voice becoming less harsh, more stable, and less dull.

Studies performed in the Institute of Physiology and Pathology of Hearing in Warsaw have provided data on voice quality in partial deafness before and after cochlear implantation. The results show that both children and adults with partial deafness develop dysphonia of different degrees, although the number of altered acoustic parameters is higher in adults than in children. After cochlear implantation, however, the voice quality of both children and adults improves, and this is reflected in both objective and subjective assessments.

5. Conclusions

Contemporary medicine gives more and more treatment opportunities for different groups of patients, including those who suffer congenital or acquired hearing impairment. Cochlear implantation is now a treatment of choice for patients with deafness or hypoacusis (including partial deafness), giving them a chance to regain hearing and improve quality of living.

Problems faced by hearing impaired people are seen in many areas of life, including communication, professional life, mental conditions and self-esteem. Voice disorders resulting from hearing impairment is one of the factors underlying patients distress.

Therefore, the procedure of cochlear implantation by enabling better hearing and voice quality improvement, helps to improve patients' comfort and life quality in many aspects.

Author details

Karol Myszel[1*] and Piotr Henryk Skarżyński[1,2,3,4,5]

1 Center of Hearing and Speech MEDINCUS, Poland

2 Department of Teleaudiology and Screening, World Hearing Center, Institute of Physiology and Pathology of Hearing, Warsaw, Poland

3 Heart Failure and Cardiac Rehabilitation Department, Faculty of Dental Medicine, Medical University of Warsaw, Warsaw, Poland

4 Institute of Sensory Organs, Poland

5 University of Maria-Curie Sklodowska, Lublin, Poland

*Address all correspondence to: karol@myszel.pl

References

[1] Szkiełkowska A. Voice Disorders Caused by Hearing Impairment. University Handbook: Rudiments of Neurologopedics. Opole: University of Opole; 2005. pp. 629-653

[2] Moulin-Frier C, Nguyen S, Oudeyer P. Self-organization of early vocal development in infants and machines: The role of intrinsic motivation. Frontiers in Psychology. 2014;**4**:1006

[3] Guenther FH. Cortical interactions underlying the production of speech sounds. Journal of Communication Disorders. 2006;**39**:350-365

[4] Maskarinec A, Cairns E, Weamer D. Longitudinal observations of individual infant's vocalizations. Journal of Speech and Hearing Disorders. 1981;**46**:267-273

[5] Moeller M, Hoover B, Putman C, Arbataitis K, Bohnenkamp G, Peterson B, et al. Vocalizations of infants with hearing loss compared with infants with normal hearing: Part I – Phonetic development. Ear & Hearing. 2007;**28**:605-627

[6] Moeller M, Hoover B, Putman C, Arbataitis K, Bohnenkamp G, Peterson B, et al. Vocalizations of infants with hearing loss compared with infants with normal hearing: Part II – Transition to words. Ear & Hearing. 2007;**28**:628-642

[7] Stoel-Gammon C, Otomo K. Babbling development of hearing-impaired and normally hearing subjects. The Journal of Speech and Hearing Disorders. 1986;**51**:33-41

[8] Mowrer O. Learning Theory and the Symbolic Processes. New York: John Wiley & Sons; 1960

[9] Fagan M. Frequency of vocalization before and after cochlear implantation: Dynamic effect of auditory feedback on infant behavior. Journal of Experimental Child Psychology. 2014;**126**:328-338

[10] Von Hapsburg D, Davis B. Auditory sensitivity and the prelinguistic vocalizations of early-amplified infants. Journal of Speech and Hearing Research. 2006;**49**:809-822

[11] Oller D, Eilers R, Bull D, Carney A. Prespeech vocalizations of a deaf infant: A comparison with normal metaphonological development. Journal of Speech and Hearing Research. 1985;**28**:47-63

[12] Campisi P, Low A, Papsin B, Mount R, Harrison R. Multidimensional voice program analysis in profoundly deaf children: Quantifying frequency and amplitude control. Perceptual and Motor Skills. 2006;**103**:40-50

[13] Pruszewicz A, Demenko G, Wika T. Variability analysis of Fo parameter in the voice of individuals with hearing disturbances. Acta Oto-Laryngologica. 1993;**113**(3):450-454

[14] Evans M, Deliyski D. Acoustic voice analysis of prelingually deaf adults before and after cochlear implantation. Journal of Voice. 2007;**21**(6):669-682

[15] Holler T, Campisi P, Allegro J, Chadha N, Harrison R, Papsin B, et al. Abnormal voicing in children using cochlear implants. Archives of Otolaryngology – Head & Neck Surgery. 2010;**136**(1):17-21

[16] Szkiełkowska A, Ratyńska J, Skarżyński H, Michalak T. Acoustic structure of voice in children considered

for partial deafness treatment (PDT). The Journal of Health Science. 2012;**2**(2):75-80

[17] Campisi P, Low A, Papsin B, Mount R, Cohen-Kerem R, Harrison R. Acoustic analysis of the voice in pediatric cochlear implant recipients: A longitudinal study. Laryngoscope. 2005;**115**(6):1046-1050

[18] Manning W, Moore J, Dunham M, Lu F, Domico E. Vowel production in a prelinguistic child following cochlear implantation. Journal of the American Academy of Audiology. 1992;**3**(1):16-21

[19] Perrin E, Berger-Vachon C, Topouzkhanian A, Truy E, Morgon A. Evaluation of cochlear implanted children's voices. International Journal of Pediatric Otorhinolaryngology. 1999;**47**(2):181-186

[20] Seifert E, Oswald M, Bruns U, Vischer M, Kompis M, Haeusler R. Changes of voice and articulation in children with cochlear implants. International Journal of Pediatric Otorhinolaryngology. 2002;**66**(2):115-123

[21] Szyfter W, Pruszewicz A, Woznica B, Swidzinski P, Szymiec E, Karlik M. The acoustic analysis of voice in patients with multi-channel cochlear implant. Revue de Laryngologie Otologie Rhinologie. 1996;**117**(3):225-227

[22] Szkiełkowska A. Rehabilitation of children with cochlear implants. Audiofonologia. 1999;**15**:133-141

[23] Skrypnik I, Grzanka A, Puuronen S, Szkiełkowska A. Selection of voice features to diagnose hearing impairments of children. IEEE CS Press. 2001:427-432

[24] Szkiełkowska A. Influence of Sensorineural Hearing Impairment on Voice Quality in Children. PhD Dissertation. Warsaw, Poland: Warsaw Medical University; 2001

[25] Lock R, Seaver E. Nasality and velopharyngeal function in five hearing impaired adults. Journal of Communication Disorders. 1984;**17**(1):47-64

[26] Baudonck N, Lierde V, D'haeseleer E, Dhooge I. Nasalence and nasality in children with cochlear implants and children with hearing aids. International Journal of Pediatric Otorhinolaryngology. 2015:7449

[27] Swapna S, Sreedevi N, Lepcha A, Mathew J. Nasalence in cochlear implantees. Clinical and Experimental Otorhinolaryngology. 2015;**8**(3):202-205

[28] Ysunza A, Vazquez M. Velopharyngeal sphincter physiology in deaf individuals. The Cleft Palate-Craniofacial Journal. 1993;**30**(2):141-143

[29] Fletcher S, Mahfuzh F, Hendarmin H. Nasalence in the speech of children with normal hearing and children with hearing loss. American Journal of Speech-Language Pathology. 1999;**8**(3):241-248

[30] Colton R, Cooker H. Perceived nasality in the speech of the deaf. Journal of Speech and Hearing Research. 1968;**11**:553-559

[31] Stevens K, Nickerson R, Boothhroyd A, Rollins A. Assessment of nasalization in the speech of deaf children. Journal of Speech, Language, and Hearing Research. 1976;**19**:393-416

[32] Fletcher S, Higgins J. Performance of children with severe to profound auditory impairment in instrumentally guided reduction of nasal resonance. The Journal of Speech and Hearing Disorders. 1980;**45**:181-194

[33] Chen M. Acoustic parameters of nasalized vowels in hearing-impaired and normal-hearing speakers. The Journal of the Acoustical Society of America. 1995;**98**:2443

[34] Das B, Chatterjee I, Kumar S. Laryngeal aerodynamics in children with hearing impairment versus age and height matched normal hearing peers. Otolaryngology. 2013:394604

[35] Forner L, Hixon T. Respiratory kinematics in profoundly hearing impaired speakers. Journal of Speech and Hearing Research. 1977;**20**(2):373-408

[36] Myszel K, Szkiełkowska A. Development of voice in hearing-impaired individuals: Overview of physio-pathological aspects. Journal of Hearing Science. 2020;**10**(3):19-23

[37] Szkiełkowska A, Myszel K. Acoustic voice parameters in hearing-impaired, school-aged children: Research study outcomes. Journal of Clinical Otorhinolaryngology. 2021;**3**(3)

[38] Hocevar-Boltezar I, Vatovec J, Gros A, Zargi M. The influence of cochlear implantation on some voice parameters. International Journal of Pediatric Otorhinolaryngology. 2005;**69**(12):1635-1640

[39] Kishon-Rabin L, Taitelbaum R, Tobin Y, Hildesheimer M. The effect of partially restored hearing on speech production of postlingually deafened adults with multichannel cochlear implants. The Journal of the Acoustical Society of America. 1999;**106**(5):2843-2857

[40] Szkiełkowska A, Maniecka-Aleksandrowicz B, Dolecki J. Rehabilitacja głosu dzieci z implantami ślimakowymi. Audiofonologia. 1999;**15**:132-139

[41] Kosztyła-Hojna B, Moskal D, Kasperuk J, Falkowski D, Rutkowski R. Ocena mowy i zaburzeń językowych u chorych z implantem ślimakowym – doniesienie wstępne. Pol Merkuriusz Lek. 2010;**27**(171):187-193

[42] Kosztyła-Hojna B, Rogowski M, Kasperuk M, Rutkowski R, Ryćko P. Analiza jakości głosu i mowy u pacjentów z implantem ślimakowym – doniesienie wstępne. Pol Merkuriusz Lek. 2009;**27**(160):305-310

[43] Myszel K, Skarżyński PH. Zmiany głosu i mowy u pacjentów po wszczepieniu systemu implantu ślimakowego. Analiza wybranych danych literaturowych. Now Audiofonol. 2018;**7**(1):19-24

[44] Skarzyński H, Lorens A, Piotrowska A. A new method of partial deafness treatment. Medical Science Monitor. 2003;**9**(4):20-24

[45] Skarzynski H, Lorens A, Dziendziel B, Skarzynski PH. Electro-natural stimulation (ENS) in partial deafness treatment: Pediatric case series. Otology & Neurotology. 2019;**40**(2):171-176

[46] Skarzynski H, Lorens A, Dziendziel B, Rajchel JJ, Matusiak M, Skarzynski PH. Electro-natural stimulation in partial deafness treatment of adult cochlear implant users: Long-term hearing preservation results. Journal of Otorhinolaryngology Related Specials. 2019;**81**(2-3):63-72

[47] Skarzynski H, Lorens A, Piotrowska A, Anderson I. Partial deafness cochlear implantation in children. International Journal of Pediatric Otorhinolaryngology. 2007;**71**(9):1407-1413

[48] Skarzynski H. Long-term results of partial deafness treatment. Cochlear

Implants International. 2014;**15**(Suppl. 1):21-23

[49] Skarzynski PH, Skarzynski H, Dziendziel B, Rajchel JJ, Gos E, Lorens A. Hearing preservation with the use of Flex20 and Flex24 electrodes in patients with partial deafness. Otology & Neurotology. 2019;**40**(9):1153-1159

[50] Myszel K, Szkiełkowska A. Quality of voice in patients with partial deafness before and after cochlear implantation. Journal of Voice. 2022

[51] Skarzynski H, Lorens A. Partial deafness treatment. Cochlear Implants International. 2010;**11**(Suppl. 1):29-41

Section 2

Hearing Loss and Precision Medicine

Chapter 8

Hearing Aid Directional Microphone Systems for Hearing in Noise

Charlotte T. Jespersen

Abstract

Sensorineural hearing loss is the most common type of permanent hearing loss. Most people with sensorineural hearing loss experience challenges with hearing in noisy situations, and this is the primary reason they seek help for their hearing loss. It also remains an area where hearing aid users often struggle. Directionality is the only hearing aid technology—in addition to amplification—proven to help hearing aid users hear better in noise. It amplifies sounds (sounds of interest) coming from one direction more than sounds ("noise") coming from other directions, thereby providing a directional benefit. This book chapter describes the hearing-in-noise problem, natural directivity and hearing in noise, directional microphone systems, how directionality is quantified, and its benefits, limitations, and other clinical implications.

Keywords: hearing-in-noise, natural directivity, directional microphone systems, microphone arrays, fixed and adaptive arrays, benefits, limitations, and clinical implications

1. Introduction

The inability to hear in noise is a strong driver of help-seeking among people with hearing loss. Although satisfaction with hearing aids is high among users, they are often relatively less satisfied with how well they hear in noisy backgrounds when wearing their hearing aids [1]. The most common solution to help people who use hearing aids to hear better in noise is the use of directional microphone systems, also called simply "directionality". This technology allows hearing aids to amplify sound from one direction more than sound from other directions and can thereby reduce interfering noise that arises from a different location than the sound of interest. With digital technology, the performance capabilities and automatic control of directionality has increased in complexity and sophistication with the purpose of increasing both benefit and ease of use for the hearing aid user.

2. Why do people with hearing loss have trouble hearing in noise?

People with sensorineural hearing loss (SNHL) have reduced audibility of soft sounds which means their thresholds of hearing are elevated, such that they cannot hear soft sounds that people with normal hearing can. People with mild to even moderate-severe hearing loss are known to report that they have little-to-no difficulty hearing in one-on-one conversations in quieter environments but struggle to understand speech when there are multiple people talking or when in background noise. It is often these increased difficulties hearing in noise or more adverse listening conditions that makes them pursue hearing aids.

SNHL involves damage to the cochlea and often the peripheral neural pathway of the auditory system. Because this system is nonlinear in its behavior, so are the effects of damage on perception of sound. In addition to the loss of hearing sensitivity already mentioned, those with SNHL show effects on how sound above hearing thresholds is perceived, including:

- Frequency dependent loss of audibility. SNHL tends to affect high frequencies to a greater degree than lower frequencies. Because the sensation of loudness is dominated by lower frequency sound, some people may not even recognize that they have hearing loss until their hearing loss progresses enough that it impacts more daily listening situations. Many high-frequency consonant sounds are crucial for speech understanding, especially in background noise, and loss of audibility in higher frequencies can have a disproportionate negative impact. (for a review, see Ref. [2]).

- Reduced dynamic range of hearing. In SNHL, thresholds of hearing sensitivity are elevated, while levels of discomfort are not correspondingly higher. Therefore, the dynamic range (difference between threshold of hearing and loudness discomfort) is reduced. People with SNHL may not hear soft sounds but may find loud sounds equally as bothersome as those with normal hearing. This is partly because those with hearing loss experience a more rapid growth of loudness compared to people with normal hearing, which is referred to as "loudness recruitment". How SNHL affects loudness perception is outlined in detail by Moore [3].

- Poorer frequency and temporal resolution. The ability to discriminate sounds that are closely spaced in frequency and/or in time is less in persons with SNHL compared to those with normal hearing. This can result in some sounds being "covered up" by others, which contributes to difficulties hearing in noisy environments. There are excellent descriptions of reduced frequency and temporal resolution [3].

- Reduced pitch perception. The ability to detect changes in frequency over time is poorer than normal with SNHL. This may impair, for example the ability to perceive pitch patterns of speech, to discern which are the emphasized words in an utterance, and to determine whether what is being said is a question or a statement. Pitch also conveys information about a speaker's gender, age, and emotional state. This means that people with hearing loss may have more difficulty with perception of these basic, but important aspects of understanding speech and the speaker's intention. A more detailed review of the negative impact of reduced pitch perception is available [3].

- Reduced binaural processing abilities. The ability to integrate, analyze, and compare information received from each ear is poorer with SNHL compared to those with normal hearing, and contributes to difficulties hearing in noisy environments. Differences in frequency, intensity, timing, and phase of information received by each ear in a listening environment provide the brainstem with cues needed to help determine the location a sound is coming from, and to best extract speech out of background noise. These cues are degraded in people with hearing loss. There are thorough overviews of binaural hearing abilities [3].

These effects are all contributors to the experience of difficulties hearing in noise that most people with SNHL report. Perceived difficulties with hearing in noise are also reflected in objective performance measures. SNHL results in poorer speech understanding in noise compared to normal hearing in the same situation. Many speech tests measure percent correct at a given signal-to-noise ratio (SNR). SNR indicates the relationship between the signal of interest e.g., speech, as compared to background noise. It is expressed in decibels (dB), and a SNR of 0 dB indicates that the signal level is equal to the noise level. A positive SNR value indicates that the signal is greater than the noise, and a negative SNR value indicates that the signal is less than the noise. Effectively, the greater the SNR, the easier it is to hear the signal of interest among the noise. Another useful way to quantify performance differences in addition to speech recognition in noise tests is to quantify performance differences by measuring a person's SNR loss [4]. SNR loss is defined as the increase in SNR required by a person with hearing loss to understand speech in noise, relative to the average SNR required for a person with normal hearing. Research has shown that people with hearing loss may require SNR improvements ranging from 2 to 18 dB, depending on the magnitude of the hearing loss, to hear as well as people with normal hearing under the same listening conditions [3–8]. The reduced ability to understand speech in noise seems to mainly be caused by decreased audibility for people with mild and mild-moderate hearing losses. For people with severe and profound losses, and for some people with more moderate loss, decreased frequency and temporal resolution seem to play a larger role in their reduced ability to understand speech in noise [2, 3].

SNHL occurs with various degrees and combinations of decreased audibility, reduced dynamic range, deficits in frequency/pitch and temporal resolution, and poor binaural hearing processing. Regardless of the specific deficits for a person with hearing loss, SNHL results in poorer speech understanding compared to normal hearing in the same situation even when the person with hearing loss uses hearing aids. The reduced ability to understand speech in noise seems to mainly be caused by decreased audibility for people with mild and mild-moderate hearing losses. For people with severe and profound losses, and for some people with more moderate loss, decreased frequency and temporal resolution seem to play a larger role in their reduced ability to understand speech in noise [2, 3].

If the hearing loss is not too severe, loss of audibility can be compensated for by hearing aids, because amplification can focus on those frequencies where speech has the softest components e.g., typically the high frequencies, which is likewise where hearing loss is typically the greatest. On the other hand, it is more challenging to compensate for the other auditory processing deficits that cause difficulties hearing in background noise with hearing aids. For example, reduced frequency and temporal resolution degrade important speech cues, effectively decreasing the SNR of the auditory information processed at the auditory periphery before it ascends to the auditory cortex where it is "heard" [2]. All hearing aids can do to minimize the problems caused by reduced frequency resolution is to keep noise from being amplified by the hearing aids as much as possible, and to provide appropriate variation of gain by frequency so that low-frequency parts of speech or noise do not mask the high-frequency parts of speech and so that frequency regions dominated by noise are not louder than frequency regions dominated by speech.

A proven solution to compensate for hearing difficulties in noise beyond what can be obtained with hearing aid amplification is to use directional microphone systems [9, 10]. These work by amplifying sounds coming from one direction more than sounds from other directions, and thereby reducing interfering noise that arises from a different location than the desired sound and providing an SNR benefit. Directionality is the only hearing aid technology, apart from amplification itself, that has been shown to improve speech recognition in noisy situations [9, 10].

3. Natural directivity and hearing in noise

People with normal hearing use naturally provided directional and spatial perception cues to hear in both quiet and noisy environments. It is useful to understand how this is accomplished as directional microphone systems may interfere with, or conversely, attempt to preserve or replicate these natural perceptual advantages.

Listening with two ears (binaural hearing) compared to with only one ear (monaural hearing), has benefits that arise from several monaural and binaural cues that contribute to an improved ability to hear in noise [11, 12].

Sound from each ear creates a cohesive auditory image in the central auditory system of the surroundings in terms of the number, distance, direction, and orientation of sound sources, and the amount of reverberation [3]. Binaural hearing provides perceptual advantages in terms of localization of sound, an increase in loudness, noise suppression effects, and improved speech clarity and sound quality. Binaural hearing enables us to selectively attend to something of specific interest, like a single voice among many talkers [2].

3.1 Localization via binaural and monaural cues

One thing that listening with two ears helps us to do is to determine which direction sound comes from. This is because the sound arriving at each ear will be different in terms of loudness, time of arrival, and spectral shape, and our brains can decode these cues.

Sound originating closer to one ear will reach that ear sooner and with higher intensity than the other more distant ear. Low-frequency sound has long wavelengths that are longer than the curved distance between the two ears and will bend around the head, maintaining the intensity of the sound between the ears. However, sound originating on one side of the head will arrive at the ear on that side before it reaches the ear on the other side. This difference in time of arrival between the ears is called the interaural time difference (ITD) and is the most salient cue for determining whether sound comes from the right or left side.

High-frequency sound has short wavelengths that are shorter than the dimensions of the head resulting in high-frequency sound being diffracted by the head. This diffraction of high-frequency sound results in more intense sound in the ear on the side of the head closest to the sound and an attenuation of sound going around the head to the other ear, with the latter being a phenomenon known as the "head shadow effect".

This difference in intensity of sound between the two ears is called the interaural level difference (ILD) [12]. Cues for ITD are most efficient at frequencies 1500 Hz and below, while cues for ILD are most pronounced above 1500 Hz [13]. The ITD and ILD cues are binaural cues that help with localizing which side a sound is coming from (lateralization).

The main cues for localizing sound in terms of elevation (up-down localization) and in the front or back are provided by diffraction patterns of sound striking the head, pinnae, and upper body [11]. High-frequency sound is boosted by the pinnae, head, and upper body when arriving from the front, and is attenuated when arriving from behind. Although this spectral shaping of sound is a monaural cue, listeners require both monaural and binaural cues to localize correctly [2, 14].

The cues upon which sound localization is based (i.e., ITDs, ILDs, and spectral shaping) also enable spatial hearing, which is the ability to localize and externalize sounds in terms of direction and distance. Spatial hearing provides a broader sense of the environment, thereby helping segregate sounds to choose what to focus on [2, 11, 12].

People with normal hearing uses redundancy in these binaural and monaural cues. When they are in more difficult listening conditions where some of the cues are masked, they can still make use of those that are not. A low-frequency noise "covering up" the ITD cues of a desired sound can for instance easily be compensated by the high-frequency ILD cues. People with hearing loss usually cannot as easily take advantage of this redundancy [12, 15].

3.2 Hearing in noise

When in noise, a person can hear speech more effectively with two ears than with one because of the ability to localize sound, but also because of the head shadow effect, binaural redundancy, and binaural squelch. These binaural cues become advantageous when people leverage them to achieve their listening goals in noise, even though this is somewhat unconscious.

Binaural squelch refers to the auditory system's ability to employ ITD and ILD cues to spatially separate competing sounds and to attend to the ear with the better SNR [11].

Binaural redundancy is the advantage of receiving the same signal at both ears. When the same signal is received at both ears the treatment of information is more sensitive to small differences in intensity and frequency, and speech recognition is improved in the presence of noise. Binaural redundancy includes binaural loudness summation, where the loudness of a sound is greater if it is heard with two ears as opposed to with only one [11].

Binaural listening can be described in terms of two broad strategies: the "better ear strategy" and the "awareness strategy" [16]. The better ear strategy describes the advantage of one ear having a better SNR than the other ear in noise, due to the diffraction pattern from the head that leads to a different SNR in each ear when the desired signal and noise reach the head from different directions. People using the better ear strategy will position themselves relative to the desired sound to maximize the audibility of that sound, and they will rely on the ear with the best representation or best SNR of that sound [2, 11]. The combined directivity characteristics of the two ears form a perceptually focused beam that can be taken advantage of depending on the desired sound's location. Therefore, if at least one ear has a favorable SNR, then the auditory system will take advantage of it.

The awareness strategy is an extension of the better ear strategy. This strategy includes the all-around aspects of binaural listening that allow a person to remain connected and aware of the surrounding soundscape when the head shadow effect improves the SNR in one of the two ears. Due to the geometric location of the two ears on the head, the brain can either use the head shadow to enhance the sound of interest or make the head acoustically "disappear" from the sound scene so that the person can attend to sounds all around.

Although they may be experienced to a lesser degree, binaural hearing advantages also exist in the presence of peripheral damage to the auditory system. Bilaterally-fitted hearing aids can maintain and enhance binaural hearing advantages by making auditory cues audible [2, 15]. However, this is provided that the way the sound is collected and processed by the hearing aids gives the appropriate input for the brain to make use of the cues. In other words, hearing aids can support binaural hearing advantages, but they can also interfere with them.

4. How directionality is quantified

Directional microphone systems help address the most fundamental problem of people with hearing loss i.e., understanding speech when there are multiple speakers or when in background noise. These systems provide a directional beam of sounds that are amplified more than sounds from other directions, thereby providing a better SNR compared to when the hearing aid amplifies sounds from all directions equally. As a prerequisite to understanding the operating principle of directional microphone systems and the factors that affect the performance, it makes sense to first discuss how performance is measured and represented.

How well a directional microphone system amplifies sounds from one direction while attenuating sounds from other directions can be quantified electro-acoustically [17] and is usually illustrated in a polar pattern. Polar patterns are displayed on a circular graph, displaying the entire 360° sensitivity response of the system, with 0° marking the frontward-facing direction. When referring to a directional microphone system's pickup pattern, sound not coming from directly in front of the microphone (0°) is referred to as off-axis. Greater attenuation equates to less sound being picked up by the directional microphone system. An omnidirectional (non-directional) microphone's polar pattern is equally sensitive to sounds from all directions and has the shape of a circle [2]. Directional microphone systems can provide an indefinite number of different polar patterns. The polar pattern can be unchangeable ("fixed") and/or flexible and adapting between multiple polar patterns depending on the listening environment. Furthermore, different polar patterns will be evident for different frequencies for any given directional microphone system. **Figure 1** shows the most prototypical polar patterns starting from the left with an omnidirectional polar pattern with a bold black line indicating a polar pattern that is equally sensitive to sounds from all directions (360°), followed by a cardioid polar pattern with the bold black line indicating a polar pattern showing excellent sensitivity to the front (0°), reduced sensitivity to the sides (90° and 270°), and minimal sensitivity to the rear (180°). Next is a super-cardioid polar pattern with the black line indicating a polar pattern that shows excellent sensitivity to the front (0°), reduced sensitivity to the sides (90° and 270°) and some sensitivity to the rear (180°). The fourth plot from the left shows a hyper-cardioid polar pattern with the black line indicating a polar pattern that is

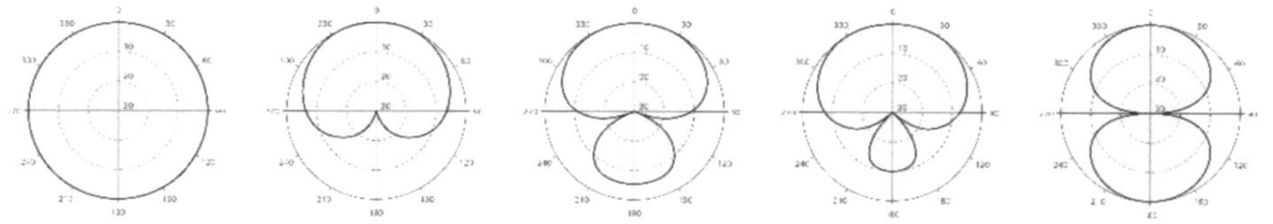

Figure 1.
The figure is showing the following polar patterns from the left: Omnidirectional-, cardioid-, super-cardioid-, hyper-cardioid-, and a bi-directional polar pattern (in dB).

very much like the hyper-cardioid, but with less sensitivity to the rear (180°). The last illustration shows a bi-directional polar pattern with the black line illustrating a polar pattern that has the same sensitivity to the front (0°) as to the rear (180°) with reduced sensitivity to either side.

The polar pattern of a directional microphone system can be measured either in free space or in/on the ear of a person. When measured in free space, the polar patterns look like those shown in **Figure 1**. The head and pinna affect the intensity of sound reaching the ear canal as described above. The acoustic effects of the head shadow and pinna also affect the intensity of the sound reaching the hearing aid microphones. Therefore, the polar patterns of a directional microphone system as worn on the head will be different than the polar patterns measured in free space. The head and pinna attenuate sounds when the head and pinna are placed between the sound and the directional microphone system (Head shadow effect) and boost the sound when the directional microphone system is next to the head and pinna and close to the sound. The attenuation and boosting effect of the head and pinna increases with frequency [2].

Another way of quantifying directionality is by use of the directivity index (in dB). The directivity index shows a directional microphone system's sensitivity to sounds from the front compared to its mean sensitivity to sounds from all other directions [17]. The comparison to the mean of sounds from all other directions can be to sounds from all other directions in a two-dimensional (2D) horizontal plane (in a circle) or in a three-dimensional (3D) space (in a sphere) [2]. The directivity index can also be weighted according to a speech importance function called the Articulation Index. This is intended to provide a better prediction of how directivity will influence actual speech recognition in noise performance. The directivity index, with and without the articulation index weighting, has been found to correlate well with speech recognition in noise performance, although the weighting function does not appear to increase the accuracy of predicting perceptual benefit [17].

A directional microphone system's directionality can also be quantified by its front-to-back ratio. This measure shows the system's sensitivity to sounds from in front (0°) relative to sounds from directly behind (180°). This measure captures less information about the directional characteristics of the system than polar patterns or directivity index. It is most useful in determining whether a system is directional or not, rather than in describing its characteristics.

Perceptual or behavioral testing is a clinical way to measure directionality, and this is very commonly reported as an outcome in the literature on directional microphone systems. Adaptive tests that determine an SNR at which listeners achieve a certain performance level, such as 50% correct recognition, are the most efficient approach and allow data from groups of listeners to be easily combined.

5. Directional microphone systems

Directional hearing aids appeared on the market in 1971 [17]. Those devices were equipped with a directional microphone, which is a single microphone with a directional polar pattern. Hearing aid directionality has evolved since and directionality is today offered via two-microphone and four-microphone arrays. Various terms are used to describe these systems. For simplicity, they are often referred to as "directional microphones" even though the systems are built from multiple omnidirectional microphones.

The basic principles of how an omnidirectional and directional microphone work will be explained before discussing today's directional microphone systems, as today's technologies are based on the same principles. In an omnidirectional microphone, sound waves enter through a single sound port and reach one side of a very thin and flexible diaphragm within the microphone as shown in **Figure 2** (left panel). The sound waves cause the diaphragm to deflect and, by different means depending on the microphone type, the deflections are converted into an analogous electrical signal. An omnidirectional microphone is, as previously mentioned, equally sensitive to sounds from all directions when in a free space i.e., when not worn on the head by a hearing aid user.

A microphone can be made directional (more sensitive to sounds from one direction than from other directions) by having two sound ports, a front and a rear sound port, that feed sounds to each their side of the diaphragm as shown in **Figure 2** (right panel). Since it is assumed that hearing aid users will be facing the sound they want to hear, directional microphones are positioned in the hearing aid to be most sensitive to sound coming from the front. Sound arising from the rear will enter the rear sound port first, and the front sound port shortly after. The time it takes sound to travel between the two sound ports is called the "external delay". An acoustic filter added to the microphone design delays the sound entering the rear sound port, this is called the "internal delay". Depending on the wavelength of the sound, and the internal and external delays, the sound striking the diaphragm from each side will either add or subtract. If the sound subtracts, the deflection of the diaphragm will be smaller or perhaps it will not deflect at all, and a less intense signal or no signal will be transduced into an electrical signal. Acoustic filters can be chosen that optimize subtraction—or phase cancelation—of sound arriving from the rear, resulting in different polar patterns. Both delays are fixed in a directional microphone. The external delay determined by the sound port spacing is fixed in the physical design. The internal delay is determined by a physical acoustic filter with a specific delay.

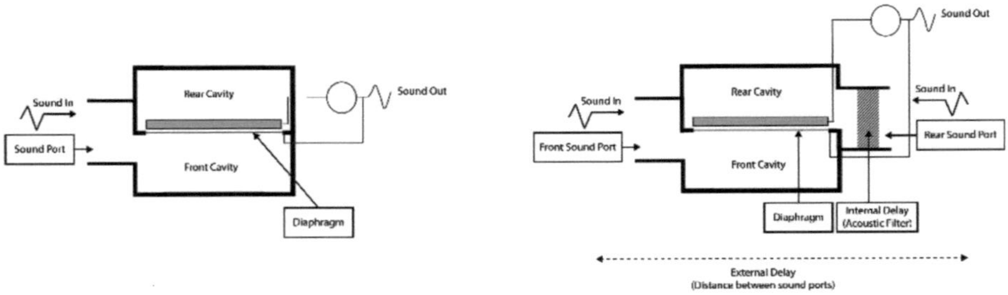

Figure 2.
Left: Illustration of an omnidirectional microphone. Right: Illustration of a directional microphone.

A directional microphone can consequently only provide one unchangeable directional polar pattern i.e., directionality is fixed.

5.1 Directional microphone arrays

Today, directionality in hearing aids is offered via microphone arrays, also called beamformers, that can be split into three categories as described below. Pertaining to directionality, the term beamformer is used to indicate that the microphone system in the hearing aid is directional. A beamformer is a type of microphone array used in hearing aids in which directional sensitivity is increased significantly in one direction, and reduced in all other directions, hence forming a "beam" in the direction of the greatest sensitivity [12, 18]. The following microphone array terminology will be used throughout this text for convenience:

- Two-microphone arrays: Consisting of two omnidirectional microphones located within the body of one hearing aid. Also referred to as "dual or twin microphone systems", unilateral beamformers, and first-order subtractive directional microphones [2, 19, 20].

- Four-microphone arrays: Consisting of the output from all four microphones of a bilaterally-fitted pair of hearing aids, each containing two microphones. Also referred to as bilateral beamformers [2, 19, 20]. This type of system requires a wired or wireless connection between the hearing aids to allow exchange of the audio signals at the two ears.

- Multi-microphone arrays: Consisting of three or more microphones on one device or multiple microphones placed on optical glasses. Also referred to as second-order directional microphones [2, 19–21]. Multi-microphone arrays are not currently used in hearing aids and will for this reason not be discussed further here.

5.1.1 Two-microphone arrays (unilateral beamformers)

The most common method of providing directionality in hearing aids is to use two omnidirectional microphones located within the body of the hearing aid. These two microphones are commonly referred to as the front and rear microphone and they serve an analogous function to the front and rear sound ports of a traditional directional microphone. When in a frontward-facing directional polar pattern, the sound from the rear microphone is subtracted from the front microphone (e.g., out of phase) to pick up sound from the front of the hearing aid user while attenuating sound from the rear. The areas of greatest sound attenuation are often referred to as "nulls". As with a traditional directional microphone, the polar pattern of the two-microphone array is determined by the ratio between the external delay and the internal delay. The external delay is the port spacing between the two microphones, while the internal delay is carried out in the digital signal processing [19]. The delay ratio defines how directional the two-microphone array will be, whether it will be a cardioid or a hyper-cardioid pattern for instance [2]. The external delay is fixed as it is dictated by the distance between the two microphones and cannot be adjusted in real time. The internal digital delay can be adjusted to provide different polar patterns. The polar patten of two-microphone arrays are in other words flexible.

5.1.2 Four-microphone arrays (bilateral beamformers)

Many hearing aids can exchange data and stream audio between a bilaterally-fitted pair of hearing aids. This has led to expanding the types of microphone arrays available in hearing aids. One such array is a four-microphone array, which utilizes all four microphones available on a bilaterally-fitted pair of hearing aids. The two hearing aids exchange audio information, which allows summing and/or subtraction of the audio signals between both hearing aids before combining the sound into one monaural output. The monaural output is then delivered to both hearing aids. Compared to a pair of hearing aids using two-microphone arrays independently, a four-microphone array can thus provide an even narrower polar pattern (beam).

Numerous methods for processing in four-microphone arrays exist and have been discussed in the literature [2, 19, 20, 22]. The most basic method is similar to two-microphone arrays, with the output of each independent two-microphone system that is treated similarly to the output from one microphone in a two-microphone array. By manipulating the internal delays in this system, the direction of maximum sensitivity is determined, along with potential frequency dependent and adaptive behavior.

5.1.3 Fixed and adaptive arrays

Two-microphone and four-microphone arrays can either duplicate the performance of a traditional directional microphone and provide one directional polar pattern only i.e., fixed directionality and/or provide flexible directional polar patterns that adapt with the acoustical environment i.e., adaptive directionality. The adaptation is based on parameters within the hearing aid system from the environmental analysis and classification [23]. The adaptive behavior of the system is intended to account for noise backgrounds that consist of noise sources that are not diffuse and/or not stationary. The adaptation will direct the nulls to the specific noise sources within the limitations of the system. A further distinction is that a given system may be broadband adaptive or show frequency-specific behavior. A broadband adaptive system can be effective in canceling a moving noise source. For example, such a system could track and reduce the sound of a car passing from right to left behind a hearing aid user. In a frequency-specific system, different sets of delays apply depending on frequency; if background noises have different frequency content and are spatially separated, they can be effectively canceled simultaneously. The benefit of the frequency specificity is that various kinds of both stationary and moving noises can each potentially be reduced maximally. For example, if the hearing aid user was in a café with a coffee grinding machine running off to the left, a higher pitched sound of a milk steamer directly behind, and a phone ringing off to the right, a frequency-specific system could cancel all of these noises simultaneously.

5.1.4 Common solutions to drawbacks in two-microphone and four-microphone arrays

All directionality, from the basic, fixed directional microphone to those with multiple arrays will feature a loss in low-frequency amplification. Low-frequency sounds have long wavelengths relative to the spacing between each microphone, resulting in similar phase alignment of sound regardless of direction of arrival. This results in greater subtraction of low-frequency sounds coming from any direction. This effect results in a predictable roll-off in the low frequencies of 6 dB/octave [24].

The loss in low-frequency amplification has typically been managed by providing additional low-frequency amplification to the directional microphone output. While this method provides make up gain in the low frequencies, it can also amplify internal noise to a degree that becomes bothersome for the hearing aid user in quiet environments [2]. A different solution to this issue is to provide band-split directionality. Band-split directionality is achieved by filtering the audio coming from the front of both microphones on each hearing aid into separate high-frequency and low-frequency channels; these separate frequency channels are then fed through individual delays. This allows the hearing aid to provide different delay times, and thus different polar patterns, to each frequency channel. Through band-split directionality, the hearing aid can provide an omnidirectional polar pattern to the low frequencies, while maintaining directivity in the high frequencies. Although this does not provide any directional attenuation of sounds that are considered noise in the low frequencies, it has the added effect of simulating the natural directivity of normal hearing [2]. It also has the advantage of preserving ITDs, which is an important binaural hearing cue. And it maintains similar sound quality to a full-band omnidirectional response, which makes it possible for automatic switching of microphone modes without the hearing aid user noticing any distracting change in the sound. Band-split directionality bypasses the issue of increased internal noise from the increased low-frequency gain that is found in hearing aids applying directionality to the low frequencies.

Behind-the-ear (BTE) and receiver-in-the-ear (RIE) hearing aid styles have a disadvantageous microphone location above and behind the pinna compromising spectral cues in these hearing aid styles. Many two-microphone and four-microphone arrays use a pinna restoration response to compensate for this. Pinna restoration mimics the natural front-facing directionality of an average pinna in the higher frequencies to compensate for the disadvantageous microphone location [18]. A pinna compensation algorithm has been shown to effectively reduce the number of front/back confusions compared with traditional omnidirectional microphones [25, 26]. In a review of studies on pinna restoration, Xu and Han suggested that individual differences in real-world performance with pinna restoration indicate that some hearing aid users may experience a localization benefit relative to omnidirectionality while others may not [27].

5.1.5 Applying directionality in daily life

Directionality has many benefits for hearing aid user, but it is not appropriate for all listening situations, and therefore full-time use of directionality is not recommended [17, 28]. It has been reported that hearing aid users prefer an omnidirectional setting in quiet environments, and while directionality is helpful in noise, it is most beneficial when sounds of interest are in front of the hearing aid user and spatially separated from the unwanted noise, which is not always the case [17, 29]. The dilemma of the capability of directionality to provide speech recognition in noise benefit, but with numerous potential drawbacks, contributed to limited fitting of directional microphones in hearing aids until the mid-1990s. Another factor was that directionality was incompatible with the small styles of in-the-ear (ITE) hearing aids that were most popular in the 1980s and 1990s. Today, most styles of hearing aids can and do house directional microphone systems, and flexibility in programming of hearing aids and in user control of hearing aid parameters provide many options for the hearing aid user to access directional benefits.

The simplest option from a technical point-of-view is to give the hearing aid user manual control of the directional setting in their hearing aids. In this case, the hearing aids have two or more settings where at least one contains directionality, and the hearing aid user can select the desired setting via a button on the hearing aid, a remote control, or a smartphone app. This solution requires the hearing aid user to recognize when directionality might be beneficial, activate the appropriate setting, and manage various aspects of their listening environment to maximize benefit. This could include, for example, asking their conversational partner to sit or stand in a well-lit area facing the unwanted noise sources so that the hearing aid user can face their partner with their back to the noise. The hearing aid user must also remember to deactivate the directional setting when it is no longer relevant.

Another option is for directionality to be activated automatically in listening conditions where it might be of benefit. This requires that the hearing aid has a way of identifying relevant acoustic environments as well as a strategy for when and how to apply the directional settings. A more detailed discussion of this concept follows.

5.1.6 Environmental analysis and classification

Hearing aids have automatic functionality that allows for changing of directional mode based on the environment. Prior to discussing the automatic aspects of directionality, it is prudent to summarize how hearing aids analyze and categorize different environments. Hearing aids determine which type of acoustic environment they are in through environmental classification algorithms, or more simply environmental classifiers.

While it is difficult to discuss specifics of environmental classifiers due to proprietary aspects of hearing aid algorithms, similarities in environmental classifiers exist across manufacturers [23]. Environmental classifiers identify pre-determined acoustic environments (e.g., quiet, noise, speech and noise, etc.) and trigger automatic changes in hearing aid settings and features in order to adjust to a given environment. Environmental classifiers can drive automatic changes in hearing aid features such as noise reduction, wind noise reduction, and directionality. Because of their role in automatic changes in hearing aids, environmental classifiers are one of the most important components of modern adaptive hearing aids.

Environmental classifiers determine environments through analyzing the acoustic features of sound, such as level or intensity, spectral shape, modulation depth and rate of the sound in the environment [2]. Directional microphone systems can also be part of the environmental analysis, as the output of the system can be used to detect the direction of arrival of speech as well as estimating the sound level coming from the front or back hemisphere. The hearing aid continually analyzes the environment and updates the classification as the environment changes or the hearing aid user moves to a new environment (e.g., from noise to quiet).

5.1.7 Automatic control of directionality

Regardless of the specific directionality, i.e., fixed or adaptive, two- or four-microphone arrays, most modern hearing aids include a steering algorithm that switches among two or more microphone modes based on environmental analysis and classification. The main purpose of an automatic steering algorithm is to make wearing the hearing aids easier for the hearing aid user, and to maximize opportunities for benefit of directionality. At a minimum, such algorithms include omnidirectional on both ears and directional on both ears when two hearing aids are fitted. Some of these algorithms work independently per device (and therefore also work on unilaterally-fitted hearing aids), while others rely on exchange of data between a pair of bilaterally-fitted hearing aids to determine the optimum microphone mode for the environment. Automatic switching of microphone modes is most commonly designed to make gradual changes even when the environment changes quickly, as hearing aid users are bothered by sudden and noticeable changes in the state of their hearing aids. This makes the hearing aids pleasant to wear but could theoretically reduce directional benefit momentarily.

The automatic control feature in a hearing aid is based on an audiological rationale, and differences in rationales result in different automatic switching behavior. A rationale for applying directionality can be very simple and trigger straightforward behavior, or it can be quite complex. The rationale is currently implemented using reactive Artificial Intelligence (AI) where an algorithm is programmed to make task specific decisions about how to apply directionality and sometimes other features such as gain and noise reduction settings. As technology advances, it is expected that AI controlled directionality and other noise reducing features will incorporate input from sensors as well as the hearing aid microphones, and that these algorithms will learn from past experience [30, 31]. **Table 1** summarizes some examples of rationales and system behavior for automatically applied directionality in order of increasing complexity. The most complex strategy is based on a binaural hearing model and combines the strengths of directionality in improving SNR and compensating for lost pinna-related cues with the binaural hearing abilities of the hearing aid user [18].

Rationale	System behavior	Potential disadvantage
Directionality is needed when noise is present because it will improve SNR for speech in front and reduce annoyance of noise even if speech is not present	Above a certain input level, directionality is applied; below that level, omnidirectionality is applied	Does not account for listening goals of the hearing aid user. Lack of audibility for important sounds in the rear; sound quality disadvantages; wind noise
Directionality is needed when noise and speech are both present because benefit will be most likely if there is a known signal of interest.	If speech is detected and the input exceeds a certain level, directionality is applied; otherwise, omnidirectionality is applied	Same as above
Directionality is needed when speech is present in front of the hearing aid user and there is also noise present; the greater specificity of listening condition will maximize benefit	If speech is detected in front of the hearing aid user and the input level exceeds a certain level, directionality is applied; otherwise omnidirectionality is applied	Same as above
The brain requires specific information to support natural ways that people listen in different types of environments. People rely on different listening strategies that are dependent on the acoustic environment including spatial hearing cues, improving SNR, and maintaining awareness of surroundings.	Depending on presence and direction of arrival of speech, presence of noise and overall input levels, one of multiple microphone modes are applied. The specific mode will either preserve cues for spatial hearing and sound quality, balance improved SNR with access to surroundings, or maximize SNR	Slow mode switching behavior could potentially cause momentary reduced access to important off-axis sounds

Table 1.
Rationales and system behavior for automatically applying directionality in order of increasing complexity.

The microphone modes that are applied support listening strategies discussed earlier such as the better ear strategy and the awareness strategy.

6. Clinical implications

6.1 Benefit

The benefit of directionality in hearing aids is well established. Directionality is the only hearing aid technology that has been shown to improve SNR in a way that significantly improves speech recognition in noisy situations where hearing aid users are listening to speech coming from in front of them with competing sound from other directions [9, 32]. This has been observed with two-microphone arrays [20, 32–36] and more recently, with four-microphone arrays. In addition, four-microphone arrays in beamforming mode have shown benefit over omnidirectional conditions in terms of rejecting stimulus from the side [20, 36–40].

Research has also shown some increased benefit using four-microphone arrays in beamforming mode compared to two-microphone arrays in beamforming mode. Picou and Ricketts [20] investigated two-microphone and four-microphone arrays in beamforming mode as compared to omnidirectional mode in a laboratory environment. The study investigated sentence recognition along with subjective responses (e.g., work, desire to control, willingness to give up, and tiredness). Results indicated both two-microphone arrays in beamforming mode and four-microphone arrays in beamforming mode significantly outperformed the omnidirectional mode in terms of sentence recognition, and there was a small, but significant improvement noted in the four-microphone array in beamforming mode over the two-microphone array in beamforming mode. Additionally, subjective benefit was noted regarding tiredness and desire to give up in the four-microphone array in beamformer mode over the two-microphone array in beamformer mode [20].

It is important to note that testing within a laboratory setting, despite the best of efforts, is not equivalent to real-world environments. Laboratory settings are frequently set up with statically-positioned signal and noise stimuli, as opposed to real-world environments with signals and noises that move. Additionally, the varying acoustic environments and reverberations experienced in the real world are difficult to faithfully reproduce in a simulated laboratory environment. It has been found that, when real-world environments mimic those of a laboratory setting, directional microphone systems can provide similar real-world benefit; however, hearing aid users do not always find themselves in laboratory-like settings [2, 41]. Despite this, we still see benefits from directionality in hearing aids as reported by hearing aid use in real-world environments.

Hearing aid users spend time in a variety of listening environments, not all of which are optimal for directional microphone systems. Previous studies have shown that listeners encounter environments that can benefit from directional microphone systems (e.g., listener in the front with noise to the sides and rear) only about one-third of the time [2, 42, 43]. This variation in listening environments is a strong argument for including automatic control of directionality in hearing aids. Automatic control of directionality provides benefit to hearing aid users in speech in noise environments, without need for manual control from the hearing aid user [18, 42]. Automatic control of directionality can also be beneficial when a talker of interest is from a direction other than the front of the hearing aid user. This benefit has been observed with the use of a specific automatic four-microphone array that switches between omnidirectional and three different directional modes based on the listening environment. The four different modes are omnidirectional/omnidirectional (both hearing aids of a pair in omnidirectional mode), four-microphone array in beamformer mode, and two asymmetric modes in which one hearing aid is in an omnidirectional mode and the other is in a directional mode [44]. The asymmetric directionality modes help to compensate for hearing aid users' environments in which the target signal is not directly from the front. When speech is detected from one side, the hearing aid on that side switches to an omnidirectional mode to allow access to the speech signal. Research involving asymmetric directionality has been shown to improve speech recognition for off-axis sounds compared to two-microphone and four-microphone arrays in beamformer mode [41, 45]. Note that this asymmetric directional rationale helps mimic the natural benefit of better ear listening used by people with normal hearing.

6.2 Directional limitations and considerations

There are multiple factors influencing the effectiveness of directional microphone systems, and it is important for both the hearing aid user and the hearing aid fitter to be knowledgeable about these factors to be able to optimize the effectiveness, and thereby benefit, of directionality. Factors that affect a directional microphone system's effectiveness include implementation, listening environment, candidacy, hearing aid factors and knowledge about when not to use directional microphone systems.

6.2.1 Implementation of directionality

Implementation of microphone arrays in hearing aids is not without inherent drawbacks, the first of which is size. As mentioned previously, physical separation of microphones is a component of creating directionality in hearing aids. If the spacing between the two microphones is too small, sensitivity is reduced, because the phase difference between the signal hitting the front microphone and the rear microphone is reduced. The reduced phase difference results in less subtraction between the two microphones, and thus less directional sensitivity [2]. As low frequencies have longer wavelengths, this reduction in sensitivity due to small spacing between the microphones mostly impacts low frequencies [2, 24]. Conversely, too large of a spacing can result in a reduction of frontal sensitivity to high frequencies. When a frequency is so high such that the distance between the microphones is half its wavelength, a reduction in high frequency directional response can occur [2]. Since there are consequences of too small or too large of a microphone spacing in hearing aids, it has been reported that a microphone spacing of between 5 and 12 mm is appropriate and commonly used for hearing aids [2, 24, 46].

Given the importance of spacing between the microphones, a hearing aid must physically be able to provide adequate microphone spacing for directionality. Thus, hearing aid style often determines whether directionality is present. It is standard to find directionality in BTE, RIE, ITE and larger in-the-canal (ITC) hearing aids. While the completely-in-the-canal (CIC) and invisible-in-the-canal (IIC) hearing aid styles do not have sufficient room on the faceplate of the hearing aid for two microphones [2], it is possible in smaller styles to use the omnidirectional microphone on each hearing aid as a two-microphone array. An issue with this is that both binaural and monaural spectral cues that are a natural acoustic advantage for these hearing aid styles are removed or disrupted, thereby diminishing the potential benefit of the directional microphone system.

Although, lack of directionality on custom devices may seem like an immediate disadvantage, it is important to consider the natural high-frequency directionality provided by pinna cues. By placing a hearing aid microphone further into the ear canal, as is the case in custom devices, the pinna shapes the sound before it reaches the hearing aid microphone, allowing an omnidirectional mode to be shaped by the natural directionality produced by the pinna. This is most noticeable on CIC and IIC hearing aids, but even ITE hearing aids with narrow microphone spacing can receive some of these benefits [47, 48]. A greater directivity index is noted as insertion depth of the hearing aid is increased [2, 24, 48].

As discussed previously, hearing aids that sit above the ear, such as BTE and RIE hearing aids, must compensate for the lack of pinna cues due to the microphone location above the ear. Proximity of the microphones to external ear anatomy, such as the helix, can obscure microphones and impact sound entering the microphones, and thus directionality [49]. Due to these factors, it is important to ensure the BTE and RIE hearing aids are positioned in such a way that they are placed as far forward on the pinna as is comfortable to reduce any positioning impacts on directionality.

As a final note regarding implementation of four-microphone arrays, they have the additional requirement for wireless functionality, so size is also a consideration, because the hearing aid must be large enough to fit the wireless antennae and batteries that can provide enough power for the wireless transmissions. As such, microphone arrays are typically found in BTE, RIE, and larger custom hearing aids.

6.2.2 Listening environment

A limitation of directional microphone systems is that the SNR benefit is realized only when certain conditions are met. First, the sounds of interest must be spatially separated from the sounds that are not of interest ("noise") [2]. Effectively, this means that noise cannot be directly next to or behind the sounds of interest, as the noise will be amplified alongside the sounds of interest.

Second, the sounds of interest must be located within the directional beam [2]. If the sounds of interest are located outside the directional polar pattern of the directional microphone system, the signal of interest will be attenuated.

Third, the sounds of interest should be within "critical distance" of the hearing aid user. The critical distance is the distance at which the sound pressure level of a sound is composed of equal parts direct sound and reverberant sound [50]. Reverberant sound, or reverberations, occurs due to the result of a sound reflecting off surfaces in the environment. Reverberations in the environment cause reflections to hit both microphones at the same time, thereby reducing the phase differences that create the intended directional response. Thus, the ability of the hearing aid to cancel the unwanted reverberant sounds are reduced [2]. Critical distance varies depending on the listening environment, and can range from 2 to 3 meters in an environment with minimal reverberation and less than 1 meter in a highly reverberant environment [50, 51]. It should be noted that sounds that fall outside of critical distance are not immediately unavailable to the hearing aid user, but rather there is a gradual reduction in benefit as sound sources cross and move further outside critical distance [2].

While hearing aid directionality provides benefits in certain environments, hearing aid users may not always find it beneficial if sounds of interest are coming from directions other than the front. As mentioned, using a hearing aid with automatic control of adaptive directionality, or providing the hearing aid user the ability to switch between settings, can provide flexibility to the user, based on their own experiences and listening environments. Thus, it is important to take hearing aid users' needs into consideration when fitting hearing aids with directionality.

6.2.3 Candidacy

All hearing aid users can benefit from directional microphone systems. With few exceptions, directional benefit does not depend on hearing loss [2, 9]. However, a person with more hearing loss, and thus SNR loss, will be more dependent on a directional microphone system than a person with less or no hearing loss [2]. Directional microphone systems cannot completely compensate for the suprathreshold auditory processing problems of some people experiencing poor aided speech recognition, such as occurs with retro-cochlear disorders of the auditory nervous system. Similarly, directional microphone systems cannot compensate in cases in which there is unaidable hearing at certain frequencies due to the extent of the SNHL [2]. While directionality can still provide the best possible SNR for these hearing aid users, it is important to establish expectations regarding the benefit of directionality and hearing aid technology.

Another aspect of candidacy to consider regarding directional benefit is whether the person with hearing loss is a candidate for open fit hearing aids. Open fit hearing aids use coupling to the ear canal (e.g., dome) that allows low-frequency sound to enter and exit the ear canal, which allows for significant venting. This provides a more natural, "open" sound, because the hearing aid user hears the low frequencies unimpeded, while the hearing aid provides amplification for the mid- and high frequencies [2]. Candidates for open fit hearing aids have relatively good low-frequency hearing, with hearing thresholds better than about 40 dB hearing level (HL) in the low frequencies. Open fit hearing aids also reduce the occlusion effect. The occlusion effect is the buildup of low-frequency sound pressure levels (SPL) in an occluded ear canal. Hearing aid user generated sounds, such as own voice, chewing, swallowing, breathing, and coughing, are conducted via the body to the ear canal [52, 53]. As an open fit does not result in the buildup of low-frequency energy, the occlusion effect is notably reduced.

However, this venting provided in open fittings has a negative impact on overall directional benefit in the low frequencies. It is only possible to provide improved SNR, and thereby a directional benefit, for frequencies where the hearing aid output is greater than the vent output [2]. Since in open fittings there is minimal low-frequency amplification, and what low-frequency amplification is provided will likely leak out of the vent, it is not possible to achieve hearing aid output greater than vent output in this frequency range. In addition, open fittings reduce the benefit of directionality because ambient noise can enter the ear canal [2, 54, 55]. These factors mean that open-fit hearing aid users will only receive directional benefit in the mid- and high frequencies [2].

Despite the drawbacks open fittings have on directional benefit, it is once again important to think about the natural directional response pattern of the ear. Recall that the open ear has a more omnidirectional response in the low frequencies compared to the high frequencies [2, 56]. Because of this, the lack of directional benefit in the lows, an open fitting with directionality can still be seen as a solution that replicates the natural directionality pattern of the open ear.

6.2.4 Hearing aid user factors

Directionality in hearing aids can provide significant benefit to hearing aid users, but as with any hearing aid technology, the hearing aid users, their own listening scenarios, and their own unique preferences must be considered. It has been shown that more than 30% of adults' active listening time is spent attending to sounds that are not in front, where there are multiple target sounds, where the sounds are moving, or any combination of these—situations where front-facing directionality can interfere with audibility of the sound of interest [2, 42, 43, 45].

Furthermore, vast assumptions are made by the hearing aid about noise and the interfering signal. While noise is assumed to be "unwanted sound," is it appropriate for hearing aids to always make assumptions on what sounds are "unwanted"? Consider that the sound of interest for a hearing aid user may not always be speech, and this can vary based on the listening environment for the same general situation e.g., in a busy airport terminal, a hearing aid user may want to hear the speech of a travel companion walking next to her/him but must also hear the announcements coming from behind.

All the above complicates a "one-size fits all" directionality, even with automatic adaptive directional microphone systems. Understanding an individual's use case scenarios can help inform the hearing aid fitting. While automatically activated adaptive directionality may be beneficial for everyday use, situations in which a fixed directional or omnidirectional mode in a hearing aid program may be beneficial may also occur. An omnidirectional program could be useful for a teacher monitoring a crowded lunchroom or a jogger who wants to be aware of their environments and traffic while jogging on a city sidewalk. Modern hearing aids allow for multiple programs, so it can be that multiple programs are set up for each hearing aid user to meet their needs, which they can then cycle through as needed.

Understanding each hearing aid user's needs is critical to ensuring that the hearing aids are programmed to provide optimal benefit in all of the user's daily environments. Additionally, it is important to provide education through counseling so that each hearing aid user knows when and how to implement program changes in their hearing aids, as well as when and how to make changes to their environments to achieve maximum directional benefit [45].

Hearing aid users must also encounter enough situations where directionality is potentially beneficial to benefit from directionality.

6.2.5 Disadvantages

Disadvantages previously discussed include reduced amplification of off-axis sounds, and reduction in the low frequencies. In environments where the signal of interest is off axis, the listener may be required to turn their head towards the signal of interest. Compensation of low-frequency loss by gain, implementation of band-split directionality, and open fitting in which no low or minimal frequency gain is applied are methods of overcoming the inherent reduction in low frequencies observed in directional microphone systems.

In addition to the above, directional microphone systems can also reduce left/right localization ability and be more susceptible to wind noise [2]. Reduced localization is most prevalent in a bilateral pair of hearing aids that do not coordinate gain settings between the ears. Modern hearing aids that synchronize both ears do not experience such reduction in localization, as they help maintain the interaural differences important for localization [2]. Furthermore, complex multiband directionality schemes can help preserve localization and provide directionality such as in band-split directionality. One example includes a hearing aid that provides omnidirectionality below an adjustable low-frequency cut-off, a monaural hyper-cardioid directionality in each hearing aid above 5000 Hz, and four-microphone array beamformer mode between the low-frequency cut-off and 5000 Hz [45, 57]. This strategy preserves the ITDs, which are the dominant cue for localization in the low frequencies, and ILDs which for sounds above 5000 Hz, help maintain high frequency localization. Lastly, the frequencies used for the beamformer mode are within the frequencies most important for speech recognition [45].

While all hearing aid microphones are susceptible to wind noise, directional microphone systems are most impacted. Wind noise occurs when wind pass over the head or pinna and creates turbulence. The turbulence creates areas of high and low pressure, which is picked up by the microphones and converted to an audible, amplified sound [58]. Wind noise is characterized by a loud low- to mid- frequency sound, depending on the speed of the wind [2, 58]. The turbulence caused by wind is unique and if the noise is uncorrelated at each microphone in a two-microphone directional system, it is not canceled out like environmental sound [58]. Instead the uncorrelated wind noise is added between the two microphones and amplified [58].

BTE and RIE hearing aids, with microphones located on the top of the ear, and larger ITE hearing aids with microphones not shielded from wind by the pinna, are especially prone to wind noise; note that these are also the hearing aids most typically used with directionality. In these hearing aids, wind noise reduction algorithms are typically used to detect and reduce wind noise. Although the exact implementation of wind noise varies between hearing aid designers, it generally includes a temporary reduction of the low-frequency gain [58–61]. Additionally, the hearing aid may switch to an omnidirectional mode that is less susceptible to wind noise or use a band-split response to create an omnidirectional pattern in the low frequencies and directional pattern in the high frequencies [58, 60, 62]. As stressed in the previous section pertaining to hearing aid user preference, it is important to understand a hearing aid user's needs and preference. A hearing aid user who is frequently in a windy environment (e.g., outside, on a boat, on bicycle, etc.) may require a dedicated program in which directionality is turned off.

All these factors influencing the potential benefit of directional microphone systems are summarized in **Table 2**.

Implementation factors
Physical distance between microphones
Hearing aid style
Hearing aid size
Listening environment factors
Sounds of interest and sounds not of interest ("noise") needs to be spatially separated
Sounds of interests need to be within the directional beam
Sounds of interest needs to be within 2–3 m of the hearing aid user (critical distance)
Reverberation reduces directional benefit
Candidacy factors
Everybody can benefit but people with more hearing loss are more dependent on directionality
Open hearing aid fittings result in loss of directional benefit in the low frequencies

Hearing aid user factors
Sound(s) of interest can vary based on listening environment and user intent, on a moment-to-moment basis
Understanding how to use the technology and possibly use multiple modes
Lifestyle e.g., opportunities to experience directional benefit
Disadvantages
Low frequency roll-off
Reduced right-left localization
Increased wind noise

Table 2.
Factors influencing the effectiveness of directional microphone systems.

7. Conclusions

People with SNHL have difficulties hearing in noise. The only hearing aid technology—in addition to amplification—proven to help hearing aid users hear better in noise is directionality, and nearly all hearing aid users can benefit from directionality [2, 17]. Modern enhancements in wireless technology have expanded the types of microphone arrays from simple two-microphone arrays on single hearing aids to four-microphone arrays in bilaterally-fitted hearing aids. Microphone arrays play an important role in improving hearing in noise for hearing aid users. Furthermore, flexibility of adaptive directionality in hearing aids, driven by environmental analysis and classification, in combination with a steering algorithm provides a customizable experience capable of meeting hearing aid users' needs to hear in multiple encountered acoustic environments.

Conflict of interest

The author declares no conflict of interest.

Author details

Charlotte T. Jespersen
GN Hearing A/S, Ballerup, Denmark

*Address all correspondence to: cjespersen@gnresound.com

References

[1] Picou EM. MarkeTrak 10 (MT10) survey results demonstrate high satisfaction with and benefits from hearing aids. Seminars in Hearing. 2020;**41**(1):21-36

[2] Dillon H. Hearing Aids. 2nd ed. Sydney: Boomerang Press; 2012

[3] Moore BC. Perceptual Consequences of Cochlear Damage. Oxford: Oxford University Press; 1995

[4] Killion MC. I can hear what people say, but I Can't understand them. Hearing Reveiw. 1997;**4**:8-14

[5] Killion MC. The SIN report: Circuits haven't solved the hearing-in-noise problem. The Hearing Journal. 1997;**50**(10):28-30

[6] Killion MC. Hearing aids: Past, present, future: Moving toward normal conversations in noise. British Journal of Audiology. 1997;**31**(3):141-148

[7] Peters RW, Moore BC, Baer T. Speech reception thresholds in noise with and without spectral and temporal dips for hearing-impaired and normally hearing people. The Journal of the Acoustical Society of America. 1998;**103**(1):577-587

[8] Plomp R. A signal-to-noise ratio model for the speech-reception threshold of the hearing impaired. Journal of Speech, Language, and Hearing Research. 1986;**29**(2):146-154

[9] Mueller GH, Ricketts TA. Directional-microphone hearing aids: An update. The Hearing Journal. 2000;**53**(5):10-19

[10] Bentler RA. Effectiveness of directional microphones and noise reduction schemes in hearing aids: A systematic review of the evidence. Journal of the American Academy of Audiology. 2005;**16**(7):473-484

[11] Avan P, Giraudet F, Büki B. Importance of binaural hearing. Audiology & Neurotology. 2015;**20**(1):3-6

[12] Derleth P, Georganti E, Latzel M, Courtois G, Hofbauer M, Raether J, et al. Binaural signal processing in hearing aids. Seminars in Hearing. 2021;**42**(3):206-223

[13] Moore BC. An Introduction to the Psychology of Hearing. 6th ed. Emerald: Bingley; 2012

[14] Musicant AD, Butler RA. Influence of monaural spectral cues on binaural localization. The Journal of the Acoustical Society of America. 1985;**77**(1):202-208

[15] Byrne D, Noble W. Optimizing sound localization with hearing aids. Trends in Amplification. 1998;**3**(2):51-73

[16] Zurek PM. Binaural advantages and directional effects in speech intelligibility. In: Studebaker GA, Hochberg I, editors. Acoustical Factors Affecting Hearing Aid Performance. Boston: Allyn & Bacon; 1993. pp. 255-275

[17] Ricketts TA. Directional hearing aids: Then and now. Journal of Rehabilitation Research and Development. 2005;**42**(4 Suppl. 2):133-144

[18] Jespersen CT, Kirkwood BC, Groth J. Increasing the effectiveness of hearing aid directional microphones. Seminars in Hearing. 2021;**42**(3):224-236

[19] Kates JM. Digital Hearing Aids. 2nd ed. San Diego: Plural Publishing; 2008

[20] Picou EM, Ricketts TA. An evaluation of hearing aid beamforming microphone

arrays in a Noisy laboratory setting. Journal of the American Academy of Audiology. 2019;**30**(2):131-144

[21] Mens LH. Speech understanding in noise with an eyeglass hearing aid: Asymmetric fitting and the head shadow benefit of anterior microphones. International Journal of Audiology. 2011;**50**(1):27-33

[22] Griffiths L, Jim C. An alternative approach to linearly constrained adaptive beamforming. IEEE Transactions on Antennas and Propagation. 1982;**30**(1):27-34

[23] Hayes D. Environmental classification in hearing aids. Seminars in Hearing. 2021;**42**(3):186-205

[24] Ricketts TA. Directional hearing aids. Trends in Amplification. 2001;**5**(4):139-176

[25] Groth J. Binaural Directionality II with Spatial Sense. Report No.: M201175-GB-14.12-Rev.A. Ballerup, Denmark: ReSound; 2015. 9 p

[26] Jespersen CT, Kirkwood B, Schindwolf I. M&RIE Receiver Preferred for Sound Quality and Localisation. Report No.: M201502GB-20.07-Rev.A. Ballerup, Denmark: ReSound; 2020. 8 p

[27] Xu J, Han W. Improvement of adult BTE hearing aid Wearers' front/Back localization performance using digital pinna-Cue preserving technologies: An evidence-based review. Korean Journal of Audiology. 2014;**18**(3):97-104

[28] Soede W, Berkhout AJ, Bilsen FA. Development of a directional hearing instrument based on array technology. The Journal of the Acoustical Society of America. 1993;**94**(2):785-798

[29] Soede W, Bilsen FA, Berkhout AJ. Assessment of a directional microphone array for hearing-impaired listeners. The Journal of the Acoustical Society of America. 1993;**94**(2):799-808

[30] Branda E, Wurzbacher T. Motion sensors in automatic steering of hearing aids. Seminars in Hearing. 2021;**42**(3):237-247

[31] Gusó E, Luberadzka J, Baig M, Sayin Saraç U, Serra X. An objective evaluation of hearing aids and DNN-based speech enhancement in complex acoustic scenes. In: AA. VV. IEEE Workshop on Applications of Signal Processing to Audio and Acoustics (WASPAA 2023). 1 ed. New Paltz, New York: IEEE; 2023. pp. 1-5

[32] Bentler R, Palmer C, Mueller GH. Evaluation of a second-order directional microphone hearing aid: I. Speech perception outcomes. Journal of the American Academy of Audiology. 2006;**17**(3):179-189

[33] Valente M, Fabry D, Potts LG. Recognition of speech in noise with hearing aids using dual microphones. Journal of the American Academy of Audiology. 1995;**6**(6):440-449

[34] Preves DA, Sammeth CA, Wynne MK. Field trial evaluations of a switched directional/omnidirectional in-the-ear hearing instrument. Journal of the American Academy of Audiology. 1999;**10**(5):273-284

[35] Compton-Conley CL, Neuman AC, Killion MC, Levitt H. Performance of directional microphones for hearing aids: Real-world versus simulation. Journal of the American Academy of Audiology. 2004;**15**(6):440-455

[36] Aspell E, Picou E, Ricketts T. Directional benefit is present with audiovisual stimuli: Limiting ceiling effects. Journal of the American Academy of Audiology. 2014;**25**(7):666-675

[37] Picou EM, Aspell E, Ricketts TA. Potential benefits and limitations of three types of directional processing in hearing aids. Ear and Hearing. 2014;**35**(3):339-352

[38] Groth J. The Evolution of the Resound Binaural Hearing Strategy: All Access Directionality and Ultra Focus. Report No.: M201493GB-20.05-Rev.A. Ballerup, Denmark: ReSound; 2020. 8 p

[39] Wang L, Best V, Shinn-Cunningham BG. Benefits of beamforming with local spatial-Cue preservation for speech localization and segregation. Trends in Hearing. 2020;**24**:2331216519896908

[40] Jespersen CT, Groth J. Enhanced Directional Strategy with New Binaural Beamformer Leads to Vastly Improved Speech Recognition in Noise. Report No.: M201620GB-22.06-Rev.A. Ballerup, Denmark: ReSound; 2022. 6 p

[41] Cord MT, Walden BE, Surr RK, Dittberner AB. Field evaluation of an asymmetric directional microphone fitting. Journal of the American Academy of Audiology. 2007;**18**(3):245-256

[42] Blamey PJ, Fiket HJ, Steele BR. Improving speech intelligibility in background noise with an adaptive directional microphone. Journal of the American Academy of Audiology. 2006;**17**(7):519-530

[43] Walden BE, Surr RK, Cord MT, Dyrlund O. Predicting hearing aid microphone preference in everyday listening. Journal of the American Academy of Audiology. 2004;**15**(5):365-396

[44] Groth J, Bridges J. An Overview of Directional Options in Resound Hearing Aids. Report No.: M201521GB-21.01-Rev.A. Ballerup, Denmark: ReSound; 2021. 9 p

[45] Jespersen CT, Kirkwood B, Groth J. Effect of directional strategy on audibility of sounds in the environment for varying hearing loss severity. Canadian Audiologist. 2017;**4**(6):1-11

[46] Ludvigsen C, Baekgaard L, Kuk F. Design Considerations in Directional Microphones. Widex Press; 2001. p. 18

[47] Ricketts T. Impact of noise source configuration on directional hearing aid benefit and performance. Ear and Hearing. 2000;**21**(3):194-205

[48] Fortune TW. Real-ear polar patterns and aided directional sensitivity. Journal of the American Academy of Audiology. 1997;**8**(2):119-131

[49] Ricketts T. Directivity quantification in hearing aids: Fitting and measurement effects. Ear and Hearing. 2000;**21**(1):45-58

[50] Ricketts TA, Hornsby BWY. Distance and reverberation effects on directional benefit. Ear and Hearing. 2003;**24**(6):472-484

[51] Hawkins DB, Yacullo WS. Signal-to-noise ratio advantage of binaural hearing aids and directional microphones under different levels of reverberation. The Journal of Speech and Hearing Disorders. 1984;**49**(3):278-286

[52] French-Saint George M, Barr-Hamilton RM. Relief of the occluded ear sensation to improve earmold comfort. Journal of the American Audiology Society. 1978;**4**(1):30-35

[53] Zachman TA, Studebaker GA. Investigation of the acoustics of earmold vents. The Journal of the Acoustical Society of America. 1970;**47**(4):1107-1115

[54] Bentler R, Wu Y-H, Jeon J. Effectiveness of directional technology

in open-canal hearing instruments. The Hearing Journal. 2006;**59**(11):40-47

[55] Mueller HG, Ricketts TA. Open-canal fittings: Ten take-home tips. The Hearing Journal. 2006;**59**(11):24-39

[56] Christensen LA. The evolution of directionality: Have developments led to greater benefit for hearing aid users? Canadian Audiologist. 2017;**4**(4):1-15

[57] Groth J, Laureyns M. Preserving localization in hearing instrument fittings. The Hearing Journal. 2011;**64**(2):34-38

[58] Korhonen P. Wind Noise Management in Hearing Aids. Seminars in Hearing. 2021;**42**(3):248-259

[59] Bentler R, Chiou L-K. Digital noise reduction: An overview. Trends in Amplification. 2006;**10**(2):67-82

[60] Stender T, Hielscher M. Windguard: Bringing Listening Comfort to Windy Conditions. Report No.: M200765-GB-12.05-Rev.A. Ballerup, Denmark: ReSound; 2012. 6 p

[61] Weile J, Andersen M. Wind Noise Management. Oticon Tech Paper; 2016

[62] Kuk F, Keenan D, Lau C-C, Ludvigsen C. Performance of a fully adaptive directional microphone to signals presented from various azimuths. Journal of the American Academy of Audiology. 2005;**16**(6):333-347

Chapter 9

Presbycusis: A Coordinated and Personalized Approach According to Different Frailty Phenotypes

Qingwei Ruan, Jian Ruan, Xiuhua Hu, Aiguo Liu and Zhuowei Yu

Abstract

Age-related hearing loss (ARHL) is the most common sensory impairment. Older people with ARHL may vary in their profiles and usually manifest heterogeneous phenotypes, including in combination with presbyastasis, tinnitus, different frailty phenotypes, and multi-morbidity. Patients with these phenotypes generally have a decreased intrinsic capacity, high health burden, and poor prognosis, such as disability, fall, and other adverse events. However, the absence of an evidence-based guidance leads to a significant limitation of current approaches to ARHL care. Here, we present a framework for the rapid and in-depth geriatric assessment, and a recommendation for the coordinated and personalized management of older adults according to their etiology of hearing loss, imbalance, tinnitus, the status of frailty phenotype, and multi-morbidity. The main purpose is to recover functional health, reduce complications, and improve the quality of life for older people with ARHL and frailty phenotypes.

Keywords: age-related hearing loss, presbyastasis, tinnitus, intrinsic capacity, frailty phenotype, multi-morbidity

1. Introduction

Age-related hearing loss (ARHL), or presbycusis, is highly prevalent in old age with the increase in life expectancy. It is estimated that 20–26% of adults aged 45 years and increasing to 63% in adults older than 70 years, and nearly 80% of people over 85 years have hearing loss [1–3]. ARHL is characterized by central auditory processing deficit (CAPD), including temporal processing and frequency resolution, and greater auditory speech perception challenges, apart from different degrees of peripheral hearing loss [4], and often associated with presbyastasis, subjective tinnitus or hyperacusis, and physical, cognitive, and psychological disorders [5–8]. The interaction of aging and internal and external environment factors results in different pathological alterations and heterogeneous clinical phenotypes. Aging causes gradually increasing decline of multi-system physiological reserve [7]. Some external environmental factors, such as environmental enrichment, including educational, occupational, or leisure activities, are beneficial for the improvement of cognitive and auditory reserves, and active physical exercise for the improvement of multi-system physiological reserves. More environmental factors are harmful for health, referred as to stressors, including physical, physiological, psychosocial, and unhealthy lifestyles [7]. Local audiogenic stressors and otological diseases can cause auditory reserve decline, the imbalance of auditory system homeostasis, and hearing loss with tinnitus. Chronic physiological (functional reserve decline in metabolically active organs, polypharmacy) and psychological stresses (sleep problems and noise exposure), and unhealthy lifestyles (unhealthy diet, smoking, physical inactivity) might lead to the allostatic load and maladaptation in different physiological systems or organs, and multi-morbidities, such as cognitive impairment, cancer, cardiometabolic and affective disorders. In turn, the comorbidities can cause secondary hearing loss, presbyastasis, and tinnitus.

The age-related decline of functional reserve in multiple physiological systems, and following vulnerability increase of the body to minor stressor exposures, might cause the imbalance of homeostasis, allostatic load, and multi-system dysregulation. This condition is defined as frailty that could increase susceptibility to the occurrence of adverse consequences, such as disability, falls, dependence, and death risk [9]. Frailty could be classified into physical [9], cognitive [10], social [11], psychological [12], psychosocial [13], and nutritional [14] frailty phenotypes. Physical frailty rises with age and the prevalence greatly varies because of lack of standardization of concepts or measures. The prevalence of physical frailty is 8–15% in community-dwelling older people and is higher in women than in men [15, 16]. Our community population study (aged 60 years or older) indicated that the prevalence of pre-physical and physical frailty is 35.86 and 4.41% assessed by the FRAIL scale, respectively, and reversible and potential reversible cognitive frailty is 19.86 and 6.3% [17]. The prevalence of (pre-) physical frailty in otological outpatient is 25.5%, cognitive frailty is 32.17%, and cognitive impairment is 18.2% (pre-MCI 10% and MCI 8.2%) [18]. Moreover, patients with physical frailty had a lower risk for severe ARHL, tinnitus, and the presence of ARHL with tinnitus than those with cognitive frailty or cognitive impairment. Patients with the reversible cognitive frailty subtype had a lower risk for severe ARHL, tinnitus, and the presentation of ARHL with tinnitus than those with the potential reversible cognitive frailty subtype. ARHL severity was independently associated with overall cognition, and domain-specific cognition, including executive function, delayed memory, and language function [19]. Patients with ARHL, presbyastasis, and tinnitus had a high risk for cognitive impairment. Physical frailty and ARHL accompanying presbyastasis and/or tinnitus had significant impacts on the overall and domain-specific quality of life [20, 21]. Physical frailty had a stronger and more profound effect on the quality of life, particularly on independent living and pain in the physical dimension and happiness and coping in the psychosocial dimension.

Since ARHL is heterogeneous and usually accompanies high prevalent multimorbidities, frailty phenotypes, the cooperation among audiologist, otologist, and geriatrician is required to face the aforementioned challenges. Frailty is a pre-disable status, and dynamic and potentially reversible. Apart from hearing and balance rehabilitation, to integrate person-centered geriatric assessment and personalized intervention into the diagnosis and management of ARHL could achieve healthy aging and reduce the risk of complications and adverse outcomes, including geriatric syndrome, functional disability, fall, dependence, and poor quality of life.

2. Early detection of presbycusis with different frailty phenotypes

There are guidelines for the etiological assessment of bilateral sensorineural hearing loss and comprehensive audiological management in children [22, 23]; and for the screening and management of ototoxic hearing loss [24]. There are also some protocols or proposals for the etiological assessment and management of presbyastasis [8, 21, 25] and tinnitus [26, 27]. Moreover, the United States Preventive Services Task Force concluded that the evidence is insufficient to assess the balance of benefits and harms for health outcomes of screening for hearing loss in asymptomatic adults 50 years or older (excluding conductive hearing loss, congenital hearing loss, sudden hearing loss, or hearing loss caused by recent noise exposure, or those reporting signs and symptoms of hearing loss) [28]. However, the international guideline for the screening and management of older adults with ARHL is limited. Notwithstanding, hearing loss has been considered as a critical component of sensory domain impairment of intrinsic capacity (IC) [29]. World Health Organization (WHO) proposed the guidance for the person-centered assessment of intrinsic capacity [30] and for systems and services of integrated care for older people (ICOPE) implementation framework [31]. For older people, several clinical practice guidelines for the screening, assessment, and management of frailty had been proposed by different organizations [32–34]. In order to reorient the disease-centered to function-centered care model and achieve healthy aging, we propose a coordinated care framework to optimize the early detection and management of ARHL according to the framework for integrated care for older people with intrinsic capacity decline and clinical practice guidelines for the management of frailty.

2.1. Rapid screening for the subject with presbycusis and different phenotypes in primary care

To capture the major clinical events, including declines in functions, onset of disability, frailty, and burdensome chronic diseases in older people aged 60 years and over, a general assessment approach for the subject with ARHL and different frailty phenotypes contains two steps outlined in **Figure 1**. The recommended step 1 is the rapid geriatric assessment, including rapid screening in primary care settings for the loss in IC and physical frailty phenotypes. Step 2 is the in-depth geriatric assessment in secondary care settings, including frailty phenotypes and the etiology of hearing loss, presbyastasis, and tinnitus.

For the beginning, the ICOPE step one is used to screen for loss of domain-specific IC (i.e., locomotion, cognition, vitality/nutrition, and psychological and sensorial capacities) by using a screening test (**Table 1**) [33, 35]. The screening test can be delivered by primary providers or by patient self-assessment using either a mobile application for a smartphone or an Internet conversational robot. The IC domains were monitored by a primary provider or nurse each 4 months [36].

About sensorial capacity domain, we proposed a preliminary presbyastasis and tinnitus screening also should be performed during hearing loss screening, since presbyastasis and tinnitus are the most related symptoms in older adults with hearing loss. Presbyastasis, or age-related degeneration of peripheral as well as the central part of the vestibular system, refers to dizziness and/or ataxia with apparent localizing signs and is typically attributed to the aging process [25, 37]. The clinical differentiation of presbyastasis from symptoms related to specific diseases or risk factors is required based on medical history. These diseases include specific or unilateral vestibular

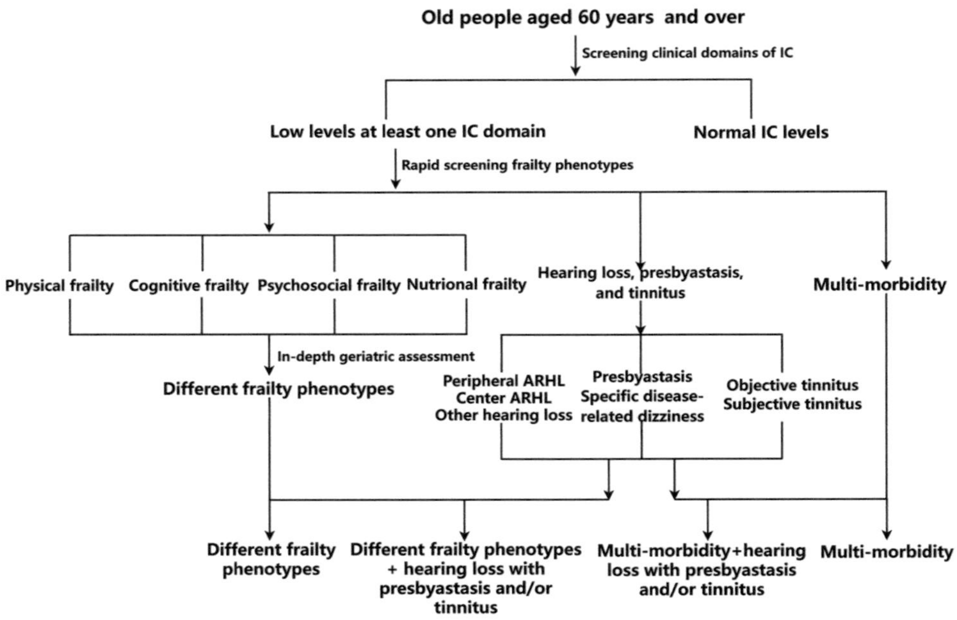

Figure 1.
An approach to rapid screening and in-depth assessment of ARHL with presbyastasis, tinnitus, frailty phenotypes, and multi-morbidity.

Intrinsic capacity domains	Recommended screening tests
Cognitive decline	1. Remember three words: for example: flower, door, rice 2. Orientation in time and space, what is the full date today? Where are you now (home, clinic, etc.) 3. Recalls the three words
Limited mobility	1. Chair rise test, Rise from chair five times without using arms 2. Did the person complete five chair rises within 14 seconds?
Malnutrition (vitality impairment)	1. Weight loss: Have you unintentionally lost more than 3 kg over the last 3 months? 2. Appetite loss: Have you experienced loss of appetite?
Depressive systems (impairment in psychological domain)	Over the past 2 weeks, have you been bothered by: feeling down, depressed or hopeless: little interest or pleasure in doing things.
Visual impairment (sensory impairment)	1. Do you have any problems you are your eyes: difficulties in seeing far, reading, eye diseases or currently under medical treatment (e.g., diabetes, high blood pressure)?
Hearing loss (sensory impairment)	1. Hears whispers (whisper test) or screening audiometry result is 35 dB or less or passes automated app-based digits-in-noise test

Table 1.
The rapid screening for the loss in intrinsic capacity [33, 35].

diseases, such as Meniere's disease, visional impairment from various etiologies, muscle weakness, neurological lesions, diabetes-related neuropathy, cognitive impairment, arthritis, narrowing of the lumbar vertebral canal, and lumbago-sciatica [21, 25, 38]. The risk factors include polypharmacy, especially drugs for hypertension (e.g., diuretics), anxiety, or depression, excessive consumption of alcohol, and extrinsic environmental factors, such as stairs and other indoor obstacles [25]. ARHL and noise exposure are the most common causes of non-pulsatile tinnitus (subjective tinnitus) [5, 6]. Other etiologically differential diagnosis of tinnitus symptoms includes pulsatile or objective (pulsatile synchronous or vascular and asynchronous or mechanical) tinnitus, and more common subjective tinnitus accompanying unilateral or bilateral hearing loss [26, 27]. The screening also includes tinnitus-related systemic morbidities, such as cardiometabolic diseases, mental health disorders, neurological diseases (e.g., multiple sclerosis and head injury), tinnitus-related otological diseases, such as Meniere's disease, middle ear infection, noise exposure, and tinnitus-related polypharmacy, such as diuretics for hypertension therapy [39], aspirin [40, 41], and other ototoxic medications [24]. Visual analog scales and questionnaires (e.g., Tinnitus handicap inventory and Tinnitus functional index) usually are used to assess tinnitus annoyance, distress, and severity [42].

Once IC decline was confirmed, individuals would have rapid physical frailty screening [33]. Although there are more than a dozen rapid frailty screening instruments, the FRAIL Scale is widely validated, simple, and rapid tool for the screening of physical frailty phenotype [32–34]. The FRAIL scale is a simple five-item questionnaire: Fatigue: Are you fatigued? Resistance: Cannot walk up one flight of stairs? Aerobic: Cannot walk one block? Illnesses: Do you have more than five illnesses? Loss of weight: Have you lost more than 5% of your weight in the last 6 months? Pre-physical frailty is defined as scoring 1 or 2; physical frailty is defined as scoring 3 or greater.

After IC and physical frailty screening, individuals were classified into with (pre-) physical frailty and without frailty. Among these with (pre-) physical frailty, individuals further were classified into psychological, nutritional, cognitive, and mixed frailty phenotypes according to the decline of domain-specific IC. The mixed frailty phenotype means accompanying a decline in two or more than two domains of IC. Individuals with cognitive frailty could be classified into reversible and potential reversible cognitive frailty [10, 17] using the rapid cognitive screening (RCS) tool [43] in combination with a pre-mild cognitive impairment (pre-MCI) questionnaire with two items [17]. The scores for dementia and MCI were ≤5 and 6-7, respectively. Individual with a score of 8-10 was considered to have pre-MCI when had a positive response to pre-MCI questionnaire. Individuals with (pre-) physical frailty and pre-MCI or MCI were defined as reversible or potentially reversible cognitive frailty.

Individuals without (pre-) physical frailty but with domain-specific decline of IC were referred to as psychological, cognitive, and sensory diseases, and other multi-morbidities (less than five chronic illnesses in the FRAIL questionnaire). These without domain-specific decline of IC and chronic diseases were considered as robust individuals. Thus, older people were classified into individuals having ARHL with different frailty phenotypes and multi-morbidity, individuals having ARHL with multi-morbidities (especially cardiometabolic morbidity), these with different frailty phenotypes, and robust individuals.

2.2. In-depth Assessment for the subject with presbycusis and different phenotypes in secondary care

Although rapid screening instruments for frailty phenotypes are sensitive, these tools often display low specificity [44]. In order to timely identify the causes of ARHL and tinnitus, individuals with ARHL and different frailty phenotypes by rapid geriatric assessment require referral to secondary care for in-depth IC-centered geriatric evaluation and frailty phenotype assessment by audiologist/geriatrician. The ICOPE care plan provides preliminary recommendations for in-depth geriatric assessment for the loss of IC [35].

Since individuals with ARHL usually accompany CAPD, presbyastasis, and subjective tinnitus, we proposed additional tests for the in-depth assessment of ARHL. For peripheral ARHL in-depth assessment, the results of audiometry should include pure-tone threshold average of the frequencies 0.5, 1.0, and 2.0 kHz (speech-frequency pure-tone average) and 4.0, 6.0, and 8.0 kHz (high-frequency pure-tone average). The word recognition (discrimination) scoring was determined by using the percentage of recognition of a list of monosyllabic phonetically balanced words at 30–40 dB above the PTA threshold for each ear. A score greater than 70% was considered normal to understand speech in a quiet environment [45, 46]. According to the WHO definition of disabling ARHL, peripheral ARHL was defined as a PTA threshold greater than 40 dB hearing level in the better ear [47].

For CAPD in-depth assessment, the eligible subject criteria for the central auditory tests include normal tympanogram, presenting ipsilateral acoustic reflexes, no history of ear surgery to exclude possible middle ear disease in the past or present, no history of hearing loss since childhood, and less than 21 dB difference among pure-tone averages (PTA) for 0.5, 1.0, and 2.0 kHz for the two ears to exclude otologic disorders (e.g., congenital or unilateral sudden deafness, tumor, or infection) other than aging [45, 46]. Moreover, individuals have no disabling peripheral ARHL (i.e., PTA threshold below 40 dB hearing level in the better ear, word recognition score at 30 dB over PTA threshold over 70%) [45, 46]. The test used to diagnose age-related CAPD includes the Synthetic Sentence Identification With Ipsilateral Competitive Message (SSI-ICM), Staggered Spondaic Word test, and other tests [48]. The SSI-ICM test consists of administering for each ear a primary signal of 10 short sentences against a background competition signal. The short sentences are presented at 50 dB over the PTA for each ear. The rate of identification of sentences is expressed as a percentage (0–100%) at various primary-competitive ratios (0, +5, +10 dB sound pressure level). Age-related CAPD was considered present when the patient scored less than 50% in the better ear with a 0-dB message-competition ratio [45, 46, 48].

Apart from medical history, the in-depth assessment for individuals with presbyastasis includes gait and stance assessment, such as "time up-and-go" test, standing on one leg, to differentiate dizziness from ataxia [25]. Hearing assessment, other accurate otoneurological evaluation, including Romberg, Unterberger, head-shaking, and Halmagyi tests, the Dix-Hallpike maneuver, and dynamic posturography; vestibular function assessment tests, such as rotational and caloric tests, videonystagmography or electronystagmography examination, and otolith function assessment usually were used to differentiate presbyastasis from disease-specific imbalance. [8, 25]. The video head impulse test was recently verified to be an effective test for the differentiation presbyastasis from Meniere's disease [38] and the prediction of fall risk in elderly patients [21]. Computed tomography imaging, MRI scanning, and ultrasonography are important auxiliary examinations.

The in-depth assessment for referring people with tinnitus includes tinnitus with acute conditions, such as a crisis of mental health, significant neurological systems or signs, uncontrolled vestibular symptoms, suspected stroke [49], tinnitus disorder (associated with emotional distress, cognitive dysfunction, and/or autonomic arousal, leading to behavioral changes, and functional disability) [50], tinnitus with sudden hearing loss, objective tinnitus, and tinnitus with unilateral or asymmetric hearing loss [26, 27, 49]. The differential diagnosis of tinnitus symptoms could be conducted by in-depth assessment, including audiological testing, psychoacoustic tests (pitch, loudness, and matching), and imaging. Idiopathic intracranial hypertension, glomus tumors, and atherosclerosis of the carotid arteries are frequent causes of pulse synchronous tinnitus [51]. Eustachian tube contraction and middle ear muscle myoclonus might cause pulse asynchronous tinnitus [27]. Unilateral tinnitus, but normal otoscopy and positive neurologic signs might be caused by cerebellopontine angle tumor, brainstem infarction, and multiple sclerosis; and by noise exposure; and these with negative neurologic signs might be Meniere's disease, semicircular canal dehiscence. Apart from ARHL and noise exposure, bilateral hearing loss and normal otoscopy findings might also be caused by acoustic trauma, otosclerosis, and ototoxic medication [26, 27].

To improve the specificity of (pre-) physical frailty, a cardiovascular health study frailty screening scale with more objective parameters (weight loss, exhaustion, low activity, slowness, and weakness) is used as an in-depth assessment instrument [9]. Individuals with a score of 1 or 2 is diagnosed as pre-physical frailty; and with a score of 3 or greater is diagnosed as physical frailty. Individuals, with (pre-) physical frailty simultaneously presenting impairment in the cognitive domain of IC, are classified as cognitive frailty. Cognitive performance could be thoroughly assessed by using demographically corrected normative z scores on the Neuropsychological Test Battery [52–54]. Reversible and potentially reversible cognitive frailty subtypes could be diagnosed according to the severity of cognitive impairment, including pre-MCI and MCI [18]. Social and psychological domains of IC are assessed by using the 21-item Social Dysfunction Rating Scale [55] and the 15-item short form of the Geriatric Depression Scale [56], respectively. Individuals with (pre-) physical frailty simultaneously presenting social or psychological dysfunction are classified as social or psychological frailty phenotype. Nutritional frailty phenotype could be diagnosed when individuals simultaneously present (pre-) physical frailty and nutritional imbalance [14]. Malnutrition also could be identified using a Mini nutritional assessment or malnutrition universal screening tool [35]. These in-depth geriatric assessments may uncover unrecognized problems following the rapid geriatric screening and provides the possibility for multi-disciplinary specialists to design and implement function-centered and personalized interventions, which can promote patient healthy aging.

3. The management of presbycusis with different frailty phenotypes

Multi-modality intervention is required for these ARHL with frailty phenotypes and/or multi-morbidity. An integrated and person-centered approach to the management of ARHL with frailty phenotypes and multi-morbidity is shown in **Table 2**.

3.1. Non-invasive treatment of ARHL with different frailty phenotypes

The integrated and person-centered management includes ARHL, presbyastasis, tinnitus, frailty phenotypes, and multi-morbidity. The primary management is to improve unfavorable lifestyles, including smoking, alcohol consumption, physical inactivity, improper nutrition, and poor social, economical, and environmental conditions, and reduction of polypharmacy, including the number and the dosage, and these increase the risk for presbyastasis, delirium, cardiovascular disease, kidney, and ototoxicity. The non-invasive intervention for ARHL is to prescribe a hearing aid, which could significantly slow short- and long-term cognitive decline [57]. The management

Hearing loss	Presbyastasis	Tinnitus	Frailty phenotypes	Multi-morbidity
Stop noise and ototoxic medication exposure	Identify risk factors and exclude potential curable causes	Exclude polypharmacy-related subjective tinnitus	Multi-component physical activity programs (resistance and aerobic exercise, balance, or coordination training) to reverse or slow the progression of (pre-)physical frailty	Proactive personalized assessment and care plan
Prescribe hearing aid	Vestibular and balance rehabilitation	Optimal pre-operative risk and toxicity assessment of invasive therapies and thorough monitoring during the treatment period to these with tinnitus of definite cause	Adequate protein, energy, and micronutrient supplementation to these with malnutrition	Optimizing the management of multi-morbidity
Optimal pre-operative risk assessment and thorough monitoring during the treatment period to these considering cochlear implant for severe-to-profound sensorineural hearing loss with poor word recognization	Drug treatment (e.g., betahistine) to increase cerebral blood flow; Other vasodilator and antivertiginous drugs	Subjective tinnitus intervention: amplification, sound, and neuromodulation	Optimizing environment and the improvement of health behavior	Reduction of polypharmacy
Optimal pre-operative risk and toxicity assessment of other invasive therapies and thorough monitoring during the treatment period to these with hearing loss of definite cause	Fall prevention, including regular physical and intellectual activities, nutritional supplement	Cognitive behavioral or comprehensive therapy to these with tinnitus disorder	Optimizing psychosocial resources to these with low mood and affective problems	Reduction of treatment burden, adverse event, and uncoordinated care
			Cognitive behavior training to these with cognitive decline	

Table 2.
The coordinated and personalized management of hearing loss with frailty phenotypes and multi-morbidity.

of presbyastasis includes the identification of risk factors and potentially curable causes, vestibular and balance rehabilitation, and drug treatment, such as H1-receptor agonist and H3-receptor anti-agonist (e.g., betahistine) and Other vasodilator and antivertiginous drugs, and fall prevention, including regular physical and intellectual activities with gradually increasing difficulty and nutritional supplement [25, 37]. Amplification by hearing aids acting as a masker by introducing more ambient noise also is used to relieve subjective tinnitus symptoms in some patients. Other non-invasive subjective tinnitus interventions include sound therapy, psychological therapies, neuromodulation, and combined therapy of these interventions [26, 27, 49, 58]. Psychological therapies, such as cognitive behavioral therapy, have been shown to improve quality of life and decrease depression for these with persistent and bothersome tinnitus, or tinnitus disorder [24, 59].

The interventions recommended by different international organizations to reverse or slow the progression of frailty include multi-component physical activity programs, adequate nutrition supplementation, and cognitive behavior training to improve physiological, psychological, and cognitive reserves [31–34, 60]. The decline of physiological, psychological, and cognitive reserves also causes multi-morbidity, and the complex overlap of frailty and morbidity, physical and mental health disorders, and frailty and polypharmacy [61]. The management of multi-morbidity includes a proactive personalized assessment and care plan, which improves the quality of life by reducing treatment burden, adverse events, and unplanned or uncoordinated care [61]. Recently, the holistic and patient-centered hearing healthcare had been proposed, including the integrated management of hearing loss with diabetes, dementia, and other comorbidities [62].

3.2. Invasive treatment in ARHL with different frailty phenotypes

Invasive treatment includes surgery, radiotherapy, chemotherapy, and multi-modal therapy. Individuals with ARHL and different frailty phenotypes may need a cochlear implant due to severe-to-profound sensorineural hearing loss with poor word recognition. Geriatric patients with dizziness-related specific diseases, or objective tinnitus-related diseases, such as idiopathic intracranial hypertension, vascular tumors, and these with subjective tinnitus-related diseases, including Meniere's disease, cholesteatoma, and otosclerosis, require complex surgery, and tinnitus-related Cerebellopontine angle tumor, acoustic neuroma, and skull base tumors require multi-modal therapy. Compared with younger patients, older people have higher surgery risk and radio- and chemotherapy toxicity. The prevalence of physical frailty in geriatric patients for elective surgery is over 10%, and individuals with physical frailty have more than two times higher risk of postoperative complications [63]. The frequent postoperative complications include death, delirium, extending stay in hospital, falls, functional deterioration, and poorer quality of life, apart from complications resulting from existing diseases such as acute coronary syndromes, stroke, thromboembolism, pneumonia, or other infections. Multi-morbidity and functional limitations are also indicated to be the main predictors of adverse prognosis and poorer tolerance of multi-modality therapy in geriatric patients with head and neck cancer [64]. However, direct evidence of adverse prognosis of the above treatments for ARHL and tinnitus with frailty phenotypes is absent. Cochlear implantation had been validated to slow cognitive decline and the progression of dementia [57, 65]. A previous study indicated that cochlear implant for older patients with frailty does not cause additional complications from existing diseases [66].

To balance the risk and benefit, the cooperation between an otolaryngologist and a geriatrician had been recommended to identify these high-risk patients and optimize the treatment with special surveillance during the treatment period [67]. A guideline for pre-operative assessment of geriatric patients had been proposed that comprehensive geriatric assessment, such as physical and mental health, daily and social function, frailty, and poly-pharmacotherapy, should be implemented during the diagnostic and therapeutic, and post-operative process [68]. The guideline is similar to our in-depth assessment of IC and frailty phenotypes. Identification of deficits in IC and frailty phenotype, and multi-morbidity in pre-operative assessment not only are used to make surgical decisions, and choose anesthesia techniques, peri-operative care, and nursing plans to minimize complications, but also allow for the patient's pre-operative preparation through nutritional support, functional improvement, and rehabilitation, and excluding surgical contraindications.

4. To prevent secondary presbycusis in subjects with different frailty phenotypes

Individuals with frailty phenotypes, or more complex overlap of frailty, multi-morbidity, and polypharmacy, usually showed an imbalance of homeostasis to additional minor stressors. The long-term allostatic load results in dysfunction in the neuroendocrine-immune system and metabolism (**Figure 2**). The maladaptation of these regulation systems results in the decline of stress-responsive capacity of the HPA axis and autonomic nervous system, chronic systemic inflammation, and over mobilization of energy metabolism. All these systemic alterations might cause secondary ARHL, tinnitus, and other widespread functional impairment or health deficits [7].

To improve IC capacity and decrease stress exposure are the basic principles for the management of these individuals. Multi-component physical activity programs, nutrition supplementation, and environmental enrichment can enhance the physical, cognitive [69], and auditory reserves [70]. The management of multi-morbidity and polypharmacy, optimal home, and psychosocial environment could slow the progress from frailty to disability, including secondary ARHL [32–34, 60].

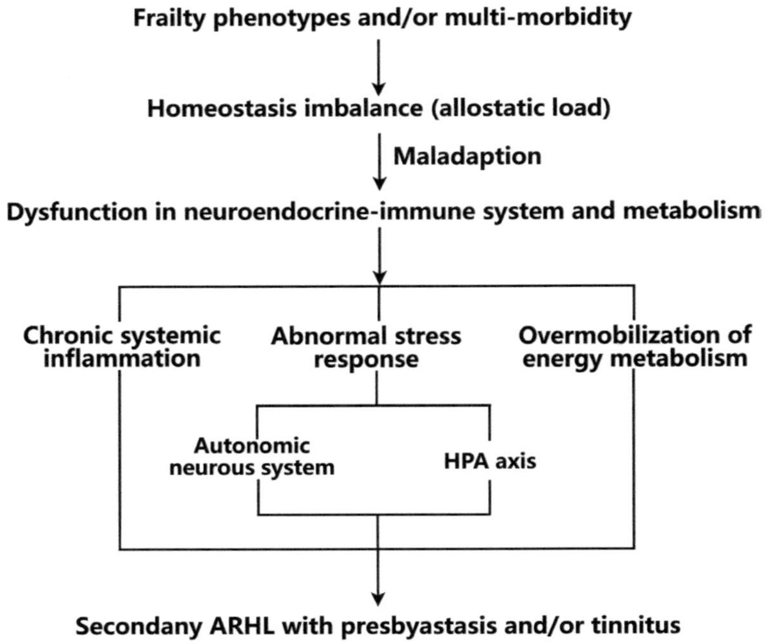

Figure 2.
The secondary ARHL with presbyastasis and/or tinnitus in subjects with frailty phenotypes and multi-morbidity.

5. Challenges of the detection and management of presbycusis with different frailty phenotypes

There are several critical challenges to optimize the diagnosis and management of presbycusis with different frailty phenotypes. One of the main challenges is frailty construct and screening instruments for clinical practice. Two well-validated and the most widely used models in clinical practice are variations of the frailty phenotype or frailty indexes based on the deficit accumulation approach [9]. However, most instruments lack extensive validation. Simple, rapid instruments for the assessment of frailty phenotypes based on physical frailty seem to meet the clinical translation demands. The evidence for frailty phenotypes, such as social frailty, nutritional frailty, and cognitive frailty, and subtypes, such as reversible and potential reversible cognitive frailty, is still limited.

Another main challenge is two parallel constructs with the same mission for healthy aging: IC and multi-morbidity. IC is endorsed by WHO but still lacks an operational definition, especially in the vitality domain [71]. Since many instruments are commonly used to diagnose frailty phenotypes and IC, it is necessary to integrate the two constructs and reduce confusion in clinical practice. Although frailty and multi-morbidity are different concepts, more than 16% of people have multi-morbidity with frailty and about three-quarters of people have frailty with multi-morbidity [72], it is difficult to separate different frailty phenotypes from comorbidities, such as cognitive frailty vs. cognitive impairment, and psychological frailty vs. psychological diseases.

There are similar challenges to differentiate peripheral from central ARHL, and tinnitus disorder from tinnitus with frailty phenotypes and multi-morbidity, especially with cognitive frailty or impairment, and psychological frailty or disorders. Therefore, further research is imperative to provide a more evidence-based proposal to improve the coordinated and personalized care to these with complex geriatric conditions.

6. Conclusions

The bidirectional association between ARHL and frailty phenotypes and multi-morbidity supports coordinated and personalized care for older people with ARHL and different frailty phenotypes. We proposed the rapid screening, in-depth assessment of IC, and frailty phenotypes as part of routine ARHL management. Albeit based predominantly on consensus and recommendation, we hope coordinated and personalized treatment strategies could be employed to reduce the complication and improve health and quality of life.

Acknowledgements

This work was supported by the Huadong Hospital project on intractable and complicated diseases (grant no. 20220101), the Medical Science and Technology Support Project of Shanghai Science, Technology Commission (grant No. 18411962200).

Conflict of interest

The authors declare no conflict of interest.

Author details

Qingwei Ruan[1,3]*, Jian Ruan[2], Xiuhua Hu[1,3], Aiguo Liu[4]* and Zhuowei Yu[1,3]*

1 Laboratory of Aging, Anti-aging and Cognitive Performance, Shanghai Institute of Geriatrics and Gerontology, Huadong Hospital, Shanghai Medical College, Fudan University, Shanghai, China

2 Department of Otolaryngology, Huadong Hospital, Shanghai Medical College, Fudan University, Shanghai, China

3 Shanghai Key Laboratory of Clinical Geriatrics, Huadong Hospital, and Research Center of Aging and Medicine, Shanghai Medical College, Fudan University, Shanghai, China

4 Department of Otolaryngology, Tongji Hospital, Tongji Medical College, Huazhong University of Science and Technology, Wuhan, China

*Address all correspondence to: 13661717346@163.com; aiguoliu309@163.com and hdyxyzw@163.com

References

[1] Agrawal Y, Platz EA, Niparko JK. Prevalence of hearing loss and differences by demographic characteristics among US adults: Data from the National Health and nutrition examination survey, 1999-2004. Archives of Internal Medicine. 2008;**168**(14):1522-1530. DOI: 10.1001/archinte.168.14.1522

[2] Lin FR, Thorpe R, Gordon-Salant S, Ferrucci L. Hearing loss prevalence and risk factors among older aduStates. The Journals of Gerontology. Series A, Biological Sciences and Medical Sciences. 2011;**66**(5):582-590. DOI: 10.1093/gerona/glr002

[3] Scholes S, Biddulph J, Davis A, Mindell JS. Socioeconomic differences in hearing among middle-aged and older adults: Cross-sectional analyses using the health survey for England. BMJ Open. 2018;**8**(2):e019615. DOI: 10.1136/bmjopen-2017-019615

[4] Kricos PB. Audiologic management of older adults with hearing loss and compromised cognitive/psychoacoustic auditory processing capabilities. Trends in Amplification. 2006;**10**(1):1-28. DOI: 10.1177/108471380601000102

[5] Jafari Z, Kolb BE, Mohajerani MH. Age-related hearing loss and tinnitus, dementia risk, and auditory amplification outcomes. Ageing Research Reviews. 2019;**56**:100963. DOI: 10.1016/j.arr.2019.100963

[6] Knipper M, Van Dijk P, Nunes I, Rüttiger L, Zimmermann U. Advances in the neurobiology of hearing disorders: Recent developments regarding the basis of tinnitus and hyperacusis. Progress in Neurobiology. 2013;**111**:17-33. DOI: 10.1016/j.pneurobio.2013.08.002

[7] Ruan J, Hu X, Liu Y, Han Z, Ruan Q. Vulnerability to chronic stress and the phenotypic heterogeneity of presbycusis with subjective tinnitus. Frontiers in Neuroscience. 2022;**16**:1046095. DOI: 10.3389/fnins.2022.1046095

[8] Berge JE, Nordahl SHG, Aarstad HJ, Goplen FK. Hearing as an independent predictor of postural balance in 1075 patients evaluated for dizziness. Otolaryngology and Head and Neck Surgery. 2019;**161**(3):478-484

[9] Hoogendijk EO, Afilalo J, Ensrud KE, Kowal P, Onder G, Fried LP. Frailty: Implications for clinical practice and public health. Lancet. 2019;**394**(10206):1365-1375. DOI: 10.1016/S0140-6736(19)31786-6

[10] Ruan Q, Yu Z, Chen M, Bao Z, Li J, He W. Cognitive frailty, a novel target for the prevention of elderly dependency. Ageing Research Reviews. 2015;**20**:1-10. DOI: 10.1016/j.arr.2014.12.004

[11] Tsutsumimoto K, Doi T, Makizako H, Hotta R, Nakakubo S, Makino K, et al. Association of social frailty with both cognitive and physical deficits among older people. Journal of the American Medical Directors Association. 2017;**18**(7):603-607. DOI: 10.1016/j.jamda.2017.02.004

[12] Gobbens RJ, van Assen MA, Luijkx KG, Wijnen-Sponselee MT, Schols JM. The Tilburg frailty indicator: Psychometric properties. Journal of the American Medical Directors Association. 2010;**11**(5):344-355. DOI: 10.1016/j.jamda.2009.11.003

[13] Solfrizzi V, Scafato E, Seripa D, Lozupone M, Imbimbo BP, D'Amato A, et al. Reversible cognitive frailty,

dementia, and all-cause mortality. The Italian longitudinal study on aging. Journal of the American Medical Directors Association. 2017;**18**(1):89.e1-89.e8. DOI: 10.1016/j.jamda.2016.10.012

[14] Zupo R, Castellana F, Guerra V, Donghia R, Bortone I, Griseta C, et al. Associations between nutritional frailty and 8-year all-cause mortality in older adults: The Salus in Apulia study. Journal of Internal Medicine. 2021;**290**(5):1071-1082. DOI: 10.1111/joim.13384

[15] Collard RM, Boter H, Schoevers RA, Oude Voshaar RC. Prevalence of frailty in community-dwelling older persons: A systematic review. Journal of the American Geriatrics Society. 2012;**60**(8):1487-1492. DOI: 10.1111/j.1532-5415.2012.04054.x

[16] Hoogendijk EO, Rijnhart JJM, Kowal P, Pérez-Zepeda MU, Cesari M, Abizanda P, et al. Socioeconomic inequalities in frailty among older adults in six low- and middle-income countries: Results from the WHO study on global ageing and adult health (SAGE). Maturitas. 2018;**115**:56-63. DOI: 10.1016/j.maturitas.2018.06.011

[17] Ruan Q, Xiao F, Gong K, Zhang W, Zhang M, Ruan J, et al. Prevalence of cognitive frailty phenotypes and associated factors in a community-dwelling elderly population. The Journal of Nutrition, Health & Aging. 2020;**24**(2):172-180. DOI: 10.1007/s12603-019-1286-7

[18] Ruan Q, Chen J, Zhang R, Zhang W, Ruan J, Zhang M, et al. Heterogeneous influence of frailty phenotypes in age-related hearing loss and tinnitus in Chinese older adults: An explorative study. Frontiers in Psychology. 2021;**11**:617610. DOI: 10.3389/fpsyg.2020.617610

[19] Zhang W, Ruan J, Zhang R, Zhang M, Hu X, Han Z, et al. Association between age-related hearing loss with tinnitus and cognitive performance in older community-dwelling Chinese adults. Psychogeriatrics. 2022;**22**(6):822-832. DOI: 10.1111/psyg.12889

[20] Zhang W, Ruan J, Zhang R, Zhang M, Hu X, Yu Z, et al. Age-related hearing loss with tinnitus and physical frailty influence the overall and domain-specific quality of life of Chinese community-dwelling older adults. Frontiers in Medicine (Lausanne). 2021;**8**:762556. DOI: 10.3389/fmed.2021.762556

[21] Politi L, Salerni L, Bubbico L, Ferretti F, Carucci M, Rubegni G, et al. Risk of falls, vestibular multimodal processing, and multisensory integration decline in the elderly-predictive role of the functional head impulse test. Frontiers in Neurology. 2022;**13**:964017

[22] McDermott JH, Molina-Ramírez LP, Bruce IA, Mahaveer A, Turner M, Miele G, et al. Diagnosing and preventing hearing loss in the genomic age. Trends in Hearing. 2019;**23**:2331216519878983. DOI: 10.1177/2331216519878983

[23] Wiseman K, Sapp C, Walker E, McCreery R. Comprehensive audiological management of hearing loss in children, including mild and unilateral hearing loss. Otolaryngologic Clinics of North America. 2021;**54**(6):1171-1179. DOI: 10.1016/j.otc.2021.08.006

[24] Lindeborg MM, Jung DH, Chan DK, Mitnick CD. Prevention and management of hearing loss in patients receiving ototoxic medications. Bulletin of the World Health Organization. 2022;**100**(12):789-796A. DOI: 10.2471/BLT.21.286823

[25] Vaz GF. Disequilibrium and its management in elderly patients.

The International Tinnitus Journal. 2009;**15**(1):83-90

[26] Langguth B, Kreuzer PM, Kleinjung T, De Ridder D. Tinnitus: Causes and clinical management. Lancet Neurology. 2013;**12**(9):920-930. DOI: 10.1016/S1474-4422(13)70160-1

[27] Wu V, Cooke B, Eitutis S, Simpson MTW, Beyea JA. Approach to tinnitus management. Canadian Family Physician. 2018;**64**(7):491-495

[28] US Preventive Services Task Force, Krist AH, Davidson KW, Mangione CM, Cabana M, Caughey AB, et al. Screening for hearing loss in older adults: US preventive services task force recommendation statement. Journal of the American Medical Association. 2021;**325**(12):1196-1201. DOI: 10.1001/jama.2021.2566

[29] Cesari M, Araujo de Carvalho I, Amuthavalli Thiyagarajan J, Cooper C, Martin FC, Reginster JY, et al. Evidence for the domains supporting the construct of intrinsic capacity. The Journals of Gerontology. Series A, Biological Sciences and Medical Sciences. 2018;**73**(12):1653-1660. DOI: 10.1093/gerona/gly011

[30] WHO. Guidance for Person-Centred Assessment and Pathways in Primary Care. Geneva: World Health Organization; 2019

[31] WHO. Integrated Care for Older People (ICOPE) Implementation Framework: Guidance for Systems and Services. Geneva: World Health Organization; 2019

[32] Dent E, Lien C, Lim WS, Wong WC, Wong CH, Ng TP, et al. The Asia-Pacific clinical practice guidelines for the Management of Frailty. Journal of the American Medical Directors Association. 2017;**18**(7):564-575. DOI: 10.1016/j.jamda.2017.04.018

[33] Ruiz JG, Dent E, Morley JE, Merchant RA, Beilby J, Beard J, et al. Screening for and managing the person with frailty in primary care: ICFSR consensus guidelines. The Journal of Nutrition, Health & Aging. 2020;**24**(9):920-927. DOI: 10.1007/s12603-020-1492-3

[34] Dent E, Morley JE, Cruz-Jentoft AJ, Woodhouse L, Rodríguez-Mañas L, Fried LP, et al. Physical frailty: ICFSR international clinical practice guidelines for identification and management. The Journal of Nutrition, Health & Aging. 2019;**23**(9):771-787. DOI: 10.1007/s12603-019-1273-z

[35] Chhetri JK, Harwood RH, Ma L, Michel JP, Chan P. Intrinsic capacity and healthy ageing. Age and Ageing. 2022;**51**(11):afac239. DOI: 10.1093/ageing/afac239

[36] de Souto BP, Guyonnet S, Ader I, Andrieu S, Casteilla L, Davezac N, et al. The INSPIRE research initiative: A program for GeroScience and healthy aging research going from animal models to humans and the healthcare system. The Journal of Frailty & Aging. 2021;**10**(2):86-93. DOI: 10.14283/jfa.2020.18

[37] Belal A Jr, Glorig A. Dysequilibrium of ageing (presbyastasis). The Journal of Laryngology and Otology. 1986;**100**(9):1037-1041

[38] Lerchundi F, Laffue AH, Olivier M, Gualtieri FJ. Bilateral posterior semicircular canal dysfunction: A new finding with video head impulse test. Journal of Neurology. 2020;**267**(8):2347-2352

[39] Borghi C, Brandolini C, Prandin MG, Dormi A, Modugno GC, Pirodda A.

Prevalence of tinnitus in patients withhypertension and the impact of different anti hypertensive drugs on the incidence of tinnitus: A prospective, single-blind, observational study. Current Therapeutic Research, Clinical and Experimental. 2005;**66**(5):420-432. DOI: 10.1016/j.curtheres.2005.10.001

[40] Salvi R, Radziwon K, Manohar S, Auerbach B, Ding D, Liu X, et al. Review: Neural mechanisms of tinnitus and Hyperacusis in acute drug-induced ototoxicity. American Journal of Audiology. 2021;**30**(3S):901-915. DOI: 10.1044/2020_AJA-20-00023

[41] Sheppard A, Hayes SH, Chen GD, Ralli M, Salvi R. Review of salicylate-induced hearing loss, neurotoxicity, tinnitus and neuropathophysiology. Acta Otorhinolaryngologica Italica. 2014;**34**(2):79-93

[42] National Guideline Centre (UK). Evidence Review for Questionnaires to Assess Tinnitus: Tinnitus: Assessment and Management: Evidence Review E. London: National Institute for Health and Care Excellence (NICE); 2020

[43] Malmstrom TK, Voss VB, Cruz-Oliver DM, Cummings-Vaughn LA, Tumosa N, Grossberg GT, et al. The rapid cognitive screen (RCS): A point-of-care screening for dementia and mild cognitive impairment. The Journal of Nutrition, Health & Aging. 2015;**19**(7):741-744. DOI: 10.1007/s12603-015-0564-2

[44] Clegg A, Rogers L, Young J. Diagnostic test accuracy of simple instruments for identifying frailty in community-dwelling older people: A systematic review. Age and Ageing. 2015;**44**(1):148-152. DOI: 10.1093/ageing/afu157

[45] Gates GA, Beiser A, Rees TS, D'Agostino RB, Wolf PA. Central auditory dysfunction may precede the onset of clinical dementia in people with probable Alzheimer's disease. Journal of the American Geriatrics Society. 2002;**50**(3):482-488. DOI: 10.1046/j.1532-5415.2002.50114.x

[46] Sardone R, Castellana F, Bortone I, Lampignano L, Zupo R, Lozupone M, et al. Association between central and peripheral age-related hearing loss and different frailty phenotypes in an older population in southern Italy. JAMA Otolaryngology. Head & Neck Surgery. 2021;**147**(6):561-571. DOI: 10.1001/jamaoto.2020.5334

[47] World Health Organization. Global costs of unaddressed hearing loss and cost-effectiveness of interventions: a WHO report. 2017. [Accessed December 20, 2019]. Available from: https://apps.who.int/iris/bitstream/handle/10665/254659/9789241512046-eng.pdf

[48] Cooper JC Jr, Gates GA. Hearing in the elderly--the Framingham cohort, 1983-1985: Part II. Prevalence of central auditory processing disorders. Ear and Hearing. 1991;**12**(5):304-311. DOI: 10.1097/00003446-199110000-00002

[49] National Guideline Centre (UK). Tinnitus: Assessment and Management. London: National Institute for Health and Care Excellence (NICE); 2020

[50] De Ridder D, Schlee W, Vanneste S, Londero A, Weisz N, et al. Tinnitus and tinnitus disorder: Theoretical and operational definitions (an international multidisciplinary proposal). Progress in Brain Research. 2021;**260**:1-25. DOI: 10.1016/bs.pbr.2020.12.002

[51] Reiss M, Reiss G. Zur Problematik des pulsierenden Tinnitus [Pulsating tinnitus]. Wiener Klinische Wochenschrift. 2000;**112**(2):84-91

[52] Thomas KR, Bangen KJ, Weigand AJ, Edmonds EC, Wong CG, Cooper S, et al. Alzheimer's disease neuroimaging initiative. Objective subtle cognitive difficulties predict future amyloid accumulation and neurodegeneration. Neurology. 2020;**94**(4):e397-e406. DOI: 10.1212/WNL.0000000000008838

[53] Ruan Q, Xiao F, Gong K, Zhang W, Zhang M, Ruan J, et al. Demographically corrected normative Z scores on the neuropsychological test battery in cognitively Normal older Chinese adults. Dementia and Geriatric Cognitive Disorders. 2020;**49**(4):375-383. DOI: 10.1159/000505618

[54] Ruan Q, Zhang W, Ruan J, Chen J, Yu Z. Clinical and objective cognitive measures for the diagnosis of cognitive frailty subtypes: A comparative study. Frontiers in Psychology. 2021;**12**:603974. DOI: 10.3389/fpsyg.2021.603974

[55] Linn MW, Sculthorpe WB, Evje M, Slater PH, Goodman SP. A social dysfunction rating scale. Journal of Psychiatric Research. 1969;**6**(4):299-306. DOI: 10.1016/0022-3956(69)90023-5

[56] Chau J, Martin CR, Thompson DR, Chang AM, Woo J. Factor structure of the Chinese version of the geriatric depression scale. Psychology, Health & Medicine. 2006;**11**(1):48-59. DOI: 10.1080/13548500500093688

[57] Yeo BSY, Song HJJMD, Toh EMS, Ng LS, Ho CSH, Ho R, et al. Association of Hearing Aids and Cochlear Implants with Cognitive Decline and dementia: A systematic review and meta-analysis. JAMA Neurology. 2023;**80**(2):134-141. DOI: 10.1001/jamaneurol.2022.4427

[58] Ruan Q, Yu Z, Zhang W, Ruan J, Liu C, Zhang R. Cholinergic hypofunction in Presbycusis-related tinnitus with cognitive function impairment: Emerging hypotheses. Frontiers in Aging Neuroscience. 2018;**10**:98. DOI: 10.3389/fnagi.2018.00098

[59] National Guideline Centre (UK). Evidence Review for Psychological Therapies: Tinnitus: Assessment and Management: Evidence Review L. London: National Institute for Health and Care Excellence (NICE); 2020 Mar

[60] Dent E, Martin FC, Bergman H, Woo J, Romero-Ortuno R, Walston JD. Management of frailty: Opportunities, challenges, and future directions. Lancet. 2019;**394**(10206):1376-1386. DOI: 10.1016/S0140-6736(19)31785-4

[61] Yarnall AJ, Sayer AA, Clegg A, Rockwood K, Parker S, Hindle JV. New horizons in multimorbidity in older adults. Age and Ageing. 2017;**46**(6):882-888. DOI: 10.1093/ageing/afx150

[62] Maidment DW, Wallhagen MI, Dowd K, Mick P, Piker E, Spankovich C, et al. New horizons in holistic, person-centred health promotion for hearing healthcare. Age and Ageing. 2023;**52**(2):afad020. DOI: 10.1093/ageing/afad020

[63] Makary MA, Segev DL, Pronovost PJ, Syin D, Bandeen-Roche K, Patel P, et al. Frailty as a predictor of surgical outcomes in older patients. Journal of the American College of Surgeons. 2010;**210**(6):901-908. DOI: 10.1016/j.jamcollsurg.2010.01.028

[64] VanderWalde NA, Fleming M, Weiss J, Chera BS. Treatment of older patients with head and neck cancer: A review. The Oncologist. 2013;**18**(5):568-578. DOI: 10.1634/theoncologist.2012-0427 Epub 2013 May 1

[65] Mosnier I, Vanier A, Bonnard D, Lina-Granade G, Truy E, Bordure P, et al. Long-term cognitive prognosis

of profoundly deaf older adults after hearing rehabilitation using Cochlear implants. Journal of the American Geriatrics Society. 2018;**66**(8):1553-1561. DOI: 10.1111/jgs.15445

[66] Gordon SA, Aylward A, Patel NS, Bowers C, Presson AP, Smith KR, et al. Does frailty or age increase the risk of postoperative complications following Cochlear implantation? OTO Open. 2021;**5**(3):2473974X211044084. DOI: 10.1177/2473974X211044084

[67] Skalska A, Składzień J. Challenges of modern medicine - geriatric otolaryngology or the advantages of cooperation between an otolaryngologist and a geriatrician. Otolaryngologia Polska. 2018;**73**(1):1-5. DOI: 10.5604/01.3001.0012.7218

[68] Chow WB, Rosenthal RA, Merkow RP, Ko CY, Esnaola NF, American College of Surgeons National Surgical Quality Improvement Program, et al. Optimal preoperative assessment of the geriatric surgical patient: A best practices guideline from the American College of Surgeons National Surgical Quality Improvement Program and the American Geriatrics Society. Journal of the American College of Surgeons. 2012;**215**(4):453-466. DOI: 10.1016/j.jamcollsurg

[69] Leon M, Woo C. Environmental enrichment and successful aging. Frontiers in Behavioral Neuroscience. 2018;**12**:155. DOI: 10.3389/fnbeh.2018.00155

[70] Skoe E, Kraus N. Musical training heightens auditory brainstem function during sensitive periods in development. Frontiers in Psychology. 2013;**19**(4):622. DOI: 10.3389/fpsyg.2013.00622

[71] Bautmans I, Knoop V, Amuthavalli Thiyagarajan J, Maier AB, Beard JR, Freiberger E, et al. WHO working definition of vitality capacity for healthy longevity monitoring. The lancet. Healthy Longevity. 2022;**3**(11):e789-e796. DOI: 10.1016/S2666-7568(22)00200-8

[72] Vetrano DL, Palmer K, Marengoni A, Marzetti E, Lattanzio F, Roller-Wirnsberger R, et al. Frailty and multimorbidity: A systematic review and meta-analysis. The Journals of Gerontology. Series A, Biological Sciences and Medical Sciences. 2019;**74**(5):659-666. DOI: 10.1093/gerona/gly110

Chapter 10

Mental Health Problems and Psychological Support for People with Hearing Loss

Noriko Katsuya and Tomoko Sano

Abstract

Hearing loss and mental health issues are very closely correlated. Hearing loss has a significant impact on daily communication and makes smooth communication difficult. For example, people with hearing loss have difficulty disclosing that they have a hearing loss and avoid communication. Because of these problems, people with hearing loss are also likely to experience difficulties in establishing and maintaining close interpersonal relationships. The difficulties in coping with interpersonal stress due to hearing loss, prejudice, and stigma against people with hearing loss may also have a significant impact on the occurrence of mental health problems such as depression, anxiety, and loneliness. Therefore, psychological support is a very necessary part of the mental health of people with hearing loss. This chapter discusses the relationship between hearing loss and mental health, practices and empirical studies of psychological support for people with hearing loss in Japan and future issues necessary to provide psychological support for people with hearing loss.

Keywords: mental health, psychological support, hearing loss, prejudice, communication

1. Introduction

Hearing loss and mental health issues are very closely related. Hearing loss has a significant impact on daily communication, making smooth communication difficult. For example, to take the first author's own example, the author also has hearing loss due to a rare disease called Auditory Neuropathy (AN) [1, 2]. The disease is characterized by bilateral low tone type deficits in pure tone audiometry, with a maximum intelligibility of less than 50% in pure tone audiometry, while the otoacoustic emission (DPOAE) is a normal response. Also, Auditory brainstem response (ABR) is unresponsive or abnormal. In daily life, the author has difficulty hearing low sounds and listening to speech but can converse normally in a quiet room. On the other hand, when there is noise, such as in a café, I instantly have difficulty hearing. This makes it difficult for me to fully participate in formal conversations, such as meetings at work, as well as informal conversations, such as chit-chat. As a result, the content of discussions is only partially understood. These experiences of daily life accumulate into minor stresses. These stressful experiences are difficult for people with normal hearing to imagine and understand [3].

This chapter discusses the relationship between hearing loss and mental health. First, we discuss the varying definitions of hearing impairment as an introduction, followed by a discussion of the mental health effects of hearing loss. Then, factors related to the mental health of persons with hearing loss will be discussed, including difficulty coping with interpersonal stress, prejudice against persons with hearing loss, and stigma against persons with hearing loss. These are thought to have a significant impact on the occurrence of mental health problems such as depression, anxiety, and loneliness. In addition, the practice and empirical research of psychological support for persons with hearing loss will be discussed, as well as future issues that need to be addressed in order to provide psychological support to persons with hearing loss. We argue that psychological support for people with hearing loss is very necessary to maintain the mental health of people with hearing loss.

2. Definitions of "deaf and hard of hearing"

Definitions of the term "deaf and hard of hearing" are diverse. First, there is the medical definition. Medical definitions of hearing impairment are based on hearing threshold, disease, and severity. Second, As for legal definitions, in Japan, there are laws related to disability such as Physically Disabled Persons Welfare Act. In Japan, the criteria to be legally recognized as hearing impaired are currently very strict. In Japan, it is necessary to obtain a physical disability certificate in order to be legally recognized as hearing impaired. Even the lowest grade, Level 6, has "Those with a hearing level of 70 dB or more in both ears, or those with a hearing level of 90 dB or more in one ear and 50 dB or more in the other ear." [4] (Ministry of Health,

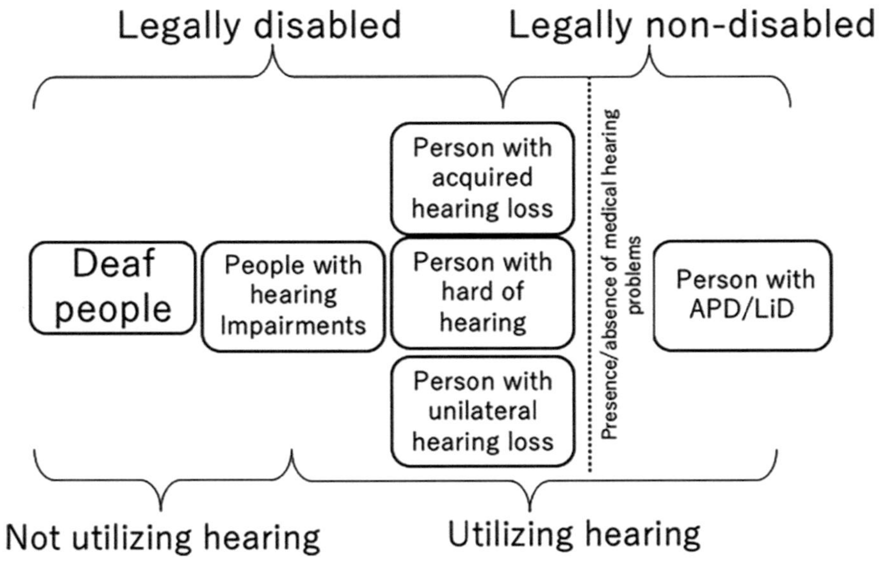

Figure 1.
Definitions of "deaf and hard of hearing".
Note. APD: Auditory Processing Disorder, LiD: Listening Difficulties.

Labor and Welfare website). This is quite a gap from the table of stages of hearing impairment and hearing thresholds in the WHO's World Report on Hearing [5]. As a result, there are people with hearing loss in Japan who cannot obtain a physical disability certificate and do not receive welfare support, even though they have difficulty hearing in daily life and experience considerable difficulties in their lives.

Third, there is the sociocultural definition. This definition is related to whether the first language is sign language or spoken language, whether or not they use their hearing, and how they define themselves in terms of their level of hearing. Based on the sociocultural definition, there are two types of people: Deaf people who use sign language and do not use their hearing, and hard-of-hearing people who use speech and use their hearing. The hard-of-hearing can be further divided into different groups according to the type of hearing loss and the time of onset of hearing loss, such as those with partial hearing loss and those with unilateral hearing loss (**Figure 1**).

3. Hearing loss and mental health

Hearing loss makes it difficult to hear speech and environmental sounds, which affects interpersonal relationships, communication, work, safety, hobbies, and many other areas [6]. According to Manchaiah and Stephens [6], hearing loss negatively or positively impacts daily life, but the negative impact is more common than the positive impact. Mental health-related effects noted include increased communication difficulties, decreased interpersonal relationships, and avoidance and withdrawal from social situations.

Hearing loss has been shown to be associated with overall mental health. A study Kobayashi's study [7] using data from the Ministry of Health, Labour and Welfare's "2007 National Survey of People's Lives" for those aged 20–39 found that the group with hard of hearing who reported hearing difficulty had worse mental health. In a study of adult hard-of-hearing people [8], the degree of mental health was lower for those with hearing loss than for those with normal hearing, but the stage of the physical disability certificate was not associated with mental health. Interestingly, in a study that examined deaf and hard-of-hearing students [9], the degree of mental health was higher for deaf students than for hard-of-hearing students. In other words, the more severe the degree of hearing loss, the worse the mental health was not necessarily. The findings suggest that other factors associated with hearing loss play a greater role in the mental health of people with hearing loss than the degree of hearing loss itself.

Next, as for other measures of mental health, various measures of depression, self-esteem, anxiety, loneliness, and general well-being have been examined for their relationship to hearing loss. The results show that hearing loss is also associated with these mental health indicators.

As for depression, adults with hearing loss have higher depression than persons without hearing loss, but there is no difference in depression between those with and without a physical disability certificate [10], older persons with hearing loss are associated with depression [11], and meta-analysis also associated hearing loss with depression [12].

It has also been shown to be associated with anxiety and stress in older people with hearing loss [11]. In addition, hearing loss has also been associated with higher loneliness [13] and anger [14] and is associated with various mental health factors.

In addition, tinnitus associated with hearing loss was also associated with depression and anxiety in a large study of a general adult sample [15]. Thus, both general and specific associations have been found between hearing loss and mental health.

As for the association with other psychiatric disorders, in a cohort study using a Korean nationwide representative sample [16], patients with sudden sensorineural hearing loss had a higher risk of affective disorders, specifically depression and anxiety disorder but not bipolar disorders. Hearing loss has been shown to be associated with mood disorders, but the degree of association is thought to vary by type of mood disorder. With regard to the association between hearing loss and developmental disabilities, some studies have examined the association with Attention Deficit Hyperactivity Disorder (ADHD). According to Solemani et al. [17], who examined the incidence of ADHD in children with hearing loss and children with normal hearing, the authors found a high prevalence of ADHD in children with hearing loss compared with normal hearing peers.

On the other hand, a study of deaf and severely hard-of-hearing patients [18] found higher rates of impulse control disorder, ADHD, and pervasive developmental disorder but lower rates of anxiety disorder, bipolar disorder, and substance abuse disorder compared to hearing patients. Although these results indicate an association between hearing loss and psychiatric disorders, it is possible that the prevalence of various psychiatric disorders may differ depending on the degree of hearing loss. The next section provides an overview of the factors involved in the mental health of persons with hearing loss.

4. Factors related to the mental health of people with hearing loss

The mental health of people with hearing loss is considered to be influenced in a multilayered manner by individual and social factors. In other words, it can be divided into factors related to the individual person with hearing loss and factors related to the society surrounding the person with hearing loss [3]. Social factors include the number and type of consultation institutions, accessibility, opportunities for contact with people with hearing loss and deafness, and social capital, as well as prejudice and stigma against people with hearing loss [3]. On the other hand, issues faced by people with hearing loss include the type and degree of hearing loss, hearing loss-specific stress experiences, stress coping strategies [3, 19], and stigma awareness [20, 21]. This section provides an overview of factors associated with the mental health of people with hearing loss and presents the authors' research examining stress specific to hearing loss, as well as prejudice and stigma consciousness.

4.1 Communication difficulties

The first factor that should be mentioned as a factor related to the mental health of people with hearing loss is the difficulty in communication due to hearing loss [22]. Hearing loss makes communication difficult because of the difficulty in hearing speech. As a result, it has a wide-ranging impact on relationships with close and important others, such as spouses and family members. Many effects of communication difficulties have been identified, including decreased social interactions, negative effects on mood, and dissatisfaction [23]. Communication difficulties also affect stress coping strategies. For example, avoidance-focused coping behavior, such as avoiding participating in conversations, is indicated to lead to depression [24].

4.2 Quality of life (QOL)

The next factor related to the mental health of persons with hearing loss is quality of life (QOL). Poor quality of life is associated with the degree of hearing loss [22]. Hearing loss affects almost every aspect of daily life, for example, forcing people to sacrifice social and leisure activities they feel they can no longer do or enjoy [23]. In addition, while there is no significant relationship between measured objective hearing loss and quality of life, activity and participation limitations due to hearing loss in daily life were significantly related to quality of life [25]. Low quality of life is thought to lower life satisfaction and affect mental health.

4.3 Stresses specific to hearing loss

The communication difficulties described above are one of the most common stress events experienced by people with hearing loss. Another stressful event is the low quality of life that results from the inability to fully participate in social and leisure activities due to hearing loss. These hearing loss-specific stress events experienced by people with hearing loss because of their hearing loss are also related to the mental health of people with hearing loss.

Katsuya investigated the stress experienced by people with hearing loss in Japan [10]. The results of a survey of 453 people with hearing loss showed that respondents with physical disability certificate due to hearing impairment had a higher number of items that they "experienced" than those without (**Table 1**).

Thus, stress events specific to hearing loss were shown to be commonly experienced by people with hearing loss in their daily lives. Although each individual

Item	Experience rate
It was difficult to hear (or not hear) someone with a low voice or who spoke too fast.	95.50
I had difficulty hearing the sound on TV or radio.	94.48
Had difficulty hearing (or could not hear) someone speaking from a distance.	93.05
Had difficulty hearing (or could not hear) broadcasts at train stations or inside buildings (department stores, event venues, etc.)	92.97
It was difficult to hear a person wearing a mask.	92.95
It was difficult to understand (or could not hear) broadcasts in trains, busses, and other vehicles.	92.79
I had difficulty understanding (or could not understand) the sound through a microphone or speakers.	92.78
I had difficulty hearing conversations in places where the surroundings were not quiet.	92.74
I had difficulty hearing (or did not understand) conversations at the reception desk, ticket counter, or cash register.	92.12

Table 1.
Stress events experienced by a high percentage of people with hearing loss [10].

event is considered relatively slight in comparison to suffering a serious illness or experiencing bereavement, the daily accumulation of these stress events is thought to exacerbate mental health.

4.4 Prejudice against people with hearing loss and stigma consciousness among people with hearing loss

Various prejudices against people with hearing loss still persist and can affect their perceptions, feelings, and behaviors. In Japan, the word "hearing loss" evokes images such as "sign language," "hearing aids," "not being able to understand conversations," "not being able to hear music," "troublesome," "pitiful," and "inconvenient" [26]. Such social images are taken up by people with hearing loss themselves, and are thought to influence their own perception and behavior. The negative image of hearing loss may affect the person with hearing loss by negatively influencing their perception of themselves and making them reluctant to engage in social activities.

In addition, stigma is one of the elements of social image that can cause negative reactions. The one of important issue of stigma has been pointed out as stigma consciousness [20], which is the concern that others may view them with stigma. The authors hypothesized that stigma consciousness might also be involved among people with hearing loss, so they created a Japanese version of a scale to examine stigma consciousness among people with hearing loss and investigated its actual status [21]. The Hard of Hearing version of the Stigma Consciousness Scale consists of items such as "Stereotypes about people with hearing and listening problems do not affect me personally." (reversal item). The relationship between stigma consciousness among people with hearing loss, measured by these items, and attitudes toward prejudice toward people with disabilities was examined.

The results showed that those with higher stigma consciousness were more likely to consider discrimination and prejudice against people with disabilities and people of a particular gender in general, and did not considered these discriminations and prejudices to have improved over the past five years [21]. In the future, the Japanese version of the Stigma Awareness Scale for People with Hearing Loss that was created should also be used to examine the effects on mental health.

5. Psychological support for people with hearing loss

5.1 Various forms of support for people with hearing loss

Psychological support for people with hearing loss takes various forms [3]. The first is support from specialists, that is, doctors, nurses, speech-language pathologists, licensed psychologists, and social workers. Second, support from nonprofessionals, that is, family, friends, and community members. Social support from familiar people is effective in many ways, including predicting satisfaction with hearing aids [27]. Coping behaviors [23] made between people with hearing loss and their partners [23] have been noted to play a necessary role in acceptance without denial [28] of hearing loss, participation in social activities, and commitment to the social situation.

Third, there is support from people who have the same hearing loss. Self-help group activities among people with the same problem of hearing loss are active in Japan. For example, there are consultation meetings held by associations of people with hearing loss and deaf people around Japan, workshops to understand the stress of hearing loss [19], and activities by voluntary groups of people with hearing loss and listening difficulties. The psychological and social support provided by these individuals with hearing loss functions to enable them to give and receive social support that meets their needs, to broaden their repertoire of coping behaviors for stress related to hearing loss, and to expand their interpersonal relationships.

In the next section, the authors will introduce a practical activity for people with hearing loss called "Kikoe Cafe" [29–32].

5.2 "Kikoe Cafe," a social meeting for people with hard of hearing and listening difficulties

The authors have been running the "Kikoe Cafe" [29–32], a social meeting for people with hard of hearing and listening difficulties since 2018 ("Kikoe" means "hearing" in Japanese). The aim of this group is to "share feelings and wisdom among people with hearing difficulties". The meeting is open to anyone with hard of hearing or listening difficulties, regardless of where they live, the degree or causes of their hearing loss, their age, or whether or not they have a physical disability certificate. Also, family members and siblings of persons with hard of hearing or hearing loss and supporters of persons with hearing loss have participated in the program. To date, 39 sessions have been held at different locations and in different formats (face-to-face or online). At "Kikoe Cafe," people with hearing loss do not just meet but also discuss and dialog with each other on specific themes.

"Kikoe cafe" serve two main functions [32]: First, they serve as a place to obtain social resources. In Japan, there are large regional differences in the psychological and social support and medical care systems for people with hearing loss. By sharing the wisdom, ideas, and information that people with hearing loss living in various regions have with each other, it will be possible for people with hearing loss to effectively use social resources that will enhance their quality of life.

The second point is its role as a place where informal communication is possible. People with hearing loss have difficulty participating in informal communication, such as chatting during work. This makes it difficult for them to participate in conversations, and they are likely to feel lonely and alienated. The Kikoe Café uses a real-time subtitling service to enable participants to follow the conversation, allowing them to participate in informal communication. The Kikoe Café provides an opportunity for participants with hearing loss to participate in conversations without being left out.

The authors believe that from these places where people with hearing loss gather, it could be possible to deliver a "hard-of-hearing" culture of people with hearing loss who utilize their hearing and devise ways of communication in their daily lives. In other words, a unique "hard-of-hearing" culture that shares a means of communication and a way of thinking about communication that is different from both the culture of normal-hearing people and the Deaf culture [33, 34]. "hard-of-hearing" culture may be less visible than "Deaf culture" due to the diversity of hearing characteristics, problems that they have, and coping strategies. Therefore, there is a need for a place to share and publicize the voices of people with hearing loss.

Future issues to be addressed with regard to support for people with hearing loss are as follows. First, it is necessary for specialists in psychological support and social work to expand the scope of their activities not only in hospitals that treat diseases related to hearing loss, such as otolaryngology, but also in local communities, such as elderly people's clubs. Second, it is necessary to grasp the actual situation of the support needed by people with hearing loss and to jointly create the necessary know-how and resources for support activities together with people with hearing loss. The resources necessary for support activities can then be utilized anytime and anywhere, regardless of where they live. This will serve the function of preventing hearing loss in an aging society where the number of people with hearing loss is expected to increase.

6. Conclusions

In this chapter, the authors first overviewed perspectives on the definition of hearing loss. The legal, sociocultural, and medical definitions of hearing loss are quite diverse. Therefore, people with hearing loss also have different self-perceptions of how they perceive themselves in terms of their hearing. This self-perception influence not only communication methods and characteristics of interpersonal relationships but also the stresses experienced in daily life. These factors could influence the way in which social factors, which are discussed next, affect them.

Next, the factors related to the mental health of people with hearing loss are reviewed. These factors include not only the personal factors of the person with hearing loss themselves, but also the social factors surrounding the person with hearing loss. Therefore, in order to maintain and promote the mental health of persons with hearing loss, it is necessary to consider these factors and provide multilayered support, including not only psychological support, but also support for improving the environment and support for making use of necessary social resources.

Finally, the actual situation of psychological support for people with hearing loss is reviewed, focusing on efforts in Japan, and future issues are also discussed. To prevent hearing loss as well, it is necessary to hold seminars and workshops for people who are at risk of hearing loss, such as the elderly, and to provide them with opportunities to receive a full range of health education. In addition, to address the interpersonal and communication problems associated with hearing loss, it is necessary to encourage participation in self-help groups and provide cooperative learning opportunities for people with hearing loss.

Acknowledgements

The studies presented in this chapter were supported by JSPS KAKENHI Grant Numbers, JP19K03347 and JP19K02219. We are sincerely grateful to Dr. Pinel for permission to use the Stigma Consciousness Scale. The content of this chapter is based on a presentation given at Phonak's online seminar "Well-Hearing is Well-Being—The Necessity of Good Hearing and Its Impact on Mental and Physical Health."

Conflict of interest

The authors declare no conflict of interest.

Author details

Noriko Katsuya[1*] and Tomoko Sano[2]

1 Research Center for Advanced Science and Technology, University of Tokyo, Tokyo, Japan

2 Josai International University, Chiba, Japan

*Address all correspondence to: katsuya@bfp.rcast.u-tokyo.ac.jp

References

[1] Kaga K, Nakamura M, Shinogami M, Tsuzuku T, Yamada K, Shindo M. Auditory nerve disease of both ears revealed by auditory brainstem responses, electrocochleography and otoacoustic emissions. Scandinavian Audiology. 1996;**25**(4):233-238

[2] Kaga K. Auditory nerve disease or auditory neuropathy—auditory dysfunction detected by combined DPOAE, electrocochleography, and ABR in 1996. Journal of Otolaryngology of Japan. 2011;**114**(5):520-523

[3] Katsuya N. Psychological support for people with hard of hearing, acquired hearing loss and auditory processing disorders. The Japanese Journal of Special Education. 2022;**60**(3):159-169

[4] Ministry of Health, Labour and Welfare [Internet]. 2023. Available from: https://www.mhlw.go.jp/stf/seisakunitsuite/bunya/hukushi_kaigo/shougaishahukushi/techou.html [Accessed: May 25, 2023]

[5] WHO. World Report on Hearing. [Internet]. 2021. Available from: https://www.who.int/publications-detail-redirect/9789240020481 [Accessed: May 25, 2023]

[6] Manchaiah VKC, Stephens D. Perspectives on defining 'hearing loss' and its consequences. Hearing, Balance and Communication. 2013;**11**(1):6-16

[7] Kobayashi Y, Tamiya N, Moriyama Y, Nishi A. Triple difficulties in Japanese women with hearing loss: Marriage, smoking, and mental health issues. PLoS ONE. 2015;**10**(2):e0116648

[8] Takamiya M, Fujita T. Mental health of persons with hearing loss or Acquired Deafness: Assessment with the 30-item General Health Questionnaire. The Japanese Journal of Special Education. 2005;**43**(4):279-290

[9] Takizawa H. Mental health in America and Japanese hearing impaired populations: A comparative study. Journal of the Society of Humanities. Sapporo Gakuin University. 2000;**68**:33-44

[10] Katsuya N. Stress and mental health among people with hearing loss in Japan: Toward a better understanding of hard of hearing and people with hearing loss. In: Proceedings of the 78th Annual Meeting Japan Psychological Association; 10-12 September 2014; Kyoto: JPA; 2014. p. 446

[11] Jayakody DM, Almeida OP, Speelman CP, Bennett RJ, Moyle TC, Yiannos JM, et al. Association between speech and high-frequency hearing loss and depression, anxiety and stress in older adults. Maturitas. 2018;**110**:86-91

[12] Adigun OT. Depression and individuals with hearing loss: A systematic review. Journal of Psychology & Psychotherapy. 2017;7(5):1-6

[13] Sung YK, Li L, Blake C, Betz J, Lin FR. Association of hearing loss and loneliness in older adults. Journal of Aging and Health. 2016;**28**(6):979-994

[14] Ferrari S, Monzani D, Gherpelli C, MacKinnon A, Mongelli F, Federici G, et al. Acquired hearing loss, anger, and emotional distress: The mediating role of perceived disability. The Journal of Nervous and Mental Disease. 2019;**207**(6):459-466

[15] Krog NH, Engdahl BO, Tambs K. The association between tinnitus and mental health in a general population sample: Results from the HUNT study. Journal of Psychosomatic Research. 2010;**69**(3):289-298

[16] Kim J-Y, Lee JW, Kim M, Kim MJ, Kim D. Association of idiopathic sudden sensorineural hearing loss with affective disorders. JAMA Otolaryngology–Head & Neck Surgery. 2018;**144**(7):614-621

[17] Soleimani R, Jalali MM, Faghih HA. Comparing the prevalence of attention deficit hyperactivity disorder in hearing-impaired children with normal-hearing peers. Archives de Pédiatrie. 2020;**27**(8):432-435

[18] Diaz DR, Landsberger SA, Povlinski J, Sheward J, Sculley C. Psychiatric disorder prevalence among deaf and hard-of-hearing outpatients. Comprehensive Psychiatry. 2013;**54**(7):991-995

[19] Katsuya N. An attempt to create a program to help people with hearing loss understand their own hearing loss and stress: A stress coping workshop. Journal of Special Education. 2019;**56**(5):305-314

[20] Pinel EC. Stigma consciousness: The psychological legacy of social stereotypes. Journal of Personality and Social Psychology. 1999;**76**(1):114-128

[21] Katsuya N, Sano T, Matsuo A. Stigma awareness among people with hearing loss - Do stigma concerns make people with hearing loss more reluctant to receive reasonable accommodations and social support? In: The 87th Annual Convention of the Japanese Psychological Association; 15-17 September 2023; Hyogo: JPA; 2023. (In press)

[22] Dalton DS, Cruickshanks KJ, Klein BE, Klein R, Wiley TL, Nondahl DM. The impact of hearing loss on quality of life in older adults. The Gerontologist. 2003;**43**(5):661-668

[23] Barker AB, Leighton P, Ferguson MA. Coping together with hearing loss: A qualitative meta-synthesis of the psychosocial experiences of people with hearing loss and their communication partners. International Journal of Audiology. 2017;**56**(5):297-305

[24] Williams KC, Falkum E, Martinsen EW. Fear of negative evaluation, avoidance and mental distress among hearing-impaired employees. Rehabilitation Psychology. 2015;**60**(1):51

[25] Hickson L, Allen J, Beswick R, Fulton M, Wolf D, Worrall L, et al. Relationships between hearing disability, quality of life and wellbeing in older community-based Australians. Australian and New Zealand Journal of Audiology. 2008;**30**(2):99-111

[26] Katsuya N. Lay theories of hearing loss. Bulletin Institute of Research Humanity Science Nihon University. 2011;**81**:123-130

[27] Singh G, Lau ST, Pichora-Fuller MK. Social support predicts hearing aid satisfaction. Ear and Hearing. 2015;**36**(6):664-676

[28] Armero OE. Effects of denied hearing loss on the significant other. The Hearing Journal. 2001;**54**(5):44-47

[29] Katsuya N, Sano T. Practice of "Kikoe Cafe" to connect people with hearing loss and difficulty in listening. In: Proceedings of 59th Annual Meeting of the Japanese Society for Special Education; 18-20 September 2021; Ibaraki: The Japanese Association of Special Education; 2021

[30] Sano T, Katsuya N. The usefulness and challenges of "Kikoe Café": An online self-help group for the hearing impaired and hard-of-hearing. In: Proceedings of 60th Annual Meeting of the Japanese Society for Special Education; 8-21 September 2022; Ibaraki: The Japanese Association of Special Education; 2022

[31] Sano T, Katsuya N. Characteristics and roles of the Kikoe Café – The Kikoe Café connects people with hearing loss and difficulty in listening with people with normal hearing. In: The 87th Annual Convention of the Japanese Psychological Association; 15-17 September 2023; Hyogo: JPA; 2023. (In press)

[32] Katsuya N, Sano T. Practice of "Kikoe Cafe" to connect people with hearing loss and difficulty in listening (2): Status of the cafe and future challenges. In: 61st Annual Meeting of the Japanese Society for Special Education; 25-27 August 2023; Kanagawa: The Japanese Association of Special Education; 2023. (In press)

[33] Fernandes JK, Myers SS. Inclusive deaf studies: Barriers and pathways. Journal of Deaf Studies and Deaf Education. 2010;**15**(1):17-29

[34] Kimura H, Ichida Y. Deaf Culture Declaration – Deaf people as linguistic minorities (Deaf Culture Declaration). Gendai Shiso. 1995;**23**(3):354-362

Chapter 11

A Tailored and Transdisciplinary Approach to Cochlear Implants

Tania Hanekom, Johan Hanekom, Werner Badenhorst, René Baron, Talita le Roux and André Uys

Abstract

Non-auditory stimulation (NAS) is a potential complication in cochlear implants (CIs) that can impact both the effectiveness of sound transmission and the quality of life for users. This issue can often be mitigated through remedial CI device programming strategies. In some cases, the symptoms of NAS are persistent irrespective of typical audiological interventions. To develop an intervention for NAS that is tailored to the auditory system and surrounding structures of an individual CI user requires a transdisciplinary approach. This chapter proposes a model for transdisciplinary, patient-centred care of CI users who suffer from persistent NAS complications from intracochlear electrical stimulation. The model combines aspects of anatomy, radiology, computational modelling and audiology to gain an understanding of the parameters that give rise to the occurrence of NAS and to provide an avenue for investigating novel intervention strategies. Addressing unintended facial nerve stimulation by a CI is used to demonstrate the application of the model.

Keywords: cochlear implants, facial nerve stimulation, computational modelling, person-centred care, transdisciplinary team

1. Introduction

The cochlear implant (CI) or 'bionic ear' is a technological intervention intended to treat severe to profound sensorineural hearing loss [1]. Often, hearing impairment is a result of cochlear hair cell loss where up to 80% of inner hair cells may be lost as a result of aetiological factors, such as medication or trauma [2]. More significant hearing loss resulting in profound deafness can only be treated by surgically implanting a CI. When the origin of deafness is sensorineural, a CI can stimulate the auditory nerve electrically to induce action potentials (APs) that travel along the auditory nerve to elicit a sensation of sound. The electrically induced APs are indistinguishable from naturally elicited APs, but there are a number of differences. Notably, the dynamic range between the stimulation threshold and saturation rates at which APs are generated (the firing rate) in response to increases in electrical current level is much smaller than that of natural neural excitation. CI speech perception in quiet may be close to normal, but it may deteriorate in noise [2].

IntechOpen

While designs vary across CI companies [3], all commercial CIs have the same components. Externally, the CI system consists of a microphone, speech processor and transmitter [4]. Internally, the CI consists of a surgically implanted receiver-stimulator and the electrode array within the cochlea. The speech processor acts as an artificial cochlea by taking the sound input from the microphone and emulating some of the processing known to take place in the healthy cochlea. The speech processor translates the acoustic signal into a format that may be used to stimulate the surviving auditory nerve fibres in the inner ear or cochlea *via* the electrode array. Stimulus data from the speech processor is transmitted *via* a wireless transcutaneous link to the implanted receiver-stimulator that encodes information in the original acoustic input into electrical pulse trains that are applied to electrode contacts of the electrode array. The wireless connectivity also enables the transfer of power to the implanted electronics, remote adjustments, updates and telemetric data collection to assess the status of the auditory nerve and the functionality of the implant.

Cochlear implants vary in electrode design and a variety of speech processing strategies exist. For example, electrode array designs differ in the number of electrode contacts, the spacing between electrodes, the positioning (e.g., lateral wall and perimodiolar designs) and the length of the electrode array [5]. Speech processors may, for example, focus on delivering temporal fine structure [6] or on accurate representation of sound spectra [7].

Cochlear implant outcomes are highly variable [8], with some CI users achieving open set speech recognition, and some having virtually no benefit other than being in contact with their sound environment. Variability in the hearing outcomes with a CI device is a direct result of interpersonal differences in the auditory systems of individual CI users and the integration of the CI technology with this unique system. Despite different designs that attempt to address different issues, outcomes are similar across electrode designs and speech processors [3]. For example, current focusing and current steering methods are used to mitigate the effect of current spread [9, 10], some electrode designs target deep insertions to ensure that the low-frequency region of the cochlea is stimulated [11] and electrode array positioning is either perimodiolar or against the cochlear lateral wall [12]. These different designs have not solved the problem of variable outcomes across CI users [13]. The same problems remain across implant designs: programming (or mapping) of the device for optimal hearing through optimal electrical stimulation parameter settings is unique for each user [14, 15]; neural survival patterns vary across CI users [16] but electrode arrays cannot be positioned to make provision for this; and patterns of current spread in each CI user is uniquely a function of individual anatomy [17]. To complicate matters further, programming of the CI device for adults can be done interactively, but mapping for babies or CI users with multiple disabilities needs to be done with objective methods, for example, based on electrically-evoked compound action potential (eCAP) measures [18]. Objective methods are needed for individualised mapping [19, 20]. Cochlear implant companies supply software platforms to streamline mapping and to some extent make the mapping process objective [21], but this is of use mostly for cases without additional complications.

Standard management and care approaches become inadequate once there is additional complexity, for example, where inner ear malformations exist [22], when the electrode array is not ideally placed, when neural survival is compromised, when the electrical environment deviates from the expected, for example when bone conductance is affected due to disease [23] or when non-auditory stimulation (NAS) causes complications that compromises hearing performance and/or quality of life [24].

When a CI user experiences sub-optimal performance or complications that cannot be resolved through conventional interventive mapping strategies, a multi- and transdisciplinary approach that incorporates computational modelling as an advanced analytic and diagnostic tool may be required to effectively investigate and ideally address the issue. This approach is person-specific, taking into account the unique characteristics of each CI user's cochlear environment, as well as other factors that may impact hearing outcomes.

This chapter describes a transdisciplinary approach that encompasses three disciplines or domains within CI management, differentiated here as the clinical, medical sciences and engineering domains. The aim of a transdisciplinary approach is to actively integrate and synthesise knowledge across various knowledge fields to address complex problems and produce novel solutions. This enables a person-centred care approach in the management of complex CI cases that is underpinned by the translation of computational models to clinical application.

2. The disciplines in CI management

2.1 Clinical domain

The standard model of care for CI users is typically practised in the clinical domain illustrated in **Figure 1**. The standard of care is person-centred, which aims to recognise the unique needs, preferences, values and circumstances of each CI user. A clinical model of care is typically an interdisciplinary model, where different members of the care team share information and insights across their respective disciplines.

Within the clinical domain, a CI team consists of a variety of clinical practitioners that need to operate in four interdisciplinary areas. The assessment of hearing and

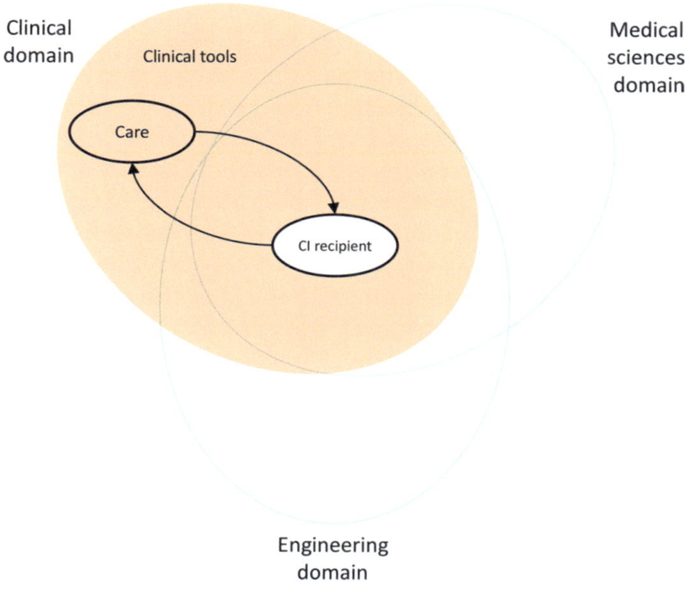

Figure 1.
Illustration of care, centred in the clinical domain.

management of hearing loss is primarily dealt with by audiologists. The surgical implantation of the CI device and maintaining auditory health is the joint responsibility of the ear, nose and throat (ENT) surgeon, radiologist, neurologist and paediatrician in paediatric cases. Counselling and supporting the CI user and their family members to optimise quality of life is the task of a psychologist and social worker, while the auditory (re)habilitation through auditory training is managed by an audiologist and/or speech-language therapist.

When a person is first diagnosed with a hearing loss that indicates CI candidacy, the person is usually referred to a CI team for clinical evaluation. The evaluation includes at least an ENT surgeon and an audiologist. Often, evaluation for candidacy also involves a psychologist and a social worker to appraise whether personal circumstances will support the decision to implant [25], along with audiological measures [26] and imaging that may include either computed tomography (CT) or magnetic resonance imaging (MRI) or both [27]. Imaging allows evaluation of the anatomic suitability for receiving a CI and may inform a yes/no decision and selection of the ear to be implanted.

Surgical implantation of the internal components of the CI device is performed by the ENT surgeon with in theatre support from an audiologist and/or a specialised clinical engineer made available by the CI company. Objective neurophysiological tests are routinely performed in-theatre as initial assessment of the neural responses to electrical stimulation and to verify the integrity of the device. For example, electrocochleography (ECochG) can be used to monitor the auditory nerve's response to electrode insertion and activation. This can provide real-time feedback to the surgeon about the electrode's positioning and its potential impact on the auditory nerve.

Subsequent activation and programming of the CI device are carried out by an audiologist. Thereafter, the CI user will have regular follow-up visits to an audiologist for updating and maintaining the CI user's map. The professional team may also include a speech-language therapist that assists with (re)habilitation with the CI device [28]. Initially, CI stimulation sounds distorted [29] and the postlingual hearing-impaired CI user needs to relearn to hear, while children with congenital deafness need to learn to hear with their CI(s) [30]. Facilitating this process is known as auditory training. (Re)habilitation and auditory training, which focus on improving speech perception, along with ongoing follow-up appointments and psychosocial support to address emotional aspects, are required to optimise CI outcomes. Lifelong management and CI device upgrades ensure access to the latest technology, aiming to enhance hearing outcomes and improve the quality of life for CI users.

An array of tools is available in the clinical domain for managing and maintaining hearing performance. From a surgical and medical practitioner perspective, this includes diagnostic tools to determine the aetiology of hearing loss, for example, genetic testing, assessment of the medical history of a patient to determine factors such as exposure to loud noise, ototoxicity, infections and underlying medical conditions, imaging that may help to identify structural abnormalities, tumours or nerve hypoplasia and physical examination. In cases where hearing loss is associated with balance problems, balance and vestibular testing may also form part of the assessments that may be conducted.

From an audiology perspective, the most important tool in the management of CI hearing performance is the CI device programming software provided by each of the CI companies. Besides mapping, this software also allows neurophysiological evaluations, such as measuring the eCAP and assessing the integrity of the device by measuring the electrical impedances of the electrode contacts. Pure tone audiometry is frequently used to monitor the unaided and aided hearing thresholds to assess both the progression of hearing loss and the aided benefit that a person receives from a hearing aid, CI or hybrid device. However, pure tone audiometry does not necessarily translate to speech understanding, and hence, tools to evaluate hearing performance as reflected by speech understanding are also employed. These include listening test batteries targeted at CI users, for example, the minimal auditory capabilities (MAC) test battery [31] and the basic auditory skills evaluation (BASE) battery [32]. Neurophysiological testing that assesses the functional level of the auditory pathway includes electrically evoked auditory brainstem responses (eABRs) and ECochGs. ECochGs can help identify conditions, such as endolymphatic hydrops (Meniere's disease) and assist in determining the site of lesion in auditory neuropathy spectrum disorder (ANSD), which may affect the success of cochlear implantation.

The default interaction between the care provided by the clinical team and the CI user, if no complications are experienced, is shown by the arrows in **Figure 1**. However, if complications arise, a second step assessment is introduced in the management strategy. **Figure 2** illustrates an array of additional tests and evaluations that may be employed in the assessment phase.

2.2 Medical sciences domain

Much of what is known about the pathology of the auditory system originates from the medical sciences domain. Medical sciences are crucial for guiding clinical interventions related to hearing loss, particularly in the context of CIs. The success of CIs relies on contributions from diverse medical science fields, including anatomy, histology and medical imaging. These contribute significantly to the foundational knowledge base, offering insight into the structure and function of the various components of the auditory system and providing tools to assess this system in order to facilitate clinical decision-making. **Figure 3** illustrates some of the expertise that

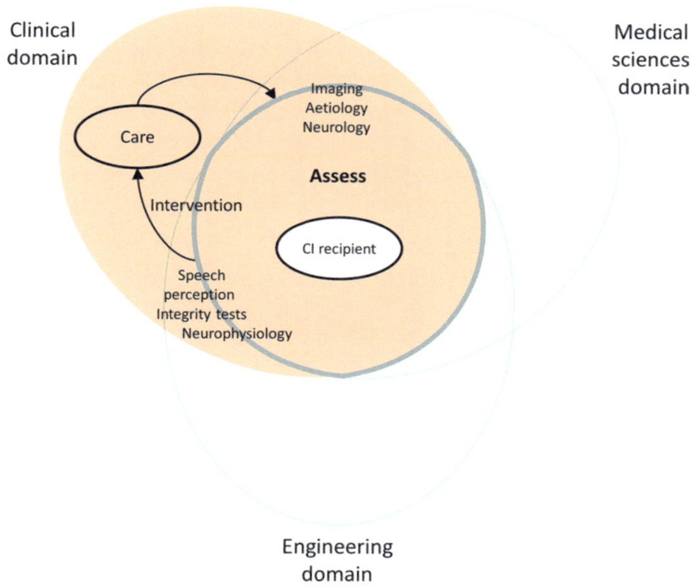

Figure 2.
Extended care that includes an assessment step for complicated CI cases.

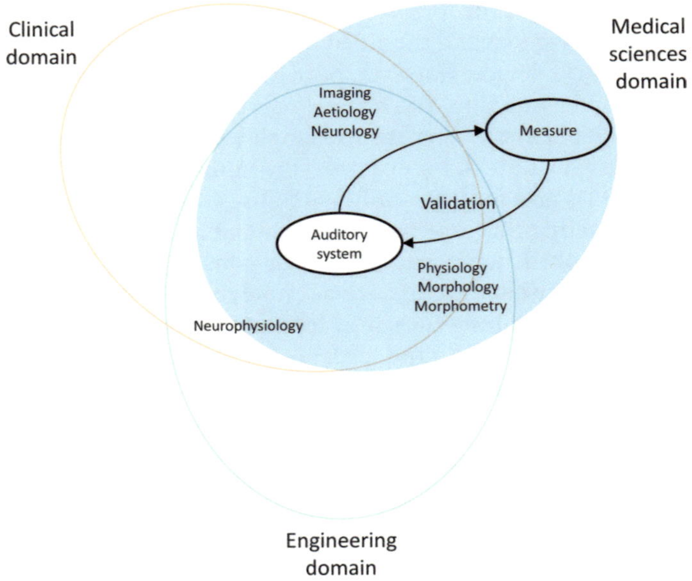

Figure 3.
The medical sciences domain offers expertise to inform and support the development of CI technology and the care and management of CI users.

the medical domain offers to inform and support the development of CI technology and the care and management of CI users.

A detailed morphological (qualitative: form and structure) and morphometric (quantitative: size and proportions) description of the cochlea, cochlear nerve and surrounding structures, provided by anatomists is necessary for the design of CI electrode arrays that would minimise implant trauma while providing an effective interface with the remaining neural structures and contribute to hearing preservation. Knowledge about the morphology is essential for surgeons to locate the cochlea during the implantation procedure and to minimise the risk of damage to surrounding structures, specifically including the facial nerve which is in close proximity to the scala tympani [33]. Understanding the anatomical variations among individual patients' cochleae and possible abnormalities is important for selecting appropriate electrode arrays [34] and customising implant procedures. Cadaver studies are an important facet of anatomy as this form the basis for characterising the detailed morphology and morphometry of the auditory system and also facilitate testing and refinement of new CI devices.

Histology provides insights into the cellular and histopathological changes that occur in the cochlea due to hearing loss. This information is invaluable for understanding the potential impact of long-term hearing loss on the cochlear structures and similarly, the ontogenesis of electric hearing over time. Histological studies can also guide researchers and clinicians in designing electrodes that effectively interface with the remaining auditory nerve fibres.

Medical imaging, specifically CT scans and MRI, provide visualisations of the inner ear anatomy, even though the resolution is low relative to the dimensions of the cochlea. Micro-computed tomography (μCT), of which the radiation levels are too high for safe clinical use, is often used in CI research to provide high-resolution images of cadaver temporal bones so that the variations in cochlear morphology and

DOI: http://dx.doi.org/10.5772/intechopen.1002920

morphometry may be studied. Cadaver studies also allow researchers to correlate imaging data with actual anatomical structures in order to validate the accuracy of measurements from imaging data. Imaging, both clinical and scientific, is crucial for preoperative planning, allowing surgeons to appreciate the general anatomy of the cochlea and surrounding structures and to assess the patient's individual cochlear anatomy [35]. Imaging provides a means to identify anatomical abnormalities and to plan the optimal trajectory for electrode insertion. Post-operative imaging provides information about the location of the electrode array within the cochlea and may also provide information about progressive changes in the cochlea and rest of the auditory system.

2.3 Engineering domain

Engineers are at the core of the design, development and improvement of CI technology, which involves several engineering disciplines, for example, biomedical engineering, electronic engineering, computer and software engineering, materials science and mechanical engineering. Engineers design and develop the hardware and software components of CI systems. This includes the external speech processor, the wireless, transcutaneous link between the external processor and the implanted system, the implanted electrode array and the powering of the implant. The development of sophisticated signal processing algorithms within the external processor that aims to enhance and optimise the quality of sound delivered to CI users is an ever-evolving engineering task. Careful design of the power supply and power management strategies are important to ensure that users can enjoy continuous hearing without frequent expensive battery replacements [36].

Apart from the development of the technology, engineers are also involved in research that probes the intricacies of the integration between biology and technology. Computational modelling is an effective tool to probe the biophysical interactions between CIs and the complex biology of the human auditory system. While untangling the factors influencing the relation between stimulus and perception in CI users is challenging because of the complexity and inaccessibility of the auditory system, computational models offer a pathway for examining how specific parameters influence aspects of hearing. The aim of a computational model is to create a digital twin of the auditory system of a specific CI user that would allow researchers to probe this system in a way that would involve excessively invasive procedures if conducted on the CI user (**Figure 4**).

There are two main types of models in CI research: models that describe the periphery, and therefore the biophysical interface between the implant and the auditory system and models that describe processing in the central auditory nervous system and perception of sound. Both of these types of models may use a physiologically-based approach, a phenomenological approach or a combination of the two. Because of the complexity of the complete auditory system, a large number of models have been created to describe distinct characteristics of this system. Often a number of different models, each describing a specific component or aspect, are combined to capture the characteristics of the auditory system more completely.

One example is modelling of the electrically stimulated auditory periphery that requires at least two models for a complete description: one to describe the volume conduction effects when stimulation current is injected into the cochlea (and surrounding tissue) and one to describe the response of the auditory nerve fibres to the injected current. Finite element volume conduction (FEVC) models of the cochlea

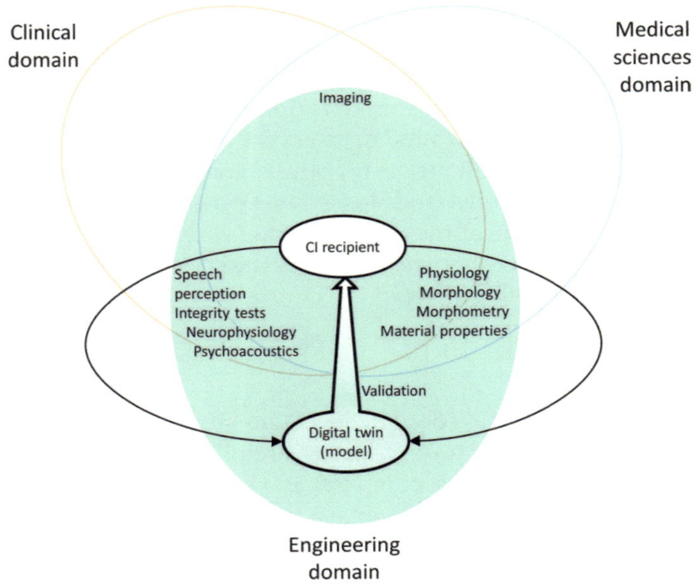

Figure 4.
Engineering domain, where computational models of a CI users' cochleae are designed and implemented. The computational model aims to be a digital twin of the CI user so that invasive test results and insights from the CI user may be gained. The arrow from the model to the CI user represents the validation route where predictions from the model are evaluated against data measured from the CI user.

attempt to capture a detailed three-dimensional (3D) description of the cochlea, auditory nerve and in many cases, the surrounding tissues and structures [17, 37–41]. The parameters that describe the anatomy and geometry of a particular CI user's cochlear structures are extracted from medical imaging data (CT or MRI scans). Different tissues in the model are assigned different electrical properties, for which the values are derived from experimental data originating in the medical sciences domain. Such a model can be used to simulate the spread of electrical current through the tissues when current is injected through the CI electrodes.

The response to the stimulation current at the output of the FEVC model is predicted by an auditory nerve fibre (ANF) model. An ANF model may take several forms, for example, it may be conductance-based, such as the Hodgkin-Huxley [39, 42, 43] or Schwartz-Eikhoff [44–46] models that comprise a set of differential equations, or it may be phenomenological [47–49] or a combination of the two [50]. ANF models are commonly developed in programming languages, such as MATLAB or Python. In combination, the FEVC and ANF models, referred to as compound models, allow prediction and analyses of the neural response to electrical stimulation [17, 23, 40, 51–53]. From these, researchers can infer how the perception of sound may be affected by different intertwined factors such as the pattern of neural survival, the location of the electrode array relative to the surviving nerve fibres and different stimulation strategies. Simulation results are typically validated by comparing them to experimental data obtained from CI users.

2.4 The need for a transdisciplinary model of care

The previous sections expanded on the roles that each of the three domains play in providing medical care, understanding the anatomy and physiology of the auditory system and how this relates to the physical characteristics of its structures and developing the various components of CIs and their supporting technologies. While the clinical model of care has been successful in providing essential services and support to CI users, a transdisciplinary team that combines the tools and techniques from the different domains may provide a deeper understanding of the complex relationship among factors that affect the unique hearing experience of individual CI users. This becomes particularly important when addressing CI complications such as NAS, where identifying the root cause might not be straightforward, or when multiple factors contribute to an issue.

Figure 5 depicts a transdisciplinary model that includes the clinical, medical sciences and engineering domains.

The model consists of a six-stage approach centred around the CI user and a digital twin of their electrically stimulated hearing system. The digital twin is created as a computational model of the cochlea, cochlear nerve and surrounding structures and allows the team to investigate a particular CI user's auditory system from an invasive viewpoint. If a CI user experiences NAS, as illustrated in **Figure 5**, the first stage in the approach is clinical care where a CI user's clinical team will identify the issue, and then proceed to intervene according to the standard models of care. If the care model is not effective in mitigating the issue, the second stage is entered, where the transdisciplinary team considers the different facets of the case and formulates data collection requirements. To be able to create a computational model of the CI user's cochlea, morphological and morphometric data must be measured for the specific individual in the third stage to complement data that was already collected during the care stage. The fourth stage involves parameterisation of the relevant data to create a person-specific computational model of components of the CI user's auditory system. The fifth stage involves creating the model and validating it against empirical data obtained from the medical history of the user, as well as from clinical tests,

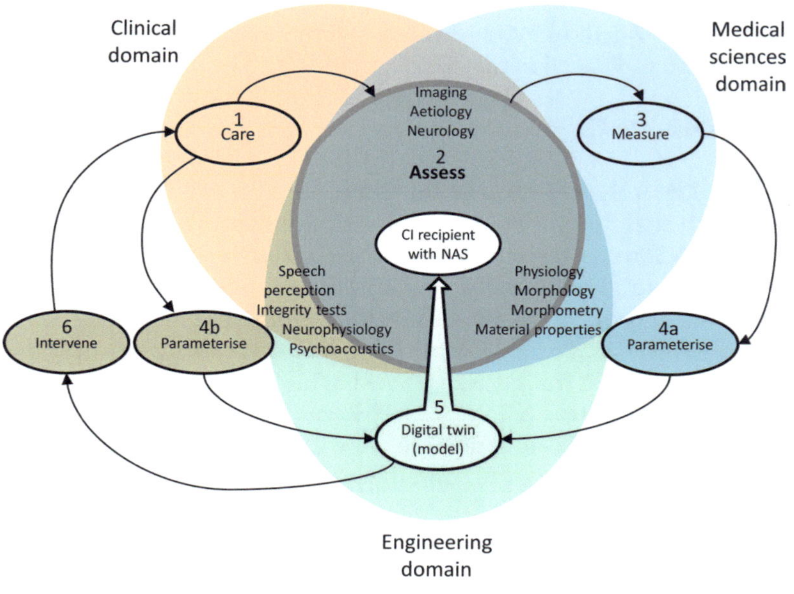

Figure 5.
A diagrammatic representation of model-based person-centred care through a six-stage transdisciplinary approach.

experiments and image data. The model is then used to investigate possible solutions to alleviate or mitigate the complication. Interventions that may have been designed or identified are tested in stage six. The process is iterative as a first iteration might not yield desired results. It is also important to realise that it may be impossible to devise an effective solution for a particular person. However, the model provides an avenue for understanding the underlying causes of the complication, thereby informing the care strategy for this and future CI users.

In the remainder of the chapter, the application of the transdisciplinary model will be unpacked within the context of facial nerve stimulation (FNS).

3. Application of the model: a practical example

To demonstrate the application of the model of care through the complication of FNS, it is necessary to provide a conceptual framework of FNS through which the reader may appreciate the complexities of and the necessity for the transdisciplinary approach.

3.1 Facial nerve stimulation

3.1.1 What is FNS, and what does it do?

FNS occurs when electrical current from the CI intended to stimulate the ANFs, spreads to and excites the nearby labyrinthine segment of the facial nerve (FN) [24, 54–56]. Symptoms of FNS in CI users vary from user discomfort in the form of facial tingling to twitching of the facial muscle to severe, painful and disfiguring facial spasms. Other symptoms that may present are referred pain in the form of headaches, loss of taste, and sensory and secretomotor symptoms. Symptoms could negatively affect the functionality of the CI, may present directly after CI device activation or after a period of use and, in users with bilateral CIs, may present on both or only one side of the face [54, 57–59]. In extreme cases, symptoms can become so severe that explantation and reimplantation may be required [60].

3.1.2 How prevalent is FNS?

Using the PRISMA algorithm on an initial pool of over 1000 CI and FNS-related articles, Van Horn et al. [60] provide a systematic review of the rate of and factors associated with FNS in CI users followed by an assessment of FNS management strategies. In their review and meta-analysis of 37 articles representing 5936 CI users, the reported FNS rate ranged from 0.68–43%, with a cumulative incidence rate of 5.6%, or almost one in every 18 CI users. Cochlear implant users with otosclerosis showed an overall FNS rate of 26% (range, 6.25–75%) having a significantly higher odds ratio (OR) to non-otosclerosis (OR = 13.73, 95% confidence interval [CI] 3.57–52.78, $p < 0.01$). Users with lateral wall arrays are more likely to experience FNS with an OR = 3.92, 95% CI 1.6–10.47, $p < 0.01$ and those with cochlear malformations showed an overall FNS rate of 28% (range, 5.3–43%).

3.1.3 What factors affect, aggravate or increase the risk of FNS?

Factors that appear to affect the occurrence of FNS include cochlear ossification (post-meningitis and otosyphilis), otosclerosis, osteoporosis, temporal bone fracture, a narrow bony cochlear nerve canal and cochlear malformations [55–57, 61–64]. Unfortunately, these factors also often result in inadequate loudness perception by the CI user, which then requires an increase in stimulus current level, thereby aggravating the FNS because the increased stimulus current level increases the spread or leakage of current to the facial nerve [55]. The type of CI array also proved a significant factor in FNS occurrence. Straight, lateral arrays are situated closer to the outer wall of the cochlea and thus closer to the facial nerve, whereas pre-curved, perimodiolar arrays with modiolar facing contacts lie in closer proximity to and direct the current towards the modiolus and are thus less likely to leak current towards the facial nerve [59].

Another risk factor in FNS is cochlear-facial dehiscence, an opening between the cochlea and labyrinthine segment of the FN [65]. When a CI electrode is activated, electrical current from the electrode may spread through the opening to the labyrinthine segment of the FN and cause FNS. Factors that may contribute to cochlear-facial dehiscences include local thinning of the otic capsule (such as in cases of meningitis and otosclerosis), topographic anatomy of the cochlea and impingement of the otic capsule upon the labyrinthine segment of the FN causing narrowing [66].

Intraoperative electrophysiology testing, such as eABR, can be performed during the surgical procedure to assess the function of the auditory. Abnormal findings, such as the detection of facial nerve (CN VII) and vestibular potentials on eABR testing, may indicate a higher likelihood of post-operative NAS [67].

3.2 Application of model-based person-centred care

Managing complications with CI stimulation is multifaceted and requires a comprehensive approach that considers all factors, including medical history, hearing needs and CI program settings. By utilising a multi- and transdisciplinary computational model-based approach, the objective is to create a person-specific map that maximises the individual's hearing outcomes while minimising complications. In this section, a qualitative narrative of the management of five CI users, presenting with FNS, is presented to demonstrate how a transdisciplinary model of care is applied at the University of Pretoria, South Africa.

3.2.1 Case studies

Case 1. In a study by Badenhorst et al. [23], a CI user received a Med-El C40+ standard electrode array in the right ear at age 4 years and 4 months following a meningitis infection. The left cochlea was implanted 3 years later with a Med-El Pulsar ci100 short array electrode because of severe ossification of the scalae. A few years later this implant caused acute headaches and pain after which it was explanted and replaced with a dummy electrode for possible future reimplantation in the ossifying left cochlea. A year after the explantation, the user experienced FNS with the remaining right implant. FNS also presented in the left cochlea upon reimplantation with a Med-El compressed array.

Case 2. The study by Van der Westhuizen et al. [53] reports on a CI user for whom hearing was lost after gentamicin injection in the middle ear following a retrosigmoid vestibular neurectomy for intractable vertigo in Ménière's disease. The person received a Cochlear Nucleus implant with a CI24RE Contour Advance electrode in the right ear. While image analysis revealed electrodes 16 and 17 to be closest to the FN, the CI user experienced severe FNS on most of the electrodes in the array.

Case 3. The origin of this CI user's deafness is unknown and started at around 4 to 5 years of age. The right ear was implanted, and the user experienced FNS since initial stimulation. The first implant was removed and was replaced with a Cochlear Nucleus implant with a CI24RE Contour Advance electrode. The FNS persisted, causing epiphora (watery, red eye) and activation of the orbicularis oculi muscle on the side of the implant.

Case 4. This CI user's hearing was lost following a tuberculosis meningitis infection. The right ear was implanted with a Cochlear Nucleus implant with CI24RE Contour Advance electrode. The CI user experienced FNS on all electrodes.

Case 5. This CI user's biological mother contracted rubella during pregnancy. The CI user was diagnosed with bilateral hearing loss at age four and started to use a hearing aid in the right ear at age nine and only 10 years later started to use a hearing aid in the left ear. This CI user received a cochlear nucleus implant in the left ear with a CI422 electrode as an adult and experienced no FNS complications in this ear. Eight years later, this CI user was implanted with a Cochlear Nucleus implant with a CI632 electrode in the right ear. Severe FNS is experienced on all electrodes implanted on the right side.

3.2.2 Care

From the brief descriptions of the FNS cases above, it is evident that the origins and management of FNS are intricate. For all the above cases, not only is the quality of sound provided by the implant affected by FNS but also the quality of life of the CI users. Despite technological advances in cochlear implantation, the interpersonal variability in factors that affect hearing outcomes, for example, aetiology of deafness and neural survival patterns implies that auditory (re)habilitation may require a range of different management strategies.

Before the need for a transdisciplinary approach becomes evident, there are a number of standard interventions that are typically attempted within the clinical domain (**Figure 2**). The most common non-invasive intervention strategy for FNS involves reprogramming or remapping of the CI by either increasing stimulation pulse widths or increasing interphase gaps to reduce stimulation levels [60, 68]. In a recent systematic review [60], FNS management strategies were reported in 28 of the 37 included studies, with a cumulative sample of 259 CI users with FNS. All studies reported the resolution of FNS through remedial CI device programming strategies, but the exact success rate of these programming strategies was not reported [60]. Reprogramming of the CI device has been attempted for all five cases described above but failed to mitigate the adverse effects of FNS. Upon onset of FNS in case 1, a new map was programmed that initially did not cause FNS, but it returned over time because of steadily increasing current levels that were required to maintain functional hearing.

To counteract the larger current spread associated with higher current levels (and associated FNS), electrical pulse width increase may present a solution. A disadvantage of this approach may be in a processor, where the time duration of a stimulus cycle (cycling through all electrodes that need to be activated) is fixed, which (e.g.) is the case in a SPEAK processing strategy. The number of spectral maxima used in the processor relates to the spectral content of the acoustic signal that is encoded in the electrical stimuli. SPEAK uses between six and eight maxima, and the spectral representation becomes sparse if the number of maxima becomes too small. For case 4, the map that rendered the best hearing (though still unsatisfactory) could accommodate only four maxima due to large pulse widths.

Lowering the stimulation levels of offending electrodes to current levels just below the stimulus level inducing the FNS symptoms while still achieving auditory stimulation [55] was also attempted in combination with deactivation of one or more electrode contacts. Deactivation of electrodes on multichannel arrays is relatively common in clinical practice, although this tends to compromise the quality of hearing and speech perception outcomes, especially in cases where multiple electrodes of the upper basal and/ or middle turns of the cochlea need to be deactivated to manage FNS [60, 68]. In cases, where both lowered stimulation levels and electrode deactivation were required to manage severe FNS, all five CI cases reported insufficient loudness to offer a comfortable listening experience. This is in accordance with the literature that states remedial CI programming strategies to be useful in most cases to reduce FNS symptoms to some extent, though sound quality and auditory performance are often affected, especially in cases that require significantly decreased levels of electrical stimulation or aggressive electrode deactivation [54, 60].

Alternative stimulation modes and triphasic pulse stimulation have also been documented as non-invasive intervention strategies for FNS [68, 69]. For example, for case 4, after the conventional extra-cochlear stimulation modes MP1 and MP2 were explored with increased pulse widths and decreased rate, intra-cochlear stimulation modes, common ground, bipolar+3, and bipolar+5 were tested. However, the intracochlear modes failed to provide sufficient loudness growth because of the close proximity of the active and reference electrodes [70]. The largest electrical dynamic range for the most active channels was achieved with a pseudomonopolar map. However, even with this map, loudness was compromised and did not improve with pulse widths beyond 200 µs. Similar challenges were experienced in the mapping of the other four CI cases, with none of the conventional FNS intervention strategies rendering a satisfactory outcome.

If none of the non-invasive strategies prove successful in managing the FNS, there are invasive strategies that may be considered. The first is botulinum toxin (Botox) treatment [71], but the inability to use facial muscles or facial expressions may lead to reduced quality of life [53]. For case 1, Botox injections were administered as a temporary measure to alleviate the effect of the FNS. The treatment partially inhibited the FNS, but at the cost of little to no facial expression while the CI user still reported perceiving contraction of the facial muscles. Botox injections were administered in case 4, but because of the risk of affecting the motor neuron pathways required for eating and drinking, the treatment was conservative. The FNS was less visible, but the user was still aware of the muscle contractions, similar to the experience of case 1.

In some severe FNS cases, where typical audiological interventions such as reprogramming of the CI and deactivation of electrodes do not alleviate the FNS symptoms, explantation and reimplantation of the CI device may be necessary [60, 68, 72, 73]. Case 3 had the first implant removed due to persistent FNS. The CI user was re-implanted with a perimodiolar electrode array that placed the electrodes further away from the FN because of its modiolus-hugging intracochlear location. The strategy of changing the type of electrode array from a lateral wall type to a perimodiolar type at reimplantation has been documented as an effective approach to eliminate FNS [74], though this approach did not resolve FNS for case 4. Case 1 had the CI on the left removed due to acute headaches and pain, which is indicative of NAS. The left side was re-implanted with a compressed array that could only be partially inserted because of ossification. Reimplantation was, however, not effective to mitigate complications in this CI user. FNS was experienced shortly after activation.

Removal of the CI and its intracochlear electrode array can also cause explantation trauma. Since explantation is often carried out a number of years after initial implantation, reactive tissue may have formed around the electrode, which may increase the risk for explantation trauma [75] and may, therefore, compromise the outcomes that may be achieved with a subsequent implant. For this reason, explantation should be a last resort.

In a transdisciplinary team, where computational modelling expertise is available, the model presented in **Figure 5** should be applied before explantation is considered, and if the latter is seen as the only option, to predict the chances of success of reimplantation given what can be extrapolated through the tools of a transdisciplinary team and specifically computational modelling.

3.2.3 Assessment

When the methods available for mitigating FNS in the clinical domain (**Figure 2**) have been exhausted, the transdisciplinary team needs to assess the available information and data that have been collected for the CI user. The transdisciplinary team comprises a core team that includes members having expertise in the relevant domains, as well as the clinical team of the specific CI user. The team may, thus, be geographically distributed, necessitating an agreement on a remote operation strategy.

The assessment will determine how computational modelling will be used to inform management of the case. In some cases, a complete model will be constructed to assess a CI user's unique situation, while it may be possible to extrapolate from observations that were made in previous modelling studies that investigated other cases.

The primary inputs required to continue with a model-based approach are good quality imaging data that may be complemented by anatomical, neuroanatomical and neurophysiological data originating from the intersection between the clinical and medical domains, the CI user's medical history and device programming information from the clinical domain, and data from speech perception tests, CI device integrity tests, neurophysiological tests and psychoacoustic tests originating from the intersection between the clinical and engineering domains.

3.2.4 Measurement

3.2.4.1 Imaging

The foundation for the construction of the 3D computational models of a specific CI user's cochlea and surrounding structures is clinical images, for example, CT. These images are used to quantify the dimensions of cochlear structures. The human cochlea is as unique as a fingerprint [76], and it has been shown that person-specific modelling of the cochlea needs to take these variations into account [17].

Multi-slice computed tomography (MSCT), cone-beam computed tomography (CBCT) and magnetic resonance imaging (MRI) are part of the routine pre-operative evaluation of a CI candidate, while only CT-based modalities are viable for post-operative assessment due to the metal artefacts that obscure the cochlea in MRI scans.

For computational models, post-operative CT images are the most crucial as these provide information on the morphology of the individual cochlea, as well as the intracochlear location of the electrode array, the depth of insertion and possibly insertion trauma should the array appear not to follow the trajectory of the scala tympani [77]. If post-operative CT imaging is not available, it has to be acquired, for example. in case 3, where the process could not continue before the images were available.

It is also worth noting that imaging modalities may differ depending on the availability of scanner technology. **Figure 6** shows a mid-modiolar slice through the CT images for each case. Cases 1, 2 and 4 had MSCT scans available, while cases 3 and 5 had CBCT images available. The advantage of MSCT is that Hounsfield units may be used to track changes in bone density over time should multiple scans be available. This characteristic of MSCT was utilised for case 1, where the progression of changes in the bone density could be measured over time. However, the grey values in CBCT are at most moderately correlated with Hounsfield units and are dependent, among others, on the specific brand of the scanner [78]. This might make it difficult to track changes in bone density should the only image data be CBCT. On the other hand, CBCT is considered a low-radiation dose alternative to MSCT with the added advantage of superior image resolution and metal artefact reduction [79], which are beneficial to capture morphometric data for the cochlea.

3.2.4.2 Landmarking

To measure the morphometric characteristics of the cochlea and facial nerve, landmarking is used to quantify the shape of the cochlea. Landmarks are a 3D constellation of discrete anatomical locations described by Cartesian coordinates. They are points of correspondence on each specimen that are identifiable and distinguishable in every cochlea. The landmarks shown in **Figure 6** have been selected to describe the

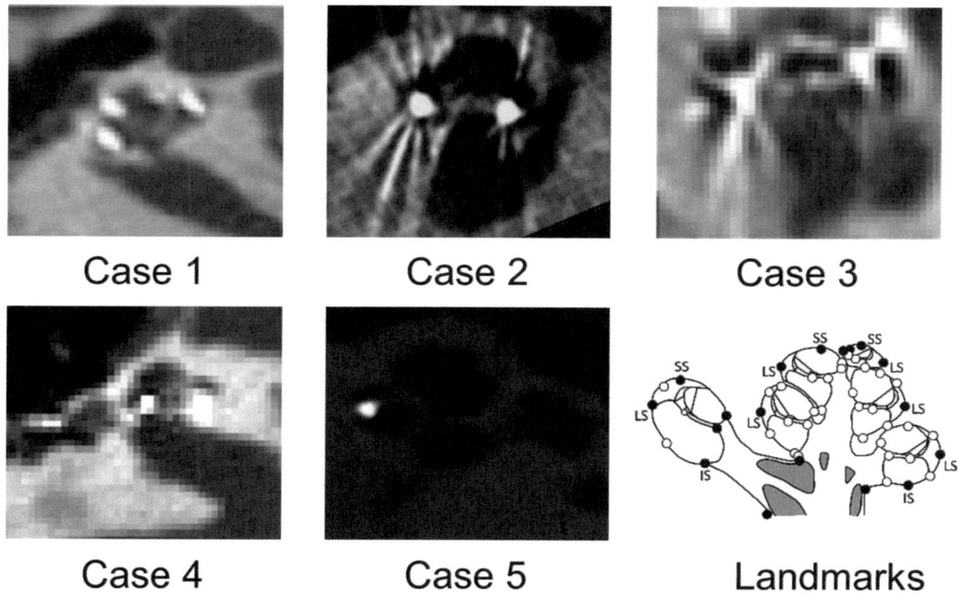

Figure 6.
Panels for cases 1 to 5. Two-dimensional mid-modiolar slices through the cochleae of cases 1 to 5 show the variation in image quality. Cases 1, 2 and 4 had MSCT scans, while cases 3 and 5 had CBCT scans. The bright areas in the images are the metal electrode contacts. The scan for case 2 is particularly affected by artefacts. Landmarks panel. A landmark set that may be used to describe the bony shape of the cochlea. Closed dots indicate landmarks that should be visible on clinical CT images, while open dots indicate landmarks that have to be derived from high-resolution images such as micro-CT scans (not used for live humans) to augment the clinical scans.

shape of the bony aspects of the cochlear canal for the purpose of 3D modelling. A minimum set of landmarks is required for the construction of 3D cochlear landmarks and for cochlear modelling; at least, the lateral spiral (LS points in **Figure 6**) must be distinguishable.

Considering the scans in **Figure 6**, case 1 shows no artefact and the lateral spiral and electrode position can be measured. Case 2 presents a scan, where the artefacts from the electrode array obscured the lateral spiral due to beam hardening. In this case, a parametric model that may be less accurate than a landmark-based model may be required [80]. While a parametric model may be constructed from a reduced landmark set, it could miss some of the person-specific local variations in cochlear shape. In case 3 no landmarks can be accurately measured and a parametric model will be required. The image for case 4, although blurry, allows the landmarks that describe the lateral (LS) and superior spirals (SS) to be delineated. Case 5 has little interference from electrode artefacts and here the superior, inferior, lateral, superolateral and inferolateral spirals can be measured. This scan can be used for 3D computational modelling of the implanted cochlea.

The measurements that need to be taken to reconstruct the FN are the length, width and angle of the labyrinthine, tympanic and mastoid segments of the FN as described in Badenhorst et al. [23]. Because the FN is enclosed in a bony canal, these measurements can all be made on the CT images of the CI users.

3.2.5 Parameterisation

The parameters in a computational model are values, settings or variables that define the characteristics, behaviour and properties of the model.

Model parameters that define the 3D structure of the model are the size and shape of the cochlear and surrounding structures and originate from the interface between medical sciences and engineering (**Figure 5**). Parameterisation of the landmark measurements obtained from the CT images involves the transformation of the measured coordinates to the coordinate system in which the models are constructed, as well as applying appropriate scaling factors. Electrical material properties are mostly obtained from the literature since it is not possible to measure these in a living CI user. However, the electrical properties of the bone surrounding the cochlea play a crucial role in the distribution of current outside the cochlea and is, therefore, an important parameter to include in FNS models. The only way to obtain an indication of the value of this parameter for a particular CI user is by means of imaging. While there is no direct relationship between Hounsfield units, bone mineral density and the electrical properties of bone, the trends in this parameter may be inferred from CT images taken at various time intervals. In the models, a decrease in the mineral content of the bone encapsulating the cochlea is represented by decreasing the bone impedance relative to the accepted value for this parameter in modelling studies [23, 38]. For case 1, several CT scans were available over a period of 18 months where a decrease in the bone density could be observed, which could then be included in the modelling study [23].

Model parameters that attempt to capture neural health, for example, the extent of neural degeneration, loss of auditory nerve fibres or other damage to the auditory nerve fibres, originate from neurophysiological testing that is performed at the intersection between the clinical and engineering domains (**Figure 5**). This includes eCAP measurements and eABR measurements, which provide an indication of the status of the auditory nerve [81, 82].

3.2.6 Modelling

Once the measurements and parameterisation are done for a specific CI user, the person-specific 3D finite element model of the cochlea, auditory nerve, facial nerve and surrounding tissues, all having different electrical properties [17], is constructed in COMSOL and positioned in a generic head model as shown in **Figure 7** for case 1 [23]. The basal-to-middle turn of the cochlea's scala tympani was partially ossified having an order of magnitude higher resistivity compared to the normal perilymph.

Current spreads through the cochlea as shown in **Figure 8** for a monopolar electrode that injects current. Notice the close proximity of the FN's labyrinthine segment to the cochlea in the bottom-right of **Figures** 7 and **8**. The bottom left panel shows how the current emanates from electrode 5. Most current then spreads through the partially ossified cochlea with some current passing through and possibly stimulating the FN (top frame).

Using a MATLAB model, ANFs are scaled and distributed within the cochlea based on the cochlear geometry and ANF morphology such as that shown in **Figure 9** [39, 43, 51].

The distribution of the ANFs relative to the cochlear geometry and electrode array for case 1 is shown in **Figure 10** with the soma and nodes represented by the markers. The FEVC current spread output and resulting electric potential distribution in the cochlea combined with the fibre node locations provide the potential at each node for any selected stimulus strategy and level. The individual nodal potentials then serve as input to the purely conductance-based computational ANF model in MATLAB to determine which auditory and/or facial nerve fibres will activate and produce a propagating action potential along the fibre [43].

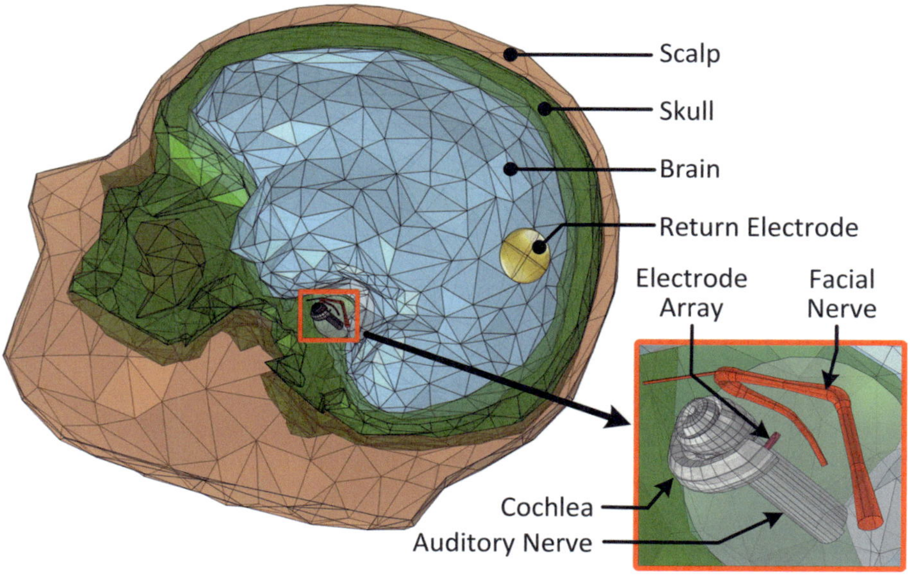

Figure 7.
Finite element volume conduction (FEVC) COMSOL model of a head, skull, brain, partially ossified cochlea, CI and facial nerve (Case 1).

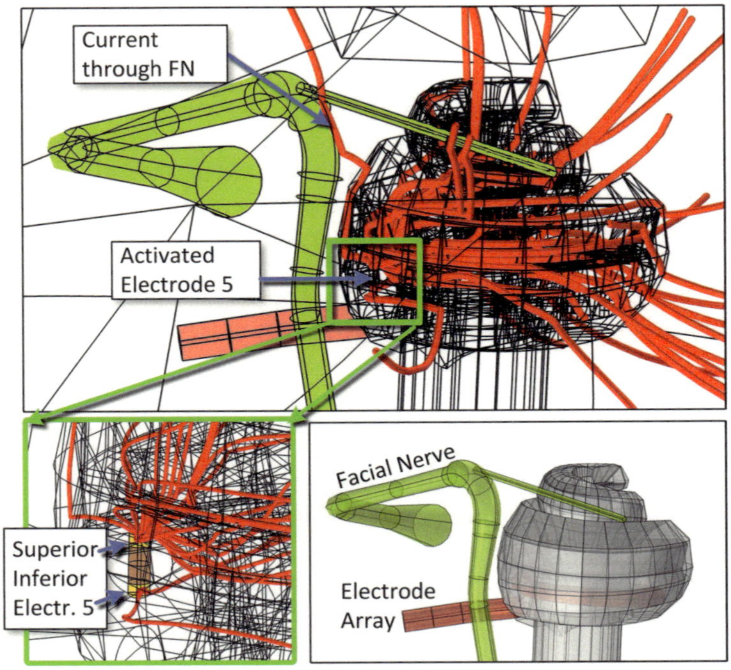

Figure 8.
Bottom-right shows asemi-transparent view of a partially ossified cochlea, electrode and FN for a FEVC simulation in COMSOL for case 1. The top panel shows the current spread (red lines) through the cochlea upon activation of electrode 5 (E5), which is nearest to the FN. The bottom left panel, an enlargement of the section indicated, shows the current originating from the superior and inferior electrodes. As expected, the top panel shows the majority of the current spreading towards the right through the cochlea, but some current finds its way through the FN causing FNS.

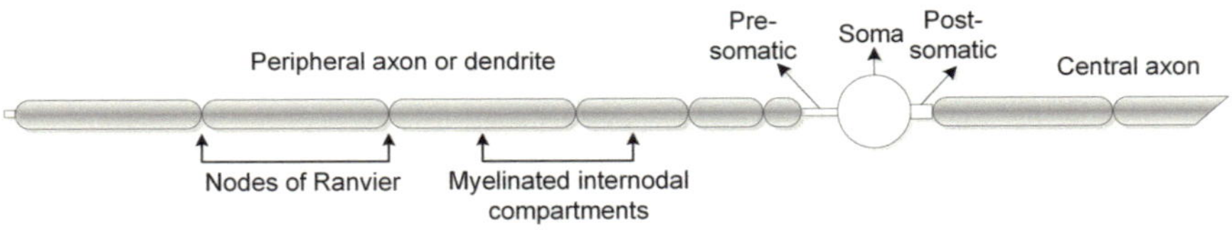

Figure 9.
Morphology of a computationally modelled auditory nerve fibre.

From the model simulations, the onset of FNS in case 1 was attributed to a decrease in resistivity of the otic capsule, likely because of the ossification of the cochlear ducts. The study suggests that the left cochlea showed a larger increase in auditory stimulation and FNS compared to the right cochlea, possibly because of increased resistivity in the cochlear ducts and decreased resistivity of the otic capsule. This could result in a decreased dynamic range in the left cochlea, which in turn could lead to decreased thresholds of the auditory and facial nerve fibres, resulting in the observed FNS.

Similar person-specific modelling and simulations for case 2 were used to investigate the implementation of apical reference (AR) stimulation as a means of reducing FNS. In using the most apical electrode as the reference electrode, the current could be contained within the cochlea and directed away from the facial nerve fibre (FNF).

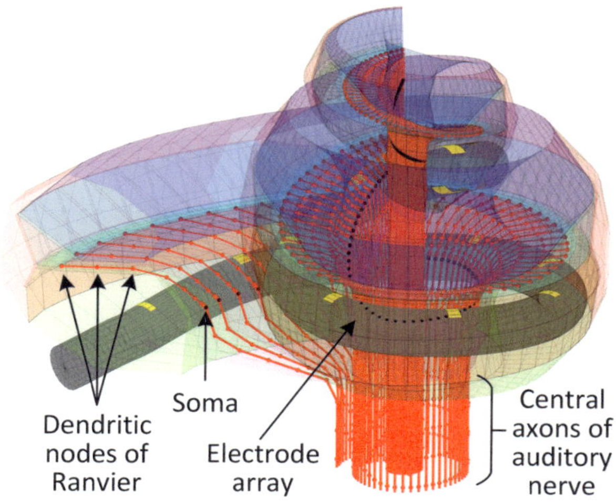

Figure 10.
A MATLAB rendering of the ANF distribution within the cochlea for case 1 indicating the dendritic nodes of Ranvier, soma, electrode array and central axons.

The hypothesis of an increased pulse width reducing the effect of FNS was tested by simulating both AR and conventional monopolar (MP1 + 2) stimulation with phase durations of 25 μs and 300 μs. For MP1 + 2 stimulation, a number of electrodes showed FNF thresholds lower than the ANF thresholds at 25 μs, with the increase in pulse width barely increasing these FNF thresholds above the ANF thresholds. For AR stimulation, however, FNF thresholds were already above ANF thresholds at 25 μs, with the increase to 300 μs further increasing the threshold difference (dynamic range) while also decreasing both FNF and ANF thresholds. This supports the hypothesis that AR stimulation is a viable strategy to alleviate FNS.

3.2.7 Intervention

The last stage of the transdisciplinary model of care is the intervention stage, where the findings of the process need to inform the subsequent management of the CI user. It is important to note that it might be necessary to iterate through the six stages of the care model based on an improved understanding of the CI user's situation from previous iterations. The following provides a brief summary of the intervention stage for the five case studies after the first iteration through the model details in this chapter.

For case 1, personal circumstances of the CI user and Med-El implants' inability to accommodate the implementation of the AR stimulation strategy with its standard clinical software limited the intervention options. Though much was learned through the modelling process that can be applied in future cases, the only intervention possible at the time was counselling for the CI user to better understand what was happening in the cochleae, how that was causing severe FNS and why the standard care procedures of remapping do not work in this specific case.

For cases 2 and 3, the outcomes were similar as both CI users have been using their CIs for an extensive period. Both MP1 + 2 and AR stimulation were tested in the laboratory. AR stimulation resulted in a decrease in threshold and an increase in comfort levels as the model predicted and the users reported a reduction in FNS symptoms.

The quality of sound with AR stimulation was, however, either poor or the CI users reported very little sound perception. Despite this, the study validated the model prediction that an AR strategy could reduce FNS.

Case 4 had not benefited from the CI as the FNS was present from initial stimulation. While a reasonable map could be fitted for this CI user, no speech perception of sound could be achieved with the AR stimulation mode.

To verify that the AR stimulation mode could provide a viable alternative stimulation mode, it was tested on two CI users who do not experience FNS. These CI users could perceive speech, though they reported their perception of sound to be much different from that provided by their original map with default parameter settings. This suggested that should a CI user be able to listen with this map, extensive auditory retraining may be required, especially if the CI user had become accustomed to another stimulation mode.

Case 5 experienced FNS almost from initial stimulation, and therefore did not have as much experience with the CI in the ear affected by FNS as cases 1 to 4. The CI user started auditory retraining with the AR map, which was effective in mitigating the FNS, but after approximately 5 weeks, the FNS returned. This suggests changes in the cochlear environment and sensitivity of the FN that have not been taken into consideration in the present models. This observation informs the next iteration through the care model to tease out the underlying mechanisms that are responsible for the FNS to reoccur.

It is worth noting that a non-invasive solution to FNS may or may not be attained through the application of a transdisciplinary model. However, the process provides a deep insight into a specific CI user's auditory system that may provide grounds for decision-making and may inform counselling. The model also contributes to the knowledge base about the factors that cause a unique listening experience for each CI user.

4. Conclusions

A transdisciplinary model of care that incorporates expertise and tools from the domains of clinical care, medical sciences and engineering is of great value for managing complex FNS cases in CI users. As discussed in the previous sections, the challenges associated with FNS complications are multifaceted and require a comprehensive approach that goes beyond traditional disciplinary boundaries. A transdisciplinary model of care offers two main advantages above a purely clinical approach to FNS management.

Firstly, it embraces a holistic person-centred care approach. Complex cases in CI require an approach that focuses on the individual's overall well-being and quality of life. A transdisciplinary model of care enables professionals from various disciplines to collaborate and provide a comprehensive assessment and tailored treatment plan. By considering medical, clinical and engineering perspectives together, the model considers the unique needs and limitations of each CI user more comprehensively than a single perspective approach.

Secondly, it offers a means to develop a detailed understanding of the effects of electrical stimulation on the particular CI user's auditory system. By involving medical sciences and bioengineering, the model can leverage expertise in fields such as computational neurophysiology and anatomy, medical imaging, signal processing and control systems theory and medical device design to devise intervention strategies for a particular CI user, or if a satisfactory intervention is not possible, to provide an understanding of the underlying causes of the FNS that may be used to manage the CI user's expectations.

It is important to acknowledge the challenges associated with implementing a transdisciplinary model of care in all CI clinics. Limited resources, geographical constraints and limited availability of experts from multiple disciplines can hinder the establishment of a transdisciplinary team. Telehealth and remote consultation technologies can be utilised to facilitate communication and collaboration among specialists located in different locations. In this way, CI users and their clinical teams may gain access to the advantages that a multidisciplinary team may offer.

Finally, while a purely clinical model of care remains the standard approach for CI users in many clinics, the inclusion of a transdisciplinary team can offer significant advantages when CI users experience complications with their CIs.

Author details

Tania Hanekom[1*], Johan Hanekom[1], Werner Badenhorst[1], René Baron[2], Talita le Roux[3] and André Uys[2]

1 Bioengineering, Department of Electrical, Electronic and Computer Engineering, University of Pretoria, Pretoria, South Africa

2 Department of Anatomy, University of Pretoria, Pretoria, South Africa

3 Department of Speech-Language Pathology and Audiology, University of Pretoria, Pretoria, South Africa

*Address all correspondence to: tania.hanekom@up.ac.za

References

[1] Carlyon RP, Goehring T. Cochlear implant research and development in the twenty-first century: A critical update. Journal of the Association for Research in Otolaryngology. 2021;**22**(5):481-508

[2] Salvi R, Sun W, Ding D, Chen GD, Lobarinas E, Wang J, et al. Inner hair cell loss disrupts hearing and cochlear function leading to sensory deprivation and enhanced central auditory gain. Frontiers in Neuroscience. 2017;**10**:1-14

[3] Zeng FG. Trends in cochlear implants. Trends in Amplification. 2004;**8**(1):1-34

[4] Patrick JF, Busby PA, Gibson PJ. The development of the Nucleus®Freedom™ cochlear implant system. Trends in Amplification. 2006;**10**(4):175-200

[5] Ertas YN, Ozpolat D, Karasu SN, Ashammakhi N. Recent advances in cochlear implant electrode Array design parameters. Micromachines. 2022;**13**(7):1081, 1-20. Available from: https://www.mdpi.com/2072-666X/13/7/1081/pdf?version=1657700835

[6] Vermeire K, Punte AK, Van De Heyning P. Better speech recognition in noise with the fine structure processing coding strategy. ORL. 2010;**72**(6):305-311

[7] Donaldson GS, Nelson DA. Place-pitch sensitivity and its relation to consonant recognition by cochlear implant listeners using the MPEAK and SPEAK speech processing strategies. Journal of the Acoustical Society of America. 2000;**107**(3):1645-1658

[8] Moberly AC, Bates C, Harris MS, Pisoni DB. The enigma of poor performance by adults with cochlear implants. Otology & Neurotology. 2016;**37**(10):1522-1528

[9] Srinivasan AG, Landsberger DM, Shannon RV. Current focusing sharpens local peaks of excitation in cochlear implant stimulation. Hearing Research. 2010;**270**(1-2):89-100

[10] Roux J, Hanekom JJ. Effect of stimulation parameters on sequential current-steered stimuli in cochlear implants. Journal of the Acoustical Society of America. 2022;**152**(1):609-623

[11] Hochmair I, Hochmair E, Nopp P, Waller M, Jolly C. Deep electrode insertion and sound coding in cochlear implants. Hearing Research. 2015;**322**:14-23

[12] Risi F. Considerations and rationale for cochlear implant electrode design-past, present and future. Journal of International Advanced Otology. 2018;**14**(3):382-391

[13] Cosetti MK, Waltzman SB. Outcomes in cochlear implantation: Variables affecting performance in adults and children. Otolaryngologic Clinics of North America. 2012;**45**(1):155-171

[14] Shapiro WH, Bradham TS. Cochlear implant programming. Otolaryngologic Clinics of North America. 2012;**45**(1):111-127

[15] Chang CJ, Sun CH, Hsu CJ, Chiu T, Yu SH, Wu HP. Cochlear implant mapping strategy to solve difficulty in speech recognition. Journal of the Chinese Medical Association. 2022;**85**(8):874-879

[16] Zimmermann CE, Burgess BJ, Nadol J. Patterns of degeneration in

the human cochlear nerve. Hearing Research. 1995;**90**(1-2):192-201

[17] Malherbe TK, Hanekom T, Hanekom JJ. Constructing a three-dimensional electrical model of a living cochlear implant user's cochlea. International Journal for Numerical Methods in Biomedical Engineering. 2016;**32**(7):e02751, 1-23. Available from: https://pubmed.ncbi.nlm.nih.gov/26430919/

[18] Scorpecci A, D'Elia A, Malerba P, Cantore I, Consolino P, Trabalzini F, et al. Maps created using a new objective procedure (C-NRT) correlate with behavioral, loudness-balanced maps: A study in adult cochlear implant users. European Archives of Oto-Rhino-Laryngology. 2016;**273**(12):4167-4173

[19] Ali H, Noble JH, Gifford RH, Labadie RF, Dawant BM, JHL H, et al., editors. Image-guided customization of frequency-place mapping in cochlear implants. In: ICASSP, IEEE International Conference on Acoustics, Speech and Signal Processing – Proceedings. Brisbane, Australia; 2015. pp. 5843-5847

[20] Kurz A, Müller-Graff FT, Hagen R, Rak K. One click is not enough: Anatomy-based fitting in experienced cochlear implant users. Otology and Neurotology. 2022;**43**(10):1176-1180

[21] Wathour J, Govaerts PJ, Lacroix E, Naïma D. Effect of a CI programming fitting tool with artificial intelligence in experienced cochlear implant patients. Otology and Neurotology. 2023;**44**(3):209-215

[22] Sennaroglu L. Cochlear implantation in inner ear malformations – A review article. Cochlear Implants International. 2010;**11**(1):4-41

[23] Badenhorst W, Hanekom T, Gross L, Hanekom JJ. Facial nerve stimulation in a post-meningitic cochlear implant user: Using computational modelling as a tool to probe mechanisms and progression of complications on a case-by-case basis. Cochlear Implants International. 2021;**22**(2):68-79

[24] Broomfield S, Mawman D, Woolford TJ, O'Driscoll M, Luff D, Ramsden RT. Non-auditory stimulation in adult cochlear implant users. Cochlear Implants International. 2000;**1**(1):55-66

[25] Entwisle LK, Warren SE, Messersmith JJ. Cochlear implantation for children and adults with severe-to-profound hearing loss. Seminars in Hearing. 2018;**39**(4):390-404

[26] Reddy P, Dornhoffer JR, Camposeo EL, Dubno JR, McRackan TR. Using clinical Audiologic measures to determine cochlear implant candidacy. Audiology and Neurotology. 2022;**27**(3):235-242

[27] Vaid S, Vaid N. Imaging for cochlear implantation: Structuring a clinically relevant report. Clinical Radiology. 2014;**69**(7):e307-ee22

[28] Van Bogaert L, Machart L, Gerber S, Lœvenbruck H, Vilain A. Speech rehabilitation in children with cochlear implants using a multisensory (French Cued Speech) or a hearing-focused (Auditory Verbal Therapy) approach. Frontiers in Human Neuroscience. 2023;**17**:1-17

[29] Caldwell MT, Jiam NT, Limb CJ. Assessment and improvement of sound quality in cochlear implant users. Laryngoscope Investigative Otolaryngology. 2017;**2**(3):119-124

[30] Roman S, Rochette F, Triglia JM, Schön D, Bigand E. Auditory training improves auditory performance in

cochlear implanted children. Hearing Research. 2016;**337**:89-95

[31] Owens E, Kessler DK, Raggio MW, Schubert ED. Analysis and revision of the minimal auditory capabilities (MAC) battery. Ear and Hearing. 1985;**6**(6):280-290. DOI: 10.1097/00003446-198511000-00002

[32] Shafiro V, Hebb M, Walker C, Oh J, Hsiao Y, Brown K, et al. Development of the basic auditory skills evaluation battery for online testing of cochlear implant listeners. American Journal of Audiology. 2020;**29**(3s):577-590

[33] Kruschinski C, Weber BP, Pabst R. Clinical relevance of the distance between the cochlea and the facial nerve in cochlear implantation. Otology and Neurotology. 2003;**24**(5):823-827

[34] Eshraghi AA, Ocak E. Cochlear implant electrode choice in challenging surgical cases: Malformation, residual hearing, ossification, or Reimplantation. Current Otorhinolaryngology Reports. 2017;**5**(4):315-322

[35] Walker N, Pham N, Ledbetter L. Cochlear implantation: Current and future roles of imaging before, during, and after implantation. Current Radiology Reports. 2023;**11**(7):97-107

[36] de Nobel J, Kononova AV, Briaire JJ, Frijns JHM, Bäck THW. Optimizing stimulus energy for cochlear implants with a machine learning model of the auditory nerve. Hearing Research. 2023;**432**:108741. Available from: https://www.sciencedirect.com/science/article/pii/S0378595523000539?via%3Dihub

[37] Malherbe TK, Hanekom T, Hanekom JJ. Can subject-specific single-fibre electrically evoked auditory brainstem response data be predicted from a model? Medical Engineering and Physics. 2013;**35**:926-936

[38] Malherbe TK, Hanekom T, Hanekom JJ. The effect of the resistive properties of bone on neural excitation and electric fields in cochlear implant models. Hearing Research. 2015;**327**:126-135

[39] Badenhorst W, Hanekom T, Hanekom JJ. Analysis of a purely conductance-based stochastic nerve fibre model as applied to compound models of populations of human auditory nerve fibres used in cochlear implant simulations. Biological Cybernetics. 2017;**111**(5-6):439-458

[40] Hanekom T, Hanekom JJ. Three-dimensional models of cochlear implants: A review of their development and how they could support management and maintenance of cochlear implant performance. Network: Computation in Neural Systems. 2016;**27**(2-3):67-106

[41] Kalkman RK, Briaire JJ, Frijns JH. Stimulation strategies and electrode design in computational models of the electrically stimulated cochlea: An overview of existing literature. Network (Bristol, England). 2016;**27**(2-3):107-134

[42] Hodgkin AL, Huxley AF. A quantitative description of membrane current and its application to conduction and excitation in nerve. Journal of Physiology. 1952;**117**:500-544

[43] Rattay F, Lutter P, Felix H. A model of the electrically excited human cochlear neuron. I. Contribution of neural substructures to the generation and propagation of spikes. Hearing Research. 2001;**153**(1-2):43-63

[44] Schwartz JR, Eikhof G. Na currents and action potentials in rat myelinated

nerve fibres at 20 and 30 degrees. Archives. 1987;**409**:569-577

[45] Frijns JHM, Mooij J, ten Kate JH. A quantitative approach to modeling mammalian myelinated nerve fibres for electrical prosthesis design. IEEE Transactions on Biomedical Engineering. 1994;**41**(6):556-566

[46] Frijns JHM, Mooij J, Schoonhoven R. Have mammalian myelinated nerve fibres diameter dependent nodal properties? A model study. In: Frijns JHM, editor. Cochlear Implants a Modelling Approach. Den Haag: CIP-Data Koninklijke Bibliotheek; 1995. pp. 69-92

[47] Takanen M, Bruce IC, Seeber BU. Phenomenological modelling of electrically stimulated auditory nerve fibers: A review. Network: Computation in Neural Systems. 2016;**27**(2-3):157-185

[48] Bruce IC, Erfani Y, Zilany MSA. A phenomenological model of the synapse between the inner hair cell and auditory nerve: Implications of limited neurotransmitter release sites. Hearing Research. 2018;**360**:40-54

[49] Tabibi S, Boulet J, Dillier N, Bruce IC. Phenomenological model of auditory nerve population responses to cochlear implant stimulation. Journal of Neuroscience Methods. 2021;**358**:109212, 1-12

[50] van Gendt MJ, Briaire JJ, Kalkman RK, Frijns JHM. A fast, stochastic, and adaptive model of auditory nerve responses to cochlear implant stimulation. Hearing Research. 2016;**341**:130-143

[51] Kalkman RK, Briaire JJ, Dekker DMT, Frijns JHM. The relation between polarity sensitivity and neural degeneration in a computational model of cochlear implant stimulation. Hearing Research. 2022;**415**:108413, 1-14. Available from: https://www.sciencedirect.com/science/article/pii/S0378595521002471/pdfft?md5=f7e5acecb2878bb928091aead5010391&pid=1-s2.0-S0378595521002471-main.pdf

[52] Biesheuvel JD, Briaire JJ, Kalkman RK, Frijns JHM. The effect of stimulus level on excitation patterns of individual electrode contacts in cochlear implants. Hearing Research. 2022;**420**:108490, 1-12

[53] van der Westhuizen J, Hanekom T, Hanekom JJ. Apical reference stimulation: A possible solution to facial nerve stimulation. Ear and Hearing. 2022;**43**(4):1189-1197

[54] Ahn JH, Oh SH, Chung JW, Lee K-S. Facial nerve stimulation after cochlear implantation according to types of nucleus 24-channel electrode arrays. Acta Otolaryngologica. 2009;**129**(6):588-591

[55] Bigelow DC, Kay DJ, Rafter KO, Montes M, Knox GW, Yousem DM. Facial nerve stimulation from cochlear implants. American Journal of Otology. 1998;**19**(2):163-169

[56] Niparko JK, Oviatt DL, Coker NJ, Sutton L, Waltzman SB, Cohen NL. Facial nerve stimulation with cochlear implantation. VA cooperative study group on cochlear implantation. Otolaryngology and Head and Neck Surgery. 1991;**104**(6):826-830

[57] Kelsall DC, Shallop JK, Brammeier TG, Prenger EC. Facial nerve stimulation after nucleus 22-channel cochlear implantation. The American Journal of Otology. 1997;**18**(3):336-341

[58] Berrettini S, Vito de A, Bruschini L, Passetti S, Forli F. Facial nerve stimulation after cochlear implantation: Our experience. Acta

Otorhinolaryngologica Italica. 2011;**31**(1):11-16

[59] Seyyedi M, Herrmann BS, Eddington DK, Nadol JB Jr. The pathologic basis of facial nerve stimulation in otosclerosis and multi-channel cochlear implantation. Otology & Neurotology. 2013;**34**(9):1603-1609

[60] Van Horn A, Hayden C, Mahairas AD, Leader P, Bush ML. Factors influencing aberrant facial nerve stimulation following cochlear implantation: A systematic review and meta-analysis. Otology and Neurotology. 2020;**41**(8):1050-1059

[61] Muckle RP, Levine SC. Facial nerve stimulation produced by cochlear implants in patients with cochlear otosclerosis. The American Journal of Otology. 1994;**15**(3):394-398

[62] Kempf HG, Tempel S, Johann K, Lenarz T. Complications of cochlear implant surgery in children and adults. Laryngo- Rhino- Otologie. 1999;**78**(10):529-537

[63] Rotteveel LJ, Proops DW, Ramsden RT, Saeed SR, van Olphen AF, Mylanus EA. Cochlear implantation in 53 patients with otosclerosis: Demographics, computed tomographic scanning, surgery, and complications. Otology & Neurotology. 2004;**25**(6):943-952

[64] Bahmer A, Adel Y, Baumann U. Preventing facial nerve stimulation by triphasic pulse stimulation in cochlear implant users: Intraoperative recordings. Otology & Neurotology. 2017;**38**(10):e438-ee44

[65] Song Y, Alyono JC, Bartholomew RA, Vaisbuch Y, Corrales CE, Blevins NH. Prevalence of radiographic cochlear–facial nerve dehiscence. Otology & Neurotology. 2018;**39**(10):1319-1325

[66] Schart-Morén N, Larsson S, Rask-Andersen H, Li H. Anatomical characteristics of facial nerve and cochlea interaction. Audiology and Neurotology. 2017;**22**(1):41-49

[67] Alnafjan F, Hasan Z, Sanli H, da Cruz MJ. Risk factors for facial nerve and other non-auditory side effects following cochlear implantation. Otology & Neurotology. 2021;**42**(8):e1022-e10e9

[68] Braun K, Walker K, Sürth W, Löwenheim H, Tropitzsch A. Triphasic pulses in cochlear implant patients with facial nerve stimulation. Otology & Neurotology. 2019;**40**(10):1268-1277

[69] Wolfe J, Schafer E. Programming Cochlear Implants. San Diego, CA: Plural Publishing; 2014

[70] Arenberg J. Threshold and channel interaction in cochlear implant users: Evaluation of the tripolar electrode configuration. The Journal of the Acoustical Society of America. 2007;**121**:1642-1653

[71] Langman A, Quigley S, Heffernan J, Brazil C. Use of botulinum toxin to prevent facial nerve stimulation following cochlear implantation. The Annals of Otology, Rhinology & laryngology Supplement. 1995;**166**:426-428

[72] Polak M, Ulubil SA, Hodges AV, Balkany TJ. Revision cochlear implantation for facial nerve stimulation in otosclerosis. Archives of Otolaryngology–Head & Neck Surgery. 2006;**132**(4):398-404

[73] Alharbi FA, Spreng M, Issing PR. Facial nerve stimulation can improve after cochlear reimplantation and post-operative advanced programming techniques: Case report. 2012

[74] Battmer R, Pesch J, Stöver T, Lesinski-Schiedat A, Lenarz M, Lenarz T. Elimination of facial nerve stimulation by reimplantation in cochlear implant subjects. Otology & Neurotology. 2006;**27**(7):918-922

[75] Asfour L, Risi F, Miah H, Roland JT Jr. Cochlear implant explantation: An in vitro model to evaluate electrode explant force and trauma. Cochlear Implants International. 2022;**23**(4):189-194

[76] Erixon E, Högstorp H, Wadin K, Rask-Andersen H. Variational anatomy of the human cochlea: Implications for cochlear implantation. Otology and Neurotology. 2009;**30**(1):14-22

[77] Van Wermeskerken GKA, Prokop M, Van Olphen AF, Albers FWJ. Intracochlear assessment of electrode position after cochlear implant surgery by means of multislice computer tomography. European Archives of Oto-Rhino-Laryngology. 2007;**264**(12):1405-1407

[78] Selvaraj A, Jain RK, Nagi R, Balasubramaniam A. Correlation between gray values of cone-beam computed tomograms and Hounsfield units of computed tomograms: A systematic review and meta-analysis. Imaging Science in Dentistry. 2022;**52**(2):133

[79] Scarfe WC, Farman AG. What is cone-beam CT and how does it work? Dental Clinics of North America. 2008;**52**(4):707-730

[80] Pietsch M, Aguirre Dávila L, Erfurt P, Avci E, Lenarz T, Kral A. Spiral form of the human cochlea results from spatial constraints. Scientific Reports. 2017;**7**(1):7500

[81] Bierer JA, Faulkner KF, Tremblay KL. Identifying cochlear implant channels with poor electrode-neuron interfaces: Electrically evoked auditory brain stem responses measured with the partial tripolar configuration. Ear and Hearing. 2011;**32**(4):436-444. DOI: 10.1097/AUD.0b013e3181ff33ab

[82] Jahn KN, Arenberg JG. Identifying cochlear implant channels with relatively poor electrode-neuron interfaces using the electrically evoked compound action potential. Ear and Hearing. 2020;**41**(4):961-973. DOI: 10.1097/AUD.0000000000000844